PSYCHIATRY IN MEDICAL PRACTICE

PSYCHIATRY IN MEDICAL PRACTICE

David Goldberg

Sidney Benjamin

Francis Creed

London and New York

First published in 1987 by Tavistock Publications
Reprinted 1989 (twice), 1991 by Routledge
11 New Fetter Lane, London EC4P 4EE

Printed in Great Britain by
Richard Clay Ltd, Bungay, Suffolk

British Library Cataloguing in Publication Data
Goldberg, David, 1934–
Psychiatry in medical practice.
1. Psychiatry   2. Family medicine
I. Title   II. Benjamin, Sidney   III. Creed,
Francis
616.89   RC454.4

ISBN 0–415–03453–1

CONTENTS

PREFACE

This book has been written from the standpoint of a medical student setting foot for the first time in a department of psychiatry: however, we have anticipated his or her needs until well after Finals and prepared him or her for psychological aspects of medical practice as it is carried out both in primary care and general medical settings.

We have therefore focused on somatic manifestations of psychological ill health, since these are the commonest syndromes encountered in both primary care and general medical settings. We have given major emphasis to the medical interview and included forms of assessment that can be used in general medical settings. A special chapter, entitled 'Psychiatry for the houseman', covers important psychological aspects of a young doctor's work which tend to be neglected since they are certainly not examined in Finals. Our book is unusual in having given students a simple and clear framework in which to understand psychological illness. We have distinguished between syndromes which are not age related, and those which are peculiar to particular stages of the life cycle, since in our view much unnecessary confusion occurs in the minds of students because this distinction is not clearly made. Our classification does not include the concept of 'neurosis', although we explain to students what this term has meant in the past.

The sciences that underpin clinical psychiatry are neurochemistry, epidemiology, and psychology: our book gives an up-to-date account of all three, as well as emphasizing the relationships which exist between psychological and physical ill health.

Our chapter on 'Treatment' gives far more detail than is usual in an undergraduate textbook of psychiatry, since we are aware that after qualification doctors need much better information than they received as undergraduates about interventions which will help their patients. We do not intend that medical students should familiarize themselves with the detail of this chapter, since we expect them to return to it in the future. Finally, we have provided them with a card small enough to be carried in a pocket or handbag, which will serve to remind them of some basic questions to be borne in mind in their day-to-day clinical work.

We wish to extend special thanks to 'guest authors' who have contributed special sections of the text: Professor David Taylor, Chapters 16 and 17; Dr David Jolley, Chapter 19; and Dr Angus Campbell, Chapter 21. Dr Elemir Szabadi contributed sections on drug treatment and neurochemistry, and Dr Chris Bradshaw and Mr Michael Wang the section on behavioural treatments. Numerous colleagues have been kind enough to read other sections of text and give us suggested amendments: these include Professor Neil Kessel, Professor H. R. Beech, Dr W. Deakin, Dr M. Duddle, Dr G. P. Maguire, and Dr F. Margison. We are grateful to all of these, but as editors must accept responsibility for any faults that may have crept into the text.

David Goldberg
Sidney Benjamin
Francis Creed

1 / INTRODUCTION

This book sets out the knowledge you will need to enable you to understand and manage the common psychiatric disorders and psychological problems that you will encounter among your patients in your pre-specialist years. It contains everything you are likely to need for your Finals examination, and then some more. It does not pretend to be a textbook for psychiatrists, but it should provide a useful introduction to the subject even for those students who intend to enter psychiatry or general practice.

THE CLINICAL APPROACH TO THE PATIENT

We start by giving an account of those **interview techniques** that are necessary in order to evaluate the importance of psychological factors in the individual case. We follow with a chapter on the **mental state examination**. Next come chapters dealing with the **classification, aetiology, assessment, and treatment** of purely psychiatric disorders; this section concludes with chapters explaining how you should decide the **prognosis** and then should set about the **formulation** of an individual patient's problems.

The chapters in this first section are fundamental to understanding what goes on in a department of psychiatry and are also relevant to work in the general wards. They will help you to elicit data relevant to a proper understanding of a patient's psychological problems, and then go on to make appropriate plans for treatment and management.

SYNDROMES OF PSYCHIATRIC DISORDER

The second section of the book gives a general account of the commoner syndromes of psychiatric disorder. We start with psychological disorders which commonly accompany physical diseases, and include sections on pain and psychiatric aspects of epilepsy. We then start at the top of a *hierarchy* of **psychiatric disorders**: starting with organic brain syndromes, going on to schizophrenia, and then considering disorders of mood. We next consider **maladaptive behaviours** such as alcohol and drug dependence, eating disorders, and obsessional states. We end with a consideration of **abnormal illness behaviours** such as hypochondriasis, hysteria, and malingering. The disorders described in this section are defined in terms of **syndromes** or collections of symptoms that commonly occur together, and in this respect they are therefore fairly similar to illnesses you will already have come across in general medicine, such as migraine or asthma.

DISORDERS RELATED TO STAGES OF THE LIFE CYCLE

In the third section we will consider disorders which either take their onset at a particular stage of human development, or are peculiar to a stage of the life cycle. We start with **mental handicap** since this group of disorders reflects problems arising at conception, during intra-uterine development, or events during or shortly after birth. We then work our way through the life cycle with chapters on **disorders of childhood and adolescence** followed by **sexual and reproductive disorders**, and finally **disorders of old age**.

PSYCHIATRY IN THE GENERAL HOSPITAL AND LEGAL ASPECTS

In the final section we return to the general wards of the hospital with a section on psychiatry for the houseman and legal aspects of the subject. We will give a **short form of clinical assessment** suitable for use in other parts of the hospital where time for such assessments may be short: we give special emphasis to the detection of three problems: affective illnesses, alcohol-related problems, and the detection of organic cerebral damage. However, we hope that those who have mastered the longer techniques described in Part 1 will readily be able to use these principles in order to make fuller assessments.

EPIDEMIOLOGY

We will be giving you figures for each illness in later chapters: here we will consider overall rates for *any psychiatric diagnosis* in various populations. In a random sample of Londoners one can expect about 6 per cent of men and 12 per cent of women to receive a psychiatric diagnosis at any point in time.

The prevalence of such illnesses is considerably higher in populations seeking medical help: general practitioners themselves consider that approximately 14 per cent of the population registered with them will consult them and be considered psychiatrically ill in the course of a year, with just over 5 per cent of these illnesses being new illnesses. If we consider consecutive attenders at general practitioners' surgeries, then somewhere between 25 and 35 per cent of them will meet research criteria for psychiatric illness.

Figures for those admitted to medical wards of general hospitals are approximately similar: recent estimates range between 20 and 40 per cent. Most of these illnesses are mood disorders or 'affective illnesses', and such disorders are usually an integral part of the various physical disorders for which help is being sought (see Chapters 10 and 13 for a fuller discussion). It is for this reason that an understanding of the assessment and management of psychiatric illness is an essential part of your medical training. Nor should it be thought that most people do not experience such illnesses: one well-conducted study in Sweden showed that a man who survived to the age of sixty-five had just over a 40 per cent chance of having an episode of a mental illness at some point in his lifetime, while the corresponding figure for a woman was just over 70 per cent!

SKILLS TO BE ACQUIRED

With the help of this book and the opportunity to interview patients, you should aim to acquire the following skills between now and the time that you qualify:

1. To **take a history** from a patient in such a way that you are able *to assess the importance of psychological factors.*
2. To **make a short assessment of a patient's personality**, and to distinguish it from illness.
3. To **carry out a mental state examination** of a patient with a psychiatric illness.
4. To **adapt your interview techniques** to special types of clinical interview, for example interviews with children, with old people, with immigrants and those with communication problems.
5. To **write a formulation** of a patient's illness.
6. To **assess an episode of self-poisoning**.
7. To **assess suicidal risk**.
8. To **take a history from a relative**.

KNOWLEDGE OF MANAGEMENT PROCEDURES

By the end of your time in the department of psychiatry you should aim to acquire knowledge of the following management procedures. It helps a great deal if you have actually seen them carried out, but there is no need for you to have done them yourself.

Medical procedures

1. The management of **delirium tremens**.

2. The management of an **acutely psychotic** patient.

3. **Electro-convulsive treatment**.

Psychological Procedures

1. (on the general wards)
   - How to break bad news.
   - Dealing with malignant disease.
   - Helping patients who have had mutilating surgery.
   - Helping the dying patient.
2. (In the paediatric department)
   How to interview a child.
3. The management of violent behaviour in hospital settings.
4. Emergency procedures under the Mental Health Act.

HOW TO READ THIS BOOK

We have written the book in the order you should read it: Part 1 deals with fundamental aspects of the psychological approach to clinical problems. Try to read Chapters 2, 3 and 4 right away: although you can skip the remaining chapters in Part 1 until you have clerked your first patient. There is more information than you need to pass Finals in the chapter on 'Treatment': however, you will need this information after you qualify in order to manage common psychological disorders – so we make no apology for the surplus!

As soon as you have interviewed a patient with a particular problem read up the appropriate chapter in Part 2, as well as relevant bits of the chapters on investigation and treatment. Aim to read the whole of the first two sections in the first week of your time in the department of psychiatry.

Parts 3 and 4 can safely be left until the earlier parts have been absorbed, although all parts are equally important.

THE CARD

We have included a card with this book which you may wish to carry about with you until you have got used to carrying out clinical assessments. On one side we have shown you, in note form, the main headings to be used in taking a *history* and carrying out a *mental state examination* with especial attention to assessments for organic damage. You will most often need this side of the card in the department of psychiatry, although you will find it useful on the general wards as well from time to time. We also give you the 'Newcastle scales' for the assessment of *cerebral impairment* in elderly patients.

On the other side we have reminded you of some of the common manifestations of *mood disorders* that accompany physical illnesses in the rest of the hospital. We also remind you of the useful screening questions for the detection of *alcoholism* in patients with medical problems. A further question reminds you of the questions that need answering when you make an assessment of *suicidal risk* in the accident room. Get into the habit of using all these questions in your routine clinical work. You will not be sorry.

In case you lose this card, we have reproduced its content at the end of the book.

PART 1
THE CLINICAL
APPROACH TO THE
PATIENT

2 / INTERVIEW TECHNIQUES AND HISTORY-TAKING

A medical interview should allow you to obtain the most accurate possible account of the patient's illness, and the events in the patient's life that are relevant to it, within a reasonably short time. If time is not to be wasted, you must create conditions from the outset so that the patient finds it easy to talk to you. To start with, you must look like a member of the medical staff. On the general wards this is quite easy since you will be wearing a white coat, but in settings like the department of psychiatry or in general practice it is important that you dress in such a way that patients who may be much older than you nevertheless see you as someone from whom help may be sought.

Start by saying who you are, and explaining the purpose of the interview. Show consideration by asking whether it is a convenient time for the patient: it usually will be, but people like to feel that they have been consulted. Let us suppose that you have been asked to see a forty-four-year-old woman called Mrs Woods, who has been referred to hospital with a severe central chest pain. You are working for a consultant called Dr Johnson:

> *Good morning, Mrs Woods. My name is Brian Mathews . . . (shake hands) . . . I'm a student doctor working with Dr Johnson. He has asked me to see you to ask you about the illness that has brought you to hospital. Is this a convenient time to talk to me?*

In the medical wards the next step is to establish some privacy by drawing the curtains so that others in the ward will not be able to eavesdrop on what the patient tells you. If you can do anything to make the patient more comfortable – for example, helping an orthopnoeic patient to sit up on his pillows – this also shows consideration, and you will be rewarded by a better history. In places where interview rooms are available you should now lead the way to the room, resisting the temptation to start the interview until you are both seated and the patient is comfortable.

You should be aware that communication between yourself and the patient will be

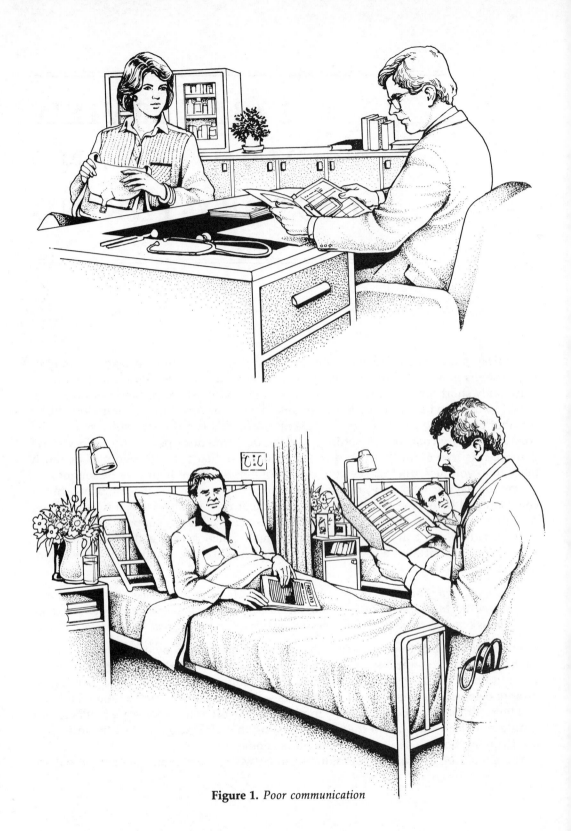

Figure 1. *Poor communication*

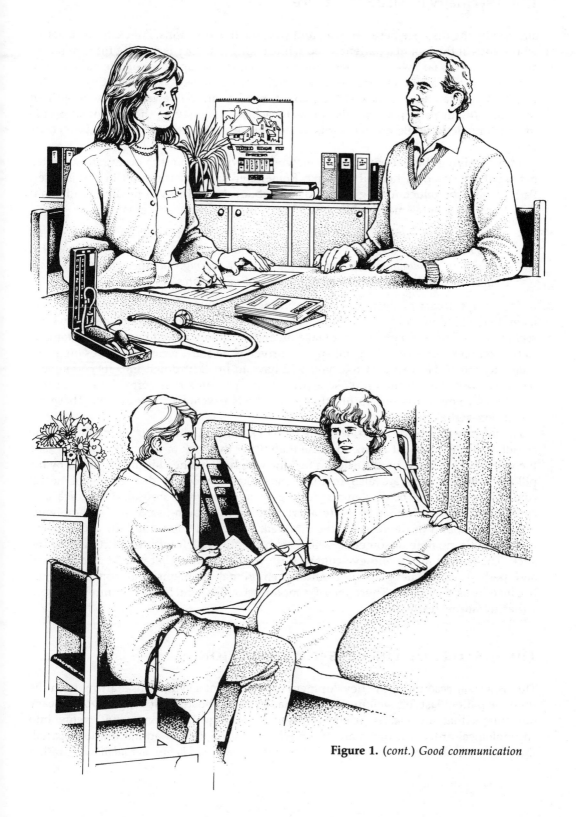

Figure 1. (*cont.*) *Good communication*

affected by the distance between you, and your relative positions. For example, a doctor who stands at the foot of a patient's bed while taking a history is making three mistakes at once: he is too far away, he is face to face, and he is looking down on the patient. You should be sitting about a metre from the patient, on the same level, and sitting in such a way that you can always look at the patient, but he can look away from you without difficulty. In out-patient work this is usually achieved by having the patient sit beside the doctor's desk, while on the wards one draws up a chair beside the bed (see *Figure 1*).

Start by giving the patient some framework for what is about to occur, and then tell her what you need to hear about first. Remember to ask permission to make notes. Patients may be reluctant to give full details about their illness to medical students if they think your notes may be left around on a bus, or in the students' union.

> *Mrs Woods, I'm going to have to ask you quite a lot of questions about yourself, but I'd like to* **start** *by asking you to tell me about the illness that has brought you into hospital. I'll need to jot down a few notes while you are talking, but the notes I make are confidential, and will be kept with your other medical notes.*

In fact, don't dream of writing down anything yet. Look at your patient and, as you listen to the first few sentences, notice as much as you can about the sick person who is seeking help. There is a great deal to take in, and eventually it will become as automatic as the complex series of actions taken by a driver as he starts a car and drives off into a busy city street. However, at first you will have to break it down into its component parts. We will concentrate on those aspects of the patient's non-verbal behaviour that should alert you to the possibility that he or she is psychologically unwell. These are called **non-verbal cues**.

The **posture** may be dejected, with the patient slumped in his chair; or it may indicate anxiety, with the patient being so tense that either the back of his chair does not take the weight of his body, or as he lies in bed the weight of his head is unsupported by his pillow. Valuable cues are also in the handshake: the warm, dry feeling of health contrasting with the cold, clammy feeling of anxious over-arousal. The **voice** also contains valuable information quite apart from what is being said: the monotonous, uninflected sound of depression; the strained, distressed sound of pain and anxiety; and the whining note of someone who feels he is always left with the dirty end of the stick. The patient may **avoid eye-contact** with you, sometimes because he is distressed and perhaps ambivalent about confiding emotional problems, but sometimes just because he is feeling ill. There may be motor activities which suggest inner tension: either **tremor** or **restlessness**.

THE HISTORY OF THE PRESENT CONDITION

This is a clear account of the development of the patient's symptoms starting from the time the patient last felt well until she was admitted to hospital. It is up to you to leave out things that are clearly irrelevant, and to arrange symptoms and events into chronological order. All times are given relative to the date of admission to hospital: thus, '*Mrs Woods began to feel a pain in her chest three weeks before her admission*', rather than '. . . *on 3rd January*, or '. . . *on the day of the Cup Final*'.

Probe questions like 'And what happened after that?' help to emphasize to the patient your interest in a sequential account of her problems.

It encourages the patient to speak in the early minutes of the interview if you utter **facilitations** – these may take the form of noises like *'uh-huh'*, words like *'yes, I see'*, or by repeating what the patient has just said with a different inflection: *'You fell down the stairs?'*. Sometimes patients start by telling us the most dramatic events, and only gradually tell us about what actually happened to them first. If you think that this is happening, say something like:

> *I need to know the order in which these things happened to you. What was the **first** thing you noticed that was wrong?.*

After each incident is described, remind her of the same need by saying:

> *And what happened after that?*

Sometimes patients start by pouring out an account of their current social problems without really mentioning medical symptoms at all. If this happens you will need to interrupt quite soon, saying something like:

> *What effect did (that) have on your health?* or

> *I'd like to come back to that in a minute. Could you start by telling me about your health (or about how you have been feeling in yourself)?*

During the course of giving the history patients will often mention key symptoms about which you will need to know many details. **Pain** is the most obvious example: you will need to know its site, quality, intensity, radiation, things that make it worse, and things that ease it. Sleep disorders, depression, and bowel disorders are other examples where there are many questions that need to be answered before you can pass on to the next topic. In your anxiety to leave nothing out, you have perhaps already got into the habit of asking patients many 'probe' questions about each of these areas, but this is not the right way of going about things. It takes too long, and patients who are suggestible often agree to things that they have not actually experienced. Get into the habit of asking **directive questions** about such important topic areas:

> *You say you developed a pain in your chest. Could you describe it to me?*

> *Tell me exactly what you have noticed wrong with your sleep.*

The student has indicated to the patient that this is an important area, but phrases his question in such a way that the patient must use her own words to convey her experience, rather than having words put into her mouth. It is often necessary to ask several directive questions. Suppose that the patient has answered the first question by saying that her pain is below her left breast and is there almost constantly. This leaves too many questions unanswered, so:

> *Try and tell me exactly what the pain is like.*

In this way although you will obtain answers to the questions in your textbook on clinical methods, you will not do so by asking them as they appear in the book. Occasionally you will ask **closed questions** which the patient can answer with a simple '*yes*' or '*no*', but generally only when the patient has told you what he can, but has left out some detail that is potentially important.

Sometimes you will notice that the patient looks emotionally unwell as she describes her physical symptoms, a **non-verbal cue** suggesting psychological illness. The thing you notice could be any of the things already mentioned, but in the case of Mrs Woods her eyes are red and swollen. As she mentions her mother's death, she dabs her eyes with her handkerchief. Instead of politely ignoring this, the student deals with it by drawing attention to it. This in effect gives the patient permission to talk about her feelings:

> *Mrs Woods, I can see you're still very upset about your mother's death. Have you found yourself crying a lot?*

This procedure is called a **reflection** of the patient's feeling, and it can be used for other feelings as well, such as anger or tension.

Sometimes patients mention their feelings at the same time as they give you important information about a physical symptom. An insensitive interviewer simply picks up the physical symptom and asks further questions about that, never returning to the abnormal mood. Remember to prick up your ears when you hear these **verbal cues** relating to psychological illness. You may well want to finish hearing about the pain first, but remember to come back to the abnormal mood, and ask a **directive question** about it:

> *You mentioned a moment ago that you've been feeling depressed. Could you tell me more about that?*

Your questioning therefore proceeds in a systematic way moving gradually forward in time, so that eventually you arrive at the day of admission. This should remind you to carry out a brief **systems review**. In the department of psychiatry some parts of this are particularly important, so be sure you remember to ask for:

1. Changes in **appetite**.
2. Changes in **weight**.
3. Changes in **sleep**.
4. Changes in **sexual feelings**.
5. Changes in **bladder and bowel habit**.
6. Decreased ability to **enjoy oneself**, including **loss of usual interests**.

Sometimes students feel embarrassed asking older people about their sexual feelings. You need not be. The patients aren't embarrassed, if you aren't. Everyone knows what sexual feelings are, whether or not they are currently having a sexual relationship with someone. If the patient isn't consulting for a sexual problem, it is usually sufficient just to ask whether there has been any *change* in their sexual feelings recently, at the same part of the interview as you are asking about other functions such as appetite and sleep.

Anyway, when you have completed the 'systems review' questions you should be thoroughly up-to-date. This should remind you to **recapitulate** the history to the patient. This only takes a few moments, and it is an excellent habit to get into. Patients frequently correct things which (often through no fault of your own) you have got wrong, and they are often reminded to put in something important that they forgot to tell you the first time:

> *Well, Mrs Woods, you seem to have been well until your mother died unexpectedly three weeks ago. You cried quite a bit on the day she died and on the day before the funeral you found you just couldn't stop crying and you began to think that it was all your fault that she had died. Members of your family told you that wasn't so, and at first you let them persuade you. However, since then you've gradually become sure that she wouldn't have died if only you had done more for her when she stayed with you six months ago. On the day of the funeral you developed a severe pain in your chest which you have had, off and on, ever since. It is just below your left breast, and feels like a dull ache. It seems to get worse when you cry a lot, and was rather better when your family doctor gave you a sedative on the day after the funeral. On the other hand, it doesn't seem to be helped by resting, or by aspirin. You have been eating very little since she died as you have lost your appetite, and have lost 12 pounds in weight. You have great difficulty falling asleep, and in the past week you have been waking three hours earlier than usual. You have lost all interest in sex, and you have been a bit constipated. You haven't been able to take any interest in your usual activities, since you have been feeling unlike your usual self: you said it was as though a black cloud had fallen over you.*

THE FAMILY HISTORY

Now that you have heard the nature of the present illness, you are in a far better position to know how much detail to take about the family history. Not everything is equally important. In Mrs Woods' case, for example, we certainly want to know about the illness that caused her mother's death, and to know something about the relationship between mother and daughter. Did her mother have a chest pain in her last illness? Had there been bad feelings between mother and daughter to help us to understand the guilt the patient now reports? Is there a tendency for depression to run in the family? These are questions in our minds, but we do not ask them right away. However, they will influence us in the amount of detail that we collect. The family history is a voyage of discovery.

However, before we embark we utter a sentence to let the patient know that we have finished one area, and are about to go on to another. These statements are called **transition statements** – think of them as a form of professional good manners – and go straight on with your first question:

> *Now that I've heard about your present problems I'd like to go on to ask you a few questions about your family. Could we start with your father? Is he still alive?*

We are aiming to get answers to the following questions about each parent:

Age, or age at death and year of death (so that you can work out how old the patient was at the time); occupation; health; whether parent suffered with 'nerves' (if so, details: were they seen by a psychiatrist; did they have any treatment?); what the parent was like; how the patient got on with them.

Go on to siblings. List them in order, showing where the patient comes in the family. If the patient uses first names, use these both in your notes and in questioning the patient, otherwise use the patient's terminology: *'So your older sister was always your mother's favourite, and you found that you never really could please her?'* You are interested in the health of all first-degree relatives, but not of relatives by marriage. The family history should tell us whether any of Mrs Woods' first-degree relatives have had mental illnesses, as well as giving us some idea of the sort of family she comes from. Do not ask about the patient's spouse or children yet: they come later.

We started our family history with some hunches about the patient: we should by now have begun to confirm or refute them, and often we now have some new insights: the voyage of discovery can continue. . . .

THE PERSONAL HISTORY

At first you will take very full and detailed personal histories, because you won't really know what is relevant and what is not. Don't worry about that, you need the practice, and you will discover some very interesting things about your patients in the process. However, once more, not everything is equally relevant. How a girl received her sex education will have great relevance if the patient is asking for help because she has not been able to consummate her marriage, but it will probably matter very little in a spinster of seventy-five who is complaining of loss of memory.

Childhood

It is helpful to take the personal history in chronological order, starting from childhood. A patient's mother may be able to tell you what her health was like in the pregnancy that produced your patient, and to give you details of the delivery and age on reaching 'milestones': however, information on the same points from the patient is likely to be unreliable. Students often begin their account of the personal histories of their patients with an air of spurious accuracy: 'Mrs Woods was born in Bermondsey as a full-term, normal delivery. Her milestones were normal, and there were no neurotic traits in childhood. . . .

Don't do this unless you can obtain information which seems to be reliable. It doesn't matter whether she was born in Bermondsey or Hoxton, and she probably doesn't really know whether her delivery was normal or not. Nor does she have much idea whether her motor milestones were normal, and it doesn't matter two pins whether or not an adult patient reports 'neurotic traits' in childhood! Although birth injury and delayed motor milestones are of great medical interest, it is better to say that you have no information than to say that things were normal when they in fact were not. However, if the patient has been told that her birth or early years were abnormal this is certainly worth recording; otherwise confine yourself to what the patient can actually remember, and which are of interest in understanding disorders in adult life.

So, start the personal history with a transition statement: *Now you've told me a bit about your family I'd like to ask a few questions about your early life. Were you ever told anything*

about your birth?
Go on to ask: *Do you remember your childhood as happy or unhappy?*

Happy childhoods can be passed over quickly, but get details about unhappiness. What was wrong, and how did it affect her? Was she separated from her parents? (If so, for how long, and how did she manage?) In patients with mixtures of physical and psychological symptoms, ask about physical health in childhood, and the attitudes of care-givers to them when physically ill. It is helpful to ask routinely whether or not there were serious physical illnesses in childhood.

School

If you are taking a detailed history start with primary school – how did they get on? What were they good at? Did they make friends? (If not, were they teased; what about?) How did they get on with teachers? Then, pass on to secondary school. The briefest school history will record age of entering and leaving full-time education, and the highest level of education achieved. Make a note of any public examination passed, since this information is especially important in the assessment of possible organic cerebral damage.

Sexual history

Move on to the sexual history by asking female patients about their age at the menarche, and go on to a menstrual history. Ask whether their mother prepared them for their menarche, and whether sexual matters could be discussed at home. Go on from there to ask about boyfriends. You are interested in their capacity to form loving relationships, as well as obtaining a detailed account of any problems encountered in the physical side of sexual relationships.

Ask male patients at what age they learned the facts of life, whether sexual matters could be freely discussed at home, and so through a similar sequence of questions. Once more, do not confine yourself to an account of the purely physical problems which the patient may describe, but try to assess the patient's capacity to form loving relationships.

Do not ask about homosexual activities unless the patient volunteers information, or unless there is some reason to suspect it and it is relevant to the patient's present problems. If you need to discuss such problems, do so without embarrassment. If anal intercourse has occurred, has the patient been worried about the possibility of AIDS?

If the patient presents with a sexual problem you will of course need to get fuller details than this brief outline suggests: these are given in Chapter 18.

Marital history

The marital history follows naturally on: once more, happy marriages can be recorded briefly. If the patient has been married more than once obtain a description of the first marriage and how that marriage ended. At what age did they meet their spouse, and get married? What is the age, health, and occupation of the spouse? Can they confide in their spouse? Have there been problems? (An example of a problem would be separations, or threatened separations.) If there have been no problems, record this briefly; otherwise obtain a description of the problems.

Is the sexual side satisfactory? Ask about children, recording separate notes about each child: age, health, any problems?

Occupational history

The occupational history gives valuable information about the patient's personality, as well as the range of his abilities. What is the patient's current occupation: if none, how long has the unemployment lasted? How many jobs have there been, and how long did the longest one last? Why do changes occur? Promotions and changes forced by circumstance require no explanation, but get someone who is constantly changing jobs to tell you what goes wrong. A list giving exact names of employers and dates is of little value: but this part of the history and the marital history gives you some idea of the patient's capacity to form enduring relationships and stick at things, as well as allowing you to judge his strengths.

Present social circumstances

Finish this part of the history by trying to assess the patient's present living circumstances. Who is there at home? How do they get on? What sort of accommodation do they live in? What patterns of friendships does the patient have?

Forensic history

Whether or not you take such a history depends largely on the patient's presenting problem. They should routinely be taken in patients with drug or alcohol problems.

Start with truancy and problems at school, both with teachers and with other students. Go on to ask if they have ever been in trouble with the police. If they have, be sure to start with the first time, not the most recent! Have they appeared before a Court, either juvenile or adult? If so, what was the charge, were they convicted, and what was the sentence?

Previous medical history

If there are important medical, surgical, or psychiatric illnesses in the **past history** these should be recorded in the usual way.

Life charts

If there appear to be relationships between life events, physical illnesses, and psychiatric illnesses it is very helpful if these are brought together as a **life chart**. An example of Mrs Woods' life chart is shown on p. 20.

THE PRE-MORBID PERSONALITY

Some personality types are at greater risk than others of developing psychiatric illnesses: for example, people with cyclothymic traits are more likely to develop manic-depressive illness, or those with obsessional traits are more likely to experience obsessional symptoms when depressed. This is discussed more fully in Chapter 5 (pp. 60–6).

However, there are two major problems in relying upon information from the patient. Unless you're very careful, patients tell you what they're like now, rather than what they used to be like. Also, people cannot tell you things that they don't know themselves, and if they are depressed they will tend to see themselves in a bad light. Always see a relative if you want accurate information. Nonetheless, there are some things that the patient can tell you about himself, and you should start, as usual, with a transition statement:

> Mrs Woods, I want to ask you some questions now about the sort of person that you were before you became ill. Could you remember how you were a year or so ago? Could you start by telling me about your interests?

Aim to collect information under headings: interests, mood, friendships, habits – including alcohol and drugs.

INTERVIEWS WITH SPECIAL GROUPS

Children and old people

Special points that should be borne in mind with patients at either end of the life cycle are discussed in Part 3: interviews with children on pp. 240–43 and interviews with old people on pp. 281–82.

Deaf people

Don't shout at them. Make sure that they can see your mouth, and speak slowly and clearly. Ask them to let you know if they cannot hear any of your questions, as you will be pleased to repeat them. If a particular question is really important, and you are unsure whether the patient really understood it, write it down.

People who do not speak English very well

Often you can manage just by speaking slowly and clearly, and *avoiding long words*. If this does not work, you will need an interpreter: these are usually available, so make proper enquiries! When the interpreter appears and you have introduced yourself, put the patient in the usual chair and address your questions to him or her, not to the interpreter. Watch the patient's face as they reply to each question: even if you do not understand a word of their language; you will learn a great deal.

Figure 2 *Example of a life chart for Mrs Vera Woods*

age	year	life events	physical illness	mental illness
	1940	Born 10.9.40		
1	1			
2	2			
3	3			
4	4			
5	5	Started school		
6	6			
7	7			
8	8	F. died;		
		M. → Dep'd	Investigated for abdo. pain	
9	9			
10	1950		Appendicectomy	
11	1			
12	2			
13	3			
14	4			
15	5	Left school; clerical job		
16	6			
17	7			
18	8			
19	9			
20	1960	1st engagement		
21	1	Broken off		Anxiety; No Rx
22	2	2nd engagement		
23	3	Marriage		
24	4			
25	5	Stopped work; daughter born		
26	6			
27	7		Hysterectomy: 'menorrhagia'	
28	8			
29	9			
30	1970			
31	1			
32	2			
33	3			
34	4			
35	5			
36	6			
37	7			
38	8			
39	9			
40	1980			
41	1			
42	2			
43	3	Daughter to univ.		Dep'd; Rx GP
44	4			
45	5	M.'s illness discovered Aug.		
46	6	M. died 18.2.86		Onset present illness

INTERVIEWING A RELATIVE

Use the same headings when you see a relative, but be sure to include your impression of your informant. Include any anecdotes that are mentioned. You should learn about the patient's capacity to form friendships, as well as patterns of relationship within the family. Look now at the following example:

Informant: husband
Mr John Woods
s/a as patient

Impression of informant

Mr Woods is a heavily built man who seems very concerned about his wife's illness. He thought carefully about some of his answers, pausing for emphasis on things he thought important. He asked particularly to be told if there was anything else that he might do to help, but appeared to have difficulty seeing how his wife's depression could have much to do with her chest pain.

Present illness

Little to add to patient's account except that she told him her mother wouldn't have died if she'd been a better daughter, and that she felt wicked.

Early life

Always trying to please her mother, but mother found fault with her. Wanted to have mother live with them last year, but informant wasn't keen as there were always arguments.

Marital history

Informant met her aged 32, a few months after she had divorced her first husband for desertion and mental cruelty. They married after about six months and were initially quite happy, although she was possessive. Intercourse satisfactory for both of them and occurred regularly until her mother's death. There was some tension in the early years because he did not get on with her mother, but in the past two years the old lady had been to stay for several long visits. They have two children – John aged 11: no problems, happy and outgoing; Dorothy aged 9: tends to be nervous and tearful. Pt. is rather over-protective, won't let them play with other children.

Previous psychiatric history

Nil.

Pre-morbid personality

Usually cheerful, but tends to be gloomy for weeks if things go wrong. During such times she is irritable, sleeps poorly, and seems listless.

Always very houseproud. 'You could eat your breakfast off her kitchen floor.' Tends to check gas-taps and switches at the best of times. Very sensitive, thought people at her work were criticizing the way they brought up their daughter: couldn't see this wasn't so.

Likes making clothes for herself and their daughter, also interested in country dancing and Help the Aged. Works tirelessly for other people: tremendous energy. Has many friends and leads an active social life. Drinks only socially; non-smoker; no recreational drugs. Tranquillizers from GP only once, about 3 years ago, he thinks.

Brian Matthews
Medical Student

3 / EXAMINATION OF THE MENTAL STATE

The examination of the mental state is an orderly and systematic procedure like that of the physical examination. It is carried out routinely for each new patient and is repeated, either in whole or in part, on every subsequent occasion that the patient is seen. A summary of the main aspects of the mental state follows this introduction. Each of these aspects is then considered in turn, with a description of the observations that are to be made and the tests that will be carried out, the interpretation of these observations, and their relevance to diagnosis. The division of the mental state into these parts is convenient, but to some extent arbitrary, because they tend to overlap.

The emphasis in this chapter is on the accurate evaluation of the most important symptoms and signs of mental illness. The student is advised to start by learning how to carry out well the tests presented here and how to evaluate the significance of the results. Many of the more esoteric phenomena, particularly those seen in schizophrenia, are not described.

As in other branches of medicine the history of the disorder should suggest the diagnosis, and the examination should help to confirm it. Although an experienced clinician will be able to concentrate on certain aspects of the mental state, the inexperienced student will only learn to carry out the mental state examination rapidly and effectively by keeping to the routine described for each patient examined. The novice can expect to take as long as an hour to carry out the examination in some cases, but by the end of a few weeks should be able to carry out at least an initial examination in about twenty minutes. (A total of one hour is the customary time allowed for a history and clinical examination of a 'long case'.)

A full and accurate account of the mental state should always be recorded in the medical notes, for both clinical and medico-legal purposes. As with all medical records each note must be dated and signed. Observations must be noted separately from opinions. For example –

The patient insists that Dr Smith is his father, refers to him as 'Dad', and describes his real father as an imposter when he comes to visit. He cannot be argued out of this belief

– should be recorded, and separately the opinion:

(This belief appears to be a delusion.)

The latter might not be the only interpretation of the finding. It might be an over-valued idea, or intentional play-acting. Records that contain only opinions, for example, 'The patient is suffering from delusions', are of little value. Another doctor, seeing the patient a few days later, may find no evidence of delusions and will probably decide that the recorded opinion is wrong and based on inexperience if he does not also have available the data on which the opinion was based.

Negative findings are as important as positive findings and should be recorded. For example, the note of orientation in time should specify the patient's replies to questions on the time, day of the week, and date, together with the correct answers, rather than the opinion 'Well-orientated in time'. Similarly 'Mood normal' is not an acceptable alternative for 'Describes his mood as "contented" and shows appropriate modulation of mood throughout the interview'.

Verbatim accounts by the patient should be recorded if they are particularly illuminating or provide an example of some morbid phenomenon and should be indicated by using inverted commas. It is especially important to record examples of speech which you consider to be abnormal: once more, a note which reads 'patient's speech grossly thought disordered' is valueless – you must record an actual example. You should also record the context in which the statement is made, or whether in response to a question.

Some of the words to be found in this chapter are also used in colloquial English, when they often have a less precise meaning. For example, 'obsession' is a term used generally to mean only a preoccupation, whereas in psychiatry it has a more specific meaning which is precisely defined and it should be used only in this way. Throughout the following account we shall use technical terms, some of which may be unfamiliar to you. Rather than break up the text each time this occurs, we have gathered these together at the back of the book in a **Glossary**, and have used asterisks to indicate that a Glossary definition is available. Thus, if you come across the word '**akathisia** (*p. 309)' this means that a full account of that term is to be found on p. 309.

APPEARANCE AND BEHAVIOUR

General description

The mental state examination should start with a brief description of what the patient looks like, so that another person hearing the account might recognize the patient in a crowded room. Include the physique, clothes, cleanliness, hair, make-up, and whether these seem appropriate to the age, sex, cultural group, and social class of the patient.

Signs of self-neglect (poor hygiene, stubbly beard, body odour, stained clothes, or loose clothes due to weight loss) occur in many mental illnesses, particularly depressive disorders, dementia, and schizophrenia, as well as being due to poverty.

Always note any evidence of disorders of the **level of consciousness**. Is the patient fully awake and alert, responding normally to stimuli, drowsy, or unrousable? Apart from normal tiredness, an impaired state of consciousness is strongly suggestive of an organic cerebral disorder, particularly delirium, but inattention also commonly occurs in affective disorders. Tests of orientation may help to differentiate these.

Reaction to interviewer

The manner of the patient towards the interviewer should be described next. Is he friendly, cooperative, complaining, suspicious, or critical? Students tend to assume either that they themselves are at fault when occasionally a patient refuses to cooperate, or alternatively that the patient is being 'difficult'. However, this is an important part of the patient's mental state and provides some indication of how the patient relates to others at the present time. One must then consider whether such behaviour is the patient's reaction to an unfamiliar and stressful experience, is a symptom of illness, or is an indication of personality problems.

Motor activity

This is sometimes referred to as 'psychomotor activity'. Included here are the facial expression, posture, and gait. Note particularly the speed of movement, the quantity, and the presence of abnormal movements. Is there any evidence of repetitive, apparently purposeless, or involuntary movements?

There may be *too little* movement. Distinguish between **akinesis** (*p. 309) in which there are reduced voluntary movements especially affecting the face, and **retardation** (*p. 313) in which all movements are slowed. **Loss of volition** (*p. 314) is where the patient generally doesn't have much go in him, and **stupor** (*p. 313) is when the patient does not move at all, although fully conscious.

There may be *too much* movement. Distinguish between a generally increased level called **over-activity** (*p. 312), or an anguished, driven restlessness which leads to **agitation** (*p. 309). **Akathisia** (*p. 309) is a state of restlessness and over-activity produced by neuroleptic drugs. Ask yourself whether any increased level of activity is associated with **disinhibition**.

There may be **involuntary movements**. Some of these are of especial interest to psychiatrists. You are probably already familiar with **tics** (*p. 314), and will have seen **choreic** movements on the neurological wards. The movements of **acute dystonia** (*p. 309) are painful spasms and **tardive dyskinesia** (*p. 313) refers to a wide variety of repetitive and distressing movements, both brought on by neuroleptic drugs.

DISORDERS OF TALKING AND THINKING

Knowledge of another person's thoughts is only available through speech or some other form of communication, such as writing or gesture. Talking and thinking are closely related; in that thought usually precedes speech; however, thoughts may remain unspoken. We therefore consider talking and thinking together.

Students often have some difficulty in understanding the essential difference between the form and the content of talk. Briefly, the **form** is how we talk, while the **content** is what we say. For example, we may talk quickly in a disjointed manner (the form), but this gives no indication of whether we are talking about the weather or our next meal (the content).

The speed of talk

The speed of talk varies greatly from one person to another, so that a moderately fast or slow rate of talk cannot be assumed to be morbid. Extremes of speed may be associated with changes in volume and also in the quantity of speech.

RETARDATION OF SPEECH

Retardation of speech (*p. 313) refers to a delay in starting to speak as well as the rate of speech.

MUTISM

Mutism (*p. 311) is total absence of speech. **Elective mutism** is characterized by mutism which occurs in some settings but not in others.

Changes in the amount of speech occur in depression and mania. A reduction in talk may sometimes be seen in dementia, where patients may say very little; alternatively, they may talk a great deal but communicate little.

PRESSURE OF SPEECH

Pressure of speech (*p. 312) describes a rapid outpouring of ideas which are often difficult to interrupt.

Continuity of talk

Note whether talk is hesitant, with longer than usual interruptions for thought, and whether it is coherent and relevant to the current conversation. Remember that this should be judged more by what is relevant to the patient, who may be preoccupied with a crisis in his life, than by what is relevant to you the interviewer. Hesitancy in speech is a common feature in those who are anxious or depressed, indecisive, or preoccupied with worries. Deafness, often unsuspected, is also a common impediment to the free flow of conversation.

Does the patient use words of his own making (**neologisms**: for example, my mind is *spired*) or strange grammatical constructions?

Does talk **follow a sequence** in which consecutive ideas follow logically, working towards an identifiable goal, or is it circumstantial, tangential, or over-inclusive? If any disorder is possibly present, record verbatim samples of speech to illustrate this, together with the question that you asked beforehand:

> *How long have you been in hospital?*

> *I came in last Wednesday: that was a fine day for mushrooms. Do you like omelettes?*

The patient may talk circumstantially, or he may wander from one subject to another, apparently with little purpose other than social contact. This must be differentiated from a breakdown of normal associations of ideas, in which talk apparently attempts, but fails, to follow a logical sequence.

SCHIZOPHRENIC THOUGHT DISORDER

In **schizophrenic thought disorder** the logical sequence of ideas may break down so that consecutive sentences are unconnected; a single sentence may contain two unrelated elements:

> *I want to go home because this hospital is nearer to the shops than the last one.*

Here there is an apparent attempt to provide an explanation in the second half of the sentence for the wish expressed in the first half, yet there is no real explanation, and the two ideas appear to be disconnected. Always ask the patient to explain the association between sentences if you are unable to discern a meaningful connection. This may result in an even greater breakdown in logical thinking or a logical explanation that was not initially evident. Asked to explain the previous statement, the patient may say:

> *Shops frighten me and if I stay here I may be expected to go to the shops. I wouldn't mind going to the other hospital.*

This now begins to make sense. Alternatively he may say:

> *I mean I want to go home because it's near the shops and the shops are near the hospital.*

This makes even less sense than previously. In extreme disorder there may be a jumble of unrelated words (**word salad**).

FLIGHT OF IDEAS

Flight of ideas describes the way in which the speech of manic patients may move rapidly from one subject to another, usually with some discernible association, which may be rather flimsy. For example:

I don't like this place. It's really rather boring. The patients keep snoring. It's just a great yawn: I'd rather have soft porn. Are you a softie, doc?

Here the ideas are associated and there is a return at the end to the initial theme. Such 'flight' is usually associated with pressure of speech, unlike schizophrenic thought disorder. However, the form of the disorders of thinking and speech in schizophrenia and mania may be so similar in practice as to defy differentiation.

If the patient suddenly seems to go blank during your examination the most likely explanation is just that he is anxious, but consider the possibility of **thought block** (*p. 314) and ask him what was happening during the pause. Another possibility is **petit mal epilepsy** (*p. 134).

PERSEVERATION

Perseveration is the repetition of a response when it is no longer appropriate. For example:

What day is it today?
Monday. (Correct)
Which day did you come into hospital?
Monday.
What is the name of the ward?
Monday.

Verbal perseveration is often associated with motor perseveration: 'Hold up your left hand.' The patient does so. 'Hold up your right hand.' The patient again raises his left hand. Perseveration is usually an indication of organic brain disease.

DISORDERS OF MOOD

The examination of mood has four main components: subjective mood, objective observation, autonomic activity, and thought content. The last of these is considered further in the next section.

Subjective mood

Always ask first about the patient's subjective mood state with an open-ended question:

How have you been feeling recently? or,
How have you been in your spirits?

If the response is non-committal, follow up with:

Have you been feeling mainly happy or sad?

If the reply indicates sadness, ask:

> *How sad? – Can you snap out of it?*

If the patient describes depressed mood, always remember to ask:

> *What do you find yourself thinking about when you feel like that?*
> *How do you feel about the future?*
> *Do you ever feel completely hopeless?*
> (If 'yes' to previous question:)
> *As though life isn't worth living?*
> (If 'yes', continue with questions about suicide, see p. 30.)

Objective observation of mood

Moods of sadness, anxiety, or happiness are conveyed through facial expression, posture, and motility. 'Normal' mood modulates frequently, depending on the thoughts and experiences of the individual.

There are two separate points to note:

1. What is the predominant mood during the course of the interview?
2. To what extent does the mood fluctuate, are fluctuations appropriate, and in what direction are these fluctuations?

Occasionally patients deny unpleasant mood states, such as depression, perplexity, or suspicion, although there may be ample alternative evidence to show this is present. In particular there may be a deliberate attempt to conceal depression by refusing to answer questions, and this should alert the interviewer to the risk of suicide.

Sadness is a feature of depressed mood, but it is not of course in itself indicative of mental illness. **Weeping** is commonly associated with sadness, although it may merely be a way of releasing pent-up tension.

In less severe depressive states the mood may improve when the patient is distracted by amusing incidents, that is to say the mood reacts to the circumstances (this is the proper meaning of '**reactive depression**'). In more severe depressive states weeping is less common, and there tends to be a more constant melancholic mood, lacking normal modulation, which may easily be mistaken for **affective blunting**. The patient may describe the experience of an inability to have feelings or to care about others, such as family members or friends.

Smiles and laughter are associated with cheerfulness and **euphoria**, in which case they usually have an 'infectious' quality. However, they can also be produced in the unhappy as an indication of irony or of social expectation, when they fail to convey real enjoyment. The manic patient is not always cheerful: he will often display irritability and impatience if frustrated by those trying to limit his activities. **Irritability** is commonly seen in all affective illnesses.

The patient may display **labile mood** (*p. 311) in that he has little control of emotion. Less commonly, you may notice examples of inappropriate or **incongruous affect** (*p. 311), or he may display **blunting of affect** (*p. 310) in that the capacity to experience emotion seems to have been lost.

Autonomic activity

Affective changes are accompanied by fluctuations in autonomic activity.

You may have noticed cold, sweaty palm as you shook hands with the patient.

Increased arousal is characterized by sweating, palpitation, dry mouth, hyperventilation, frequency of micturition which may be evident during mental state examination, while raised diastolic and systolic blood pressure, tachycardia, and increased gastro-intestinal motility may be found on physical examination. High arousal commonly occurs in all psychiatric disorders associated with anxiety, including anxiety states, depressive illness, and both acute and chronic schizophrenia.

THOUGHT CONTENT

The content of thinking is evident primarily through the patient's talk, but also through aspects of behaviour. In this respect 'actions speak louder than words'. For example, the patient may deny that he is suspicious of others, but opens the office door to see if anyone is listening outside.

Preoccupations

Themes which are predominant in a patient's thought content are likely to be revealed in his spontaneous speech. Note any topics to which he may return repeatedly during the course of the interview and the difficulty which you encounter in trying to steer him from these subjects back to other aspects of the history and mental state examination. If preoccupations are not evident, ask:

What are your main worries? or,
Do you have some thoughts that you just don't seem to be able to get out of your head?

Many people have preoccupations, but these are appropriate to the circumstances. For example, it is appropriate for a patient about to undergo major surgery to be preoccupied with the possible hazards, the likely outcome, the provision for dependants, and so on, even though there may be encouragement from others to keep these thoughts to himself. However, some preoccupations are morbid, and their content may be important in understanding the diagnosis of the disorder.

Ruminations are repetitive ideas and themes, usually having an unpleasant content, on which the patient may brood for prolonged periods. They commonly occur in anxiety states and depressive illnesses when their content reflects the **affective state**: for example, they may include ideas of guilt, low self-esteem, or hypochondriasis. These should be differentiated from delusions (see below) in which the content may be the same but the form is different. Ruminations also occur in **obsessional states** (*p. 215), in which case they reflect the state of indecision.

Suicidal ideas are of special importance, because of the risk to the patient's life. A patient who has said that life is not worth living should be asked:

> *Have you ever thought of ending your life?*
> *Have you planned what you will do?*
> *Do you intend to carry it through?*

Perhaps surprisingly most patients answer such questions honestly, but be particularly wary of the patient who avoids answering. Although commonest in depressive illness, suicidal ideas are by no means limited to that disorder.

Abnormal beliefs

Ideas which are shared by many people within a particular cultural or ethnic group may seem strange to others; for example, particular religious beliefs and practices. Individuals too may have ideas which seem idiosyncratic or eccentric, but are not necessarily symptomatic of mental illness.

Over-valued ideas are beliefs which are strongly held about matters which are of special importance and preoccupy the subject. They are not delusions, because they lack the quality of unshakeable conviction. For example, patients with anorexia nervosa may develop the characteristic belief that they are fat although they know that they are grossly underweight; indeed, they would regard others of the same weight as dangerously thin. Over-valued ideas are not necessarily indicative of illness.

Delusions are mistaken beliefs which are held with conviction, which are not shared by others of the same cultural or social background and intellect, and which persist despite all the evidence to the contrary.

For example, a patient insists that there are men plotting to kill him, hidden in the hospital grounds behind the shrubs and trees. The doctor takes him round the grounds and they look carefully in potential hiding places. Eventually they return to the ward, and the doctor points out that there is no one there:

> *'Of course not,' says the patient, 'they knew we were going to look for them and they left, but I know that they're back in the grounds now.'*

Primary delusions (also called 'true delusions') are delusions which are not secondary to other morbid processes such as abnormal moods or hallucinations. However, they may be prompted by non-morbid processes. For example, a patient may see three clouds in the sky (a normal perception) and realizes that these are a personal message to him from God telling him that he is a member of the Holy Trinity. Primary delusions are generally associated with schizophrenia provided that they occur only in a setting of clear consciousness. There are several kinds of primary delusion, but of particular importance is the **delusional perception**, of which an example is presented above. Here the perception is normal, but it is given delusional significance.

Secondary delusions (also called 'delusion-like ideas') are so called because they are delusions which occur secondary to some other morbid process. For example, a patient wrongly believes he is being persecuted by his neighbours. This belief may be secondary to an abnormal mood state of depression in which he believes he is guilty and worthy of punishment; or secondary to voices, which he identifies as belonging to the neighbours, saying 'Kill him'. Secondary delusions occur in many different disorders, but their content may be related to the diagnosis.

The possible presence of delusions usually becomes evident while taking the history. For example, the patient with delusions of persecution may tell you about the way others are acting against him, his efforts to stop them by complaining to the police or consulting solicitors, or he may appear suspicious in the course of an interview.

Do not ask about delusions routinely: only when other aspects of the history or mental state indicate that they might be present. Then ask:

> *Do you think that others are trying to harm you?*
> *Do you ever feel guilty, or to blame?*
> *Do you think that your body has changed in any way?*
> *Do you think that you have been specially chosen, or have special powers?*

If the patient agrees to any of this, detailed questioning will be necessary to discover whether such ideas, if present, satisfy the criteria of delusions. Is there evidence supporting the patient's views? Do others share his views and encourage him in them? Are his beliefs shakeable?

Delusions occur in many different mental illnesses, in fact all those commonly labelled as **psychoses** (see p. 47). Persecutory and hypochondriacal delusions occur in many disorders and are of little help with diagnosis. Others are more suggestive of diagnosis and are described in Part 2 or in the Glossary.

PERCEPTION

Most of the time we are aware of our own thoughts, our bodies and the world around us only to a limited degree, but we can focus our attention on each of these, and they have qualities and order which we recognize and take for granted. This sense of familiarity may be morbidly disrupted. Disturbances may occur in each of the modalities of our perception of ourselves and the outside world.

It is not necessary to ask every patient detailed questions about disorders of perception but it is useful to ask most patients a few 'screening' questions and to pursue these more vigorously if indicated by the history or mental state examination.

> *Have you noticed any changes in yourself or your surroundings that you can't account for?*
> *Have you heard voices of people that you couldn't see?*

The patient may have an unpleasant feeling that although his environment is the same, he or his body has changed – this is suggestive of **depersonalization** (see p. 310). Alternatively he may feel that although he is the same, the surrounding environment has altered in some way – this suggests **derealization**.

Depersonalization and derealization occur commonly in states of fatigue and high arousal, particularly in association with anxiety and depression; and less often in schizophrenia, epilepsy, and drug-induced states.

Illusions

Illusions are misinterpretations of external stimuli. They may affect each of the sensory modalities. Commonest are auditory illusions, in which the patient misinterprets what is heard, and visual illusions, in which there is a misinterpretation of visual stimuli.

Illusions are not necessarily morbid, and most people are familiar with 'optical illusions' or with the tendency to 'hear' footsteps following them when walking alone in the dark. Emotional states, such as anxiety, often result in such misinterpretation. Probably the commonest pathological cause of illusions is sensory deficit, as in partial blindness or deafness, and a similar effect may result from diminished sensory input, such as the effect of darkness. Lowering of the state of consciousness has similar effects, and illusions are particularly liable to occur in delirium. In this state it is common for the movement of shadows to be misinterpreted as, for example, the movement of dangerous animals, or the movement of bedclothes against the skin may be misinterpreted as the movement of insects. Not surprisingly, patients experiencing such illusions often appear terrified.

Hallucinations

Hallucinations are perceptions which are not based on external stimuli. For example, a voice is heard talking, but no one is there speaking, and others present hear nothing. Like illusions, hallucinations can occur in any modality of perception, but auditory hallucinations are by far the commonest.

AUDITORY HALLUCINATIONS

Ask

> *Do you ever hear voices when there is no one there, or no one is talking?*

If 'yes',

> *Are these real voices, coming from outside your head, or your own thoughts inside your head?*
> *Do you ever hear your own thoughts, spoken aloud, outside your head?*

Also ask about the content of the voices:

> *What do the voices say?*
> *Give me an example of what you heard today, or yesterday.*

Always record verbatim accounts of the patient's experiences, including the content of the hallucinations.

Auditory hallucinations can occur in many disorders, including schizophrenia, organic brain syndromes, and manic-depressive illness and their content tends to be related to the nature of the disorder. For example in manic states they may be grandiose, such as a voice telling the patient that he has special powers; whereas in depressive disorders they are likely to be abusive and consistent with the state of low self-esteem. Features suggestive of schizophrenia are described on p. 168.

VISUAL HALLUCINATIONS

These are uncommon and most likely to occur in acute organic states (for example, intoxication with drugs such as amphetamines, or other delirious states), although they occur occasionally in schizophrenia and in affective disorders. Disorganized visual hallucinations (lacking normal form) may result from occipital lobe disease.

OTHER HALLUCINATIONS

Olfactory and gustatory hallucinations may occur as symptoms of temporal lobe disease, for example, in temporal lobe epilepsy. **Tactile and somatic hallucinations**, that is perceptions arising from the body surface or internally, are described, but difficult to differentiate from illusions. All of these occasionally occur in schizophrenia.

Hallucinations occur commonly during dreams, and also in the twilight state between waking and sleeping (**hypnagogic hallucinations**), in which case they have no morbid significance. Simple hallucinations – that is to say, bangs or flashes of light – may occur in conditions of extreme fatigue. You should therefore always ask about the circumstances in which hallucinations are experienced.

> *Was it during the day or at night?*
> *Were you in bed with the lights out?*
> *Were you awake or dozing?*

It is sometimes difficult to differentiate between an illusion and a hallucination. If, for example, a patient says he heard a voice saying *'You have been specially chosen'*, ask:

> *Where did the voice come from?*
> *Was anyone else present at the time?*
> *Were they speaking?*

Pseudohallucinations lack the qualities of vividness and reality which are possessed by normal perceptions and by hallucinations: they have an 'as if' quality, and they are experienced in inner subjective space. Thus a voice is heard inside one's head, or a vision is seen as if by an 'inner eye'. Ask:

> *Did it sound just the same as a real voice, like listening to my voice now?*

Pseudohallucinations, like illusions, have little diagnostic specificity. They may occur in any mental illness, and also in those who are not mentally ill, particularly those who are highly imaginative or of dull intellect. Failure to discriminate between pseudo-hallucinations and hallucinations sometimes results in a patient being wrongly regarded as psychotic.

INTELLECTUAL FUNCTIONS

These tests should be used for most patients seen in the department of psychiatry and in particular should be carried out whenever there is a possibility that a patient is suffering from an **organic brain syndrome**. The tests described must be presented accurately if the results are to have any value. You should start by explaining what you are going to do, and why.

> *Now I am going to ask you some other questions to find out how well you are keeping up with things. It's important that you try to do your best even if you find them very easy or very difficult.*

Record correct and incorrect answers. Also note the patient's attitude to the tests. Is he really trying? Is he *unable to cooperate* because he is very anxious, or very depressed? Does he lose patience or refuse to attempt them, for example on the grounds that they are too trivial? When interpreting the results remember that to some extent they are affected by both intelligence and education, and the history of education and occupation should, therefore, be taken into account when trying to decide the significance of difficulties that are encountered.

Orientation

Orientation in time and place should be examined first. Ask:

> *What day of the week is it today?*
> *Without looking at your watch, about what time is it now?*

Can you tell me the date and the year?
What is the name of this place?

If these are inaccurate ask more detailed questions:

What sort of place is it?
What town are we in?
How would you get here from your home?
What is your name?
Who am I?

If the patient is unable to do any of these, ask:

Is it daytime or night time?
Is it nearer to 9.00 a.m. or midday?
Would you say it's Monday or Tuesday today?
The beginning or end of the month?

All patients should be able to answer the questions about identity correctly. They should also know they are in hospital and its name. They should have an accurate knowledge of the day of the week and of the time of day to within about one hour. Record verbatim replies to your questions together with the correct answers (in brackets).

Note any other observations suggesting disorientation. For example, the patient may have difficulty finding his way about a hospital ward several days after arrival or he may get into the wrong bed.

Disorientation is the cardinal sign of clouding of consciousness, which is a feature of an acute brain syndrome ('delirium'). This may be accompanied by a diminished awareness and grasp of the surroundings, and attention is also likely to be impaired. Delirious patients may be unaware of the time of day, the nature of the place, or of the function of people around them. However, inaccurate replies to questions about orientation may also be due to poor memory (in chronic brain syndrome), or to a narrowed range of interest in the affective disorders.

Attention and concentration

Defects in attention and concentration will usually be evident while the history is being taken. It may be difficult to attract the patient's attention, or once attracted it may be poorly sustained. The patient may be distracted by events in the environment which would usually be ignored during a medical consultation, such as birds singing in the garden or a book on the table, and attention may flit rapidly from one object to the next.

Attention may be diverted by experiences not shared by the interviewer, such as voices to which the patient listens. Specific tests of attention are based on the ability to keep track of sequences of material which is familiar to the patient and does not, therefore, require new learning.

Allow the patient as much time as he needs to complete each test, but note unobtrusively how long the patient takes and record this.

> *Tell me the days of the week backwards, starting with Saturday.*
> *Tell me the months of year backwards, starting with December.*

As usual record the patient's replies verbatim and the length of time taken for each task. Unimpaired subjects should be able to complete these rapidly, without mistakes.

> *Starting with one hundred, subtract seven and then continue to subtract sevens as far as you can.*

If the patient does not understand the task, ask:

> *What's seven from one hundred?*
> *And seven from ninety-three?*

Carry on like this until he's got the idea. If the patient still does not understand, or says it is too difficult, ask him to subtract threes from twenty.

Performance is more dependent on educational and intellectual attainment than the previous tests, and results must, therefore, be interpreted in the light of the history of schooling and employment. Disorders of attention are common and can occur in almost any psychiatric disorder, particularly organic states and affective disorders.

(Patients who show definite evidence of impaired attention on these tests will usually be unable to attend to the following tests of memory, in which case they will not provide any additional information and should not be carried out.)

Registration and short-term memory

DIGIT SPAN

This is a test of registration and immediate recall. Start by explaining:

> *I am going to give you some numbers to remember. When I stop I want you to repeat them to me. For example, if I say '2 4 7', you would repeat '2 4 7'.*

Give a series of three digits, at an even speed of about one per second, and avoid laying emphasis on some more than others. Ask the patient to repeat them immediately.

If he is correct, give four digits, using a new sequence, then five, and so on, until the patient makes a mistake, say at seven digits.

Finally note the maximum number of digits that can be correctly repeated in sequence. Most unimpaired adults of average intelligence can manage seven digits forwards. Five or less is strongly suggestive of impairment.

STANFORD-BINET SENTENCE

This is a test of registration and immediate recall, which makes allowance for intelligence. Explain:

I am going to ask you to remember a sentence. Listen carefully and then repeat the sentence as accurately as possible.

One of the following sentences should then be read out slowly. Select the one best suited to the patient's probable intellect. Then immediately ask him to repeat it. If he makes a mistake, try an easier sentence. If his repetition is accurate, try a more difficult sentence. Only read out a sentence *once*, slowly and clearly. Then record the response verbatim.

Sentence to be given to adults of dull intellect (completed successfully by 50 per cent of eleven-year-olds):

Yesterday we went for a ride in our car along the road that crosses the bridge.

For dull–average adults (50 per cent of thirteen-year-olds):

The aeroplane made a careful landing in the space which had been prepared for it.

For adults of average intellect:

The red-headed woodpeckers made a terrible fuss as they tried to drive the young away from the nest.

For adults of superior intelligence:

At the end of the week the newspapers published a complete account of the experiences of the great explorer.

NAME, ADDRESS AND FLOWER

This tests registration, immediate recall, and short-term memory. Explain:

I am going to give you the name and address of an imaginary person, and the name of a flower that he likes. It is a routine test of your memory which we give everyone. I want you to try to remember it and repeat it back to me as soon as I have finished. The name is:
Mr William Thompson,
118, Hamilton Terrace,
Chorlton,
Manchester 13.
The flower is a daffodil.
Now please repeat that back to me.

Record both the name and address that you give the patient and his immediate response. Note that there are nine items to be remembered, apart from 'Mr'. In selecting a name and address avoid very common names, for example, John Smith, or local addresses which are familiar to the patient. If the patient makes a mistake, read back the *same* name and address as before, and ask him to repeat it. Continue until he is entirely accurate, noting the number of trials required. When the patient is entirely correct, say:

> *I want you to try to remember that name and address and I will ask you again later on.*

Then continue with other tests, for example remote memory. After two minutes ask the patient to repeat the name and address. This time do not correct any mistakes. After a further three minutes again ask for a repetition. Record the responses each time. Was there evidence of poor registration? Once the material has been correctly registered, is there accurate recall? If mistakes are made, are they the same on each occasion, or is performance worse after five minutes than after two?

If the same test is used on subsequent occasions, use different names and addresses each time, of similar length and complexity to the example provided. Most people are able to repeat the name and address without mistakes immediately and after five minutes. Three mistakes or more at five minutes are strongly suggestive of a clinically significant deficit.

Longer-term memory

Recent memory can be tested by asking about personal experiences in the last few days: if possible ask questions to which the correct answers can be verified. For example, ask:

> *How long have you been in hospital?*
> *Who brought you here?*
> *Can you tell me about the television programme you watched last night?*
> *What's in the newspaper you were reading this morning?*

Test **remote memory** by asking about personal experiences, for example:

> *Can you tell me the name of your last school?*
> *And the name of the headmaster?*
> *What was the date when you got married?*

Past general events, for example the dates of the Second World War or the names of the last five prime ministers, are concerned with general knowledge rather than long-term memory, and answers depend on intelligence and education as well as memory. Thus, poor performance can be due to poor education as well as dull intellect or organic brain disease.

> *Can you tell me the names of five cities in England?*
> *And five sorts of fruit?*
> *What is the name of the Prime Minister?*
> *And the one before that?*

Evidence of difficulty with longer-term memory often comes to light during the process of taking the history. For example the patient may show major contradictions in his age, the year of his retirement, or when his wife died.

Defects in short-term memory alone, as revealed by the above tests, are actually defects of new learning. Memory of events prior to the onset of brain disease remains intact, but there is a disorder in the registration and retention of new experiences.

Defects in longer-term memory may involve **retrograde amnesia**, that is the loss of memories of events experienced before the onset of brain disease.

Patients with dementia often have difficulty with short-term memory, but appear to have remarkably good memory for the details of early life. However, beware of **confabulation** – the invention of replies to questions to hide poor memory. As dementia progresses, eventually even long-term memory deteriorates.

Intelligence

An impression of the patient's level of intelligence will be gained during the course of history-taking, from the extent of the vocabulary used, the complexity of the concepts expressed and from the Stanford-Binet Sentence remembered correctly. If these appear to be consistent with the patient's known history of education and employment, and if there is no evidence of impairment in tests of memory, then tests of intelligence are unlikely to be helpful.

Possible **intellectual retardation** may be assessed by simple tests of comprehension, such as:

> *What is three times nine?*
> *Sixteen divided by four?*
> *What is the difference between a fence and a wall?*
> *If a flag is being blown towards the west, from which direction is the wind coming?*

Illiteracy may be a serious handicap, which patients often fail to mention and may not be suspected. If in doubt, ask:

> *Did you learn to read and write at school?*
> *Would you mind reading to me from this newspaper?*

ABSTRACTION

Tests of abstraction can be helpful in eliciting thought disorder, and should be given only if this is suspected (see p. 26). Ask the patient to explain the meaning of one or two **proverbs**. Start by giving an example.

> *Proverbs are sayings which have general meanings. For example, 'Too many cooks spoil the broth' means 'If too many people do the same job it is likely to go wrong'. Have you heard people say 'Make hay while the sun shines'?*
> *(If yes) Could you tell me what it means?*

Record the reply and if it is satisfactory ask a more difficult proverb:

Now tell me the meaning of 'People who live in glass houses shouldn't throw stones'.

Consider the extent to which the patient's answer shows thought disorder (which may indicate schizophrenia) on the one hand, or concrete thinking (suggestive of organic damage or mental retardation) on the other.

INSIGHT AND JUDGEMENT

An understanding of the presence and nature of mental illness and of its causes is never complete and is rarely totally absent, therefore avoid generalizations, such as 'good insight' or 'bad insight'. The patient's insight may be indicated at different stages through the history and examination. The following are all quite common:

I don't need to see you. I'm not ill. It's my doctor who made me come.
My wife's the one who needs to see you.
I just need some stronger sleeping pills.

Sometimes a patient's statements about insight appear to contradict his non-verbal behaviour. For example, he may insist that he is not mentally ill, but agrees voluntarily to admission to a psychiatric unit and to take medication for mental illness. So, ask:

Do you think you are ill?
What sort of illness do you think you have?
Do you think it might be a nervous or mental illness?

To what extent does he correctly identify the relevance of his symptoms? For example, does he recognize that feelings of guilt and suicidal thoughts are due to depressive illness from which he may recover? Does he regard his auditory hallucinations as abnormal experiences, indicative of mental illness and requiring treatment; or as a normal experience, shared by others and not requiring medical attention?

Further questions may be needed to find out the patient's views about the cause of his illness and the appropriate treatment:

What do you think might have caused this illness?
Has anything happened to upset you?
What sort of help do you think you need now?

How realistic are the patient's views?

The assessment of insight has important implications for management. A patient who does not recognize that his suicidal thoughts are symptomatic of a treatable illness with good prognosis is more likely to act on such thoughts and, therefore, will require closer observation, possibly as an in-patient. The patient with persecutory delusions who is unaware that his fears are due to illness is more likely to defend himself by attacking others. A patient who shares the doctor's opinion of appropriate management is more likely to be compliant, for example either by taking medication or by involving himself in psychotherapy. Insight has, therefore, an important bearing on prognosis (see Chapter 8).

INTERVIEWER'S REACTION TO PATIENT

What is your own subjective response to the patient? Did you enjoy meeting the patient, or did he make you feel sad, frustrated, or angry? Was it easy or difficult to control the interview in order to obtain necessary information? Ask yourself what happened in the interview which caused you to feel this way. Your responses indicate something about you, as well as about the patient, and your relationship with each other. Is the patient a passive, dependent person, who induces in you frustration as much as sympathy; an aggressive, bombastic, or egocentric person, who took over the interview, prevented you from obtaining essential information and left you feeling inadequate and angry; or one who makes frequent statements about how others, particularly doctors, have let him down and, therefore, induces feelings of guilt?

If you found some difficulty in developing a working relationship with the patient, consider to what extent this is determined by the patient's behaviour and whether this is symptomatic of his present illness. Alternatively, have you elicited evidence of lifelong difficulties which the patient has had in his relationships with family, workmates, or others? It is likely that your own reaction to the patient is similar to the reactions of others and may tell you much about the patient's personality.

EXAMPLE OF A MENTAL STATE EXAMINATION

Appearance and behaviour

Mrs Woods is a rather plump, middle-aged lady who is not wearing any make-up. On introduction she shook hands limply and avoided eye contact but her manner was cooperative. She walked slowly to the interview room, then sat slumped in her chair in the same posture throughout the interview with little movement except of her hands which she clasped and rubbed together particularly when talking about her bereavement.

Speech

Talk is slow with slight delay before replying to questions and there is little spontaneous speech except about her physical health. However, her answers are coherent and to the point, and there is no evidence of formal thought disorder.

Mood

She describes her mood as 'I've got a bit low recently. I'm worrying all the time about my mother'. Says she regards life as worth living 'because of my family'. Appears sad and tense through most of the interview, weeps when talking about her mother, but smiles appropriately on several occasions.

Thought content

Describes herself as 'brooding' about her mother. On several occasions refers to her recent chest pains and asks at the end of the interview whether I think she might have had 'a heart attack'. She expresses an idea of self blame: *'If only I had done more for my mother, I'm sure she wouldn't be dead now' . . . 'I wasn't a good daughter'. Denies that there is anything specific that she could have done but this belief is firmly held. No other abnormal beliefs. She denies suicidal thoughts.*

Perception

Mrs Woods admits on direct questioning that she thought she heard the voice of her mother on three or four occasions since her death saying: 'Don't worry about me. I'm all right now'; and felt 'as if' her mother was present with her in the room. 'It must have been my imagination, but it seemed real at the time.' (These seem to have been auditory hallucinations.) She also describes a feeling of 'numbness' on the day of the funeral which has gradually diminished since then. There are no other disorders of perception.

Orientation

'Thursday, about ten o'clock, November 1985; I'm not sure, is it the 26th?'
(All correct except 28th November.)
'In the Psychiatry Department, Manchester Royal Infirmary.'
(correct.)

Attention and concentration

Generally attentive during the interview except when preoccupied with the bereavement and her own health
'Saturday, Friday, Thursday, Wednesday, Tuesday, Monday, Sunday.'
(Slow and hesitant in 25 seconds.)
'December, November, October, September . . . September, August, July, March . . . no, where was I? I'm sorry.'
(40 seconds.)
'100, 93, 86, 80, 73, 65, 60, did you say seven from a hundred? 60, 50, no 53, 45, no, I'm sorry.'
(4 mistakes; 2 minutes 10 seconds.)
'20, 17, 14, 11, 9, 7, 5 . . . no, that's not right is it?'
(25 seconds.)

Registration and short-term memory

Not tested in view of obvious problems with attention.

Long-term memory

Gives detailed and consistent account of early life.
Cities: Manchester, London, Birmingham, Liverpool, Chester, Southampton.
Knows the names of the Prime Minister and the President of the USA but cannot remember their predecessors.
Dates of world wars 1914–1918, 1939–1945.

Intelligence

Probably average in view of school to age of fifteen and semi-skilled work; consistent with present use of vocabulary.

Insight

'It's the pain in my heart . . . I don't think it's a mental illness . . . do you think I need another ECG? Well perhaps I've got a bit low since my mother died.'

SUMMARY OF THE MENTAL STATE EXAMINATION

1. **Appearance and behaviour**
   Description: reaction to interviewer; motor activity

2. **Speech**
   Speed; quantity; continuity; relevance

3. **Mood**
   Subjective account; observed mood; autonomic reactivity

4. **Thought content**
   Preoccupations; morbid thoughts; abnormal beliefs

5. **Perception**
   Illusions; hallucinations; depersonalization

6. **Intellectual function**
   6.1 Orientation
       Time, place, and person
   6.2 Attention and concentration

Days of week and months of year backwards;
Serial sevens or threes

6.3 Registration and short-term memory
Recent news; your name; consultant's name
Digit span; Stanford-Binet Sentence;
Name, address and flower

6.4 Long-term memory
Early life; six cities;
World leaders; world wars

6.5 Intelligence
Assessed from personal history

7. **Insight**
Nature of illness; causes of illness; appropriate treatment

FURTHER READING

Fish, F. (1985) *Psychopathology*. Bristol: John Wright. (Ed. M. Hamilton.)

4 / SYNDROMES AND DIAGNOSIS

THE PURPOSE AND LIMITATIONS OF DIAGNOSIS

The purpose of a diagnosis is to bring together illnesses which have the same characteristics. Ideally a diagnosis should identify disorders having the same underlying pathology, the same causes, and the same likely response to treatment. However, such an ideal is rarely achieved. Thus a diagnosis of **Huntington's chorea** identifies a necessary cause (an autosomal dominant gene), a pathology (cortical and extrapyramidal degeneration), a clinical presentation (dementia and choreiform movements with onset usually between the ages of thirty and fifty), and a course (progressive deterioration resulting in death). Ideally the diagnosis should also indicate an expected response to treatment, which in this example is at present limited to genetic counselling and symptomatic care. Although this diagnosis identifies a disease process, there are some limitations in its value, because not all those who suffer the disease will conform to this typical 'pattern. For example, some will show choreiform movements with little or no evidence of dementia. The age of onset will vary, and occasionally presentation may occur in childhood or old age. This illustrates the fact that all disease processes are subject to considerable variability.

Pulmonary tuberculosis is a diagnosis which deviates further from the ideal. All patients will have a similar basic pathology in the same organ, but the clinical presentation will vary from a chance radiological finding with no clinical features to an acute fulminating disorder. The course of these will differ widely, as will the management. All cases will have a similar necessary cause (the tubercle bacillus), but this is not a sufficient cause, and many other different factors will play a part in the aetiology of different cases (for example, the state of nutrition, accommodation, and socio-economic status).

Other 'diagnoses' tell us even less and are mainly a means of identifying clinical syndromes. A common example is **congestive cardiac failure**, which identifies a set of symptoms and signs, but provides only limited information about the underlying aetiology or pathology, and little about the course or response to particular treatments. However, even such a limited clinical label may alert us to a range of possible causes.

Most psychiatric diagnoses are syndrome diagnoses. Like the example of congestive cardiac failure, they tell us the symptoms and signs that characterize the disorder, but only a little about the aetiology, which must be considered separately. A diagnosis of **acute brain syndrome** will convey the clinical presentation, but does not tell us which of the many different causes of this syndrome is relevant to a particular case (see p. 141), and so it therefore does not tell us which specific treatment will be appropriate.

However, it does direct our attention to known causes of delirium, just as the diagnosis of depression directs our attention to known causes of depressive illness. Cause and treatment must, therefore, be considered separately from diagnosis for each patient.

A further complication arises because not only may a syndrome have a different cause in different cases, but also there are often multiple interacting factors all contributing to the aetiology of a single case. In the example of pulmonary tuberculosis, contact with a case of pulmonary tuberculosis exposes an individual to the risk of developing the disorder, but he will not necessarily become infected unless other factors are also involved. Similarly a woman's susceptibility to the development of a **depressive illness** will be increased by the death of her mother before the age of eleven, having no close supportive relationship, and having three children or more below the age of fourteen. However, not all women with these experiences will develop depressive illness. Just as malnutrition may predispose an individual to many different physical illnesses, the same aetiological factors may increase susceptibility to several psychiatric syndromes.

THE TRADITIONAL ORGANIZATION OF DIAGNOSTIC CATEGORIES

It has been traditional to differentiate between categories of psychiatric disorder in two ways. The first divides them according to clinical presentation, into **psychoses**, **neuroses**, and **personality disorders**. The second has regard to aetiology, and divides them into '**organic**' disorders that are secondary to known brain disease, and '**functional**' disorders whose physical basis is unknown.

Both the psychoses and the neuroses share a widely accepted criterion of illness, that is a deterioration from a presumed previous state of health and the development of symptoms. By contrast **personality disorders** do not involve change. They are identified by the presence of personality characteristics (traits) which are relatively constant throughout life and cause the subject and/or society to suffer (see pp. 60–5).

The differentiation between the psychoses and neuroses is essentially arbitrary, and based mainly on historical beliefs and practices. The **psychoses** include those disorders traditionally regarded as madness, in which strange beliefs and perceptions, often accompanied by violent and destructive behaviour, at one time resulted in incarceration in mental asylums. It has long been recognized that some of these illnesses are secondary to structural disease of the brain and these are therefore called **organic psychoses**, while others occur in brains that appear histologically normal, and are therefore called '**functional' psychoses**.

However, recent research shows that demonstrable structural or neurochemical changes also occur in the functional psychoses, so that the distinction between them and organic psychoses no longer has much substance.

The term **neurosis** was first used in 1769 by William Cullen to describe what were believed to be organic diseases of nerve tissue. Patients with these disorders presented to physicians with complaints generally thought to indicate physical illness, such as lassitude, dizziness, weakness, and poor appetite. They were considered to be suffering literally from 'weak nerves', and the terminology survives, even though there is usually no corresponding underlying physical disease of nerve tissue. During the nineteenth century there was an increasing awareness that these physical complaints could have their foundation in mental rather than physical mechanisms. The development of psychoanalysis from the 1890s, and behavioural psychology from the 1920s, led to increasing awareness of the way that mental mechanisms might operate to produce these symptoms.

By the beginning of the twentieth century psychiatrists saw those who presented with physical symptoms that were without known organic cause (hysterical neuroses and hypochondriasis), and also began to see patients with wholly psychological disorders such as anxiety state, obsessional neurosis, and phobic neurosis.

In the United Kingdom psychiatrists began to be appointed to the staff of general hospitals in any numbers only in the 1930s, and departments of 'psychological medicine' arose, to which patients with somatic symptoms unaccompanied by physical disease – the 'neurotics' of the previous century – were referred. However, most psychiatrists continued to work in mental hospitals, where their clinical work was mainly concerned with 'psychotic' illnesses. Thus patients with neuroses and psychoses were seen and treated in different hospital settings and often by different groups of psychiatrists. Although these barriers have almost disappeared the separation between neuroses and psychoses lingers on as a vestigial remnant.

By the middle of this century psychiatrists were working more closely with colleagues in general hospital settings, were seeing patients referred by general practitioners, and were beginning to be asked to see increasing numbers of patients with **maladaptive behaviours** which cannot be fitted into the categories of either psychosis or neurosis. These disorders include disorders such as alcoholism, anorexia nervosa, bulimia nervosa, and drug dependency; self-damaging behaviours such as self-poisoning and self-mutilation; and certain sexual disorders.

We will now consider the distinction between the various categories which we have discussed so far.

Organic versus functional psychosis

The disorders at present referred to as 'organic' should more accurately be thought of as those where we have a clear idea of an aetiology, and that aetiology is a physical disease. They include conditions where the structure of the brain is abnormal such as Alzheimer's disease or psychoses secondary to cerebro-vascular disease, and conditions where the brain is structurally normal – such as delirium associated with typhoid fever, pneumococcal pneumonia, or alcohol withdrawal ('delirium tremens'). It could be argued that the latter group are in a sense 'functional', and that as knowledge of neurochemistry advances we can expect to gain a greater understanding of many – if not all – of those psychoses at present referred to as 'functional', such as schizophrenia and manic-depressive illness.

For the present, there are clear advantages in making a distinction between those conditions where the aetiology is either coarse brain disease or physical disease elsewhere in the body, and those where the disorder arises from disordered functioning of the brain itself.

Neurosis versus psychosis

Previous claims that psychoses differ from neuroses because they are more 'severe' are not valid, because many neurotic patients also suffer from chronic, severely disabling illnesses. Although psychotic patients are said to be less in touch with reality (or to show 'defects in reality testing') and to have less insight into their illness, it will be remembered from the previous chapter that insight is never completely present or absent. Psychotic patients rarely have no insight at all, and neurotic patients never have perfect insight. It is a matter of degree, so insight cannot be a basis on which two categories of disease can be separated.

The only criterion by which these groups of disorders can be separated reliably involves an arbitrary operational definition. Psychotic illnesses are characterized by the presence of 'psychotic symptoms', specifically delusions and hallucinations. Such symptoms occur only in the psychoses, whereas 'neurotic symptoms' occur in both the neuroses and the psychoses. Thus if delusions or hallucinations are found in a particular mental illness, by definition it is a psychosis; if absent, it is a neurosis. The reason for making the distinction at all is that patients experiencing psychotic phenomena are more likely to have grossly deranged neurochemistry, and are therefore both more likely to require treatment as in-patients and to respond to physical treatments such as psychotropic drugs and ECT.

However, the word 'neurosis' applies to a kind of illness which can come and go, while the word 'neurotic' refers to long-standing attributes in a person. There are many individuals who have episodes of allegedly 'neurotic' illness such as depressive illness who are not especially 'neurotic' people. The term 'neurosis' should really be abandoned, but it will probably obstinately live on, if only because it is a pithy way of saying 'non-psychotic'. However, we shall not be using it in the remainder of this book.

Non-psychotic illnesses therefore form a large residual category of disorders. Within this category the mood disorders – those related to depression and anxiety – are most like medical syndromes such as migraine, but there are also other patterns of maladaptive behaviour such as alcoholism, self-poisoning, and patterns of abnormal illness behaviour which the doctor must understand, and these will be described in the chapters which follow.

THE HIERARCHICAL MODEL OF DIAGNOSIS

We have seen that the various syndromes of psychiatric disorder can be arranged in a rough hierarchy, where the top level (*'level one'*) represents those conditions which have a known 'organic' aetiology, the second (*'level two'*) those psychotic conditions where there are likely to be severe neurochemical derangements in cerebral functioning, and then there is a rather heterogeneous residual group. It is reasonable to make a distinction between disorders where concepts of treatment and recovery are appropriate (*'level three'*: affective disorders, maladaptive behaviours, and abnormal illness behaviours), and those which represent stable attributes of human functioning (*'level four'*: personality disorders).

The latter should not be thought of as illnesses, but they are often relevant to understanding the aetiology of illness, they may complicate treatment plans, and they are associated with suffering – either for the patient, or those with whom he lives. The scheme is shown in *Table 1*. From the student's point of view, the main advantage of such a hierarchy is to remind you that certain symptoms have more specificity than others in leading to a syndrome diagnosis.

Thus symptoms in the 'intellectual function' section of the mental state examination mean that serious consideration must be given to the possibility that the patient can be recruited to the top of the hierarchy. If we decide to do this, we will give less attention to other symptoms from lower in the hierarchy that might be present. For example, if we decide a patient has an acute brain syndrome we will pay little diagnostic attention to anxious mood since we will be preoccupied with finding (and treating) the cause of the acute brain syndrome.

Within the psychotic stratum, it is now usual to put clear manic symptoms 'above' schizophrenic symptoms, and to put these in turn 'above' depressive symptoms (see p. 186). This is because many studies have shown schizophrenia-like symptoms in manic patients who have recovered completely from such illnesses and gone on to develop clear manic-depressive (or 'bipolar') illnesses. However, providing manic symptoms are absent, 'disintegrative delusions' (thought reading, thought withdrawal, or ideas of passivity) are suggestive of schizophrenia, *providing that features indicating an organic disorder are absent*. This is because certain organic illnesses can cause schizophrenia-like symptoms (see pp. 168–9), and if these illnesses are present it is usual to diagnose them rather than schizophrenia.

In this way 'schizophrenia' becomes a name attached to disorders which have certain typical symptoms but for which no organic aetiology has been identified and which are not clearly manic: and it is in this sense that organic illnesses and mania are 'above' schizophrenia in the hierarchy. On the other hand, mood disorders such as depression and anxiety occur commonly in the setting of schizophrenia but do not alter the

Table 1 *The hierarchical model of diagnosis*

___

level one:
ORGANIC
DISORDERS

acute brain syndrome (delirium)
chronic brain syndrome (dementia)
Korsakow's syndrome

level two:
'FUNCTIONAL'
PSYCHOSES

mania
schizophrenia
psychotic depression

level three:
NON-PSYCHOTIC
DISORDERS

depressive illness

anxiety disorders
anxiety state
specific phobias
agoraphobia
panic disorder

maladaptive behaviours
obsessive compulsive disorder
alcoholism
drug dependence
anorexia nervosa and bulimia
self-poisoning
self-mutilation

abnormal illness behaviours
hypochondriasis
hysteria
malingering
factitious illness

level four:
PERSONALITY
DISORDERS

schizoid personality
cyclothymic personality
sensitive personality
'depressive' personality (low self-esteem)
passive dependent personality
obsessional personality
histrionic personality
antisocial personality

___

diagnosis of schizophrenia since they are said to be 'below' schizophrenia. Thus a depressive illness would be diagnosed only if signs of schizophrenia and of an organic state were absent.

The third level of the hierarchy contains all possible symptoms except those pathognomonic of organic disorders or strongly suggestive of psychotic illness. These symptoms are non-specific in the sense that they can also occur at the higher levels, but if they do they will not alter the diagnosis. They attract syndromal labels only when they occur on their own.

ONE DIAGNOSIS OR TWO?

In the case of 'maladaptive behaviours' it will often be useful to diagnose these *in addition to* a diagnosis based on experienced symptoms.

For example, if a patient with schizophrenia (a *level 2 diagnosis*) also has symptoms of alcoholism (a maladaptive behaviour) we should diagnose both conditions, since the second diagnosis gives important information not contained in the first. There is no underlying assumption about their relationship: they might be coincidental, or either might be a factor contributing to the aetiology of the other. It is usual to ask ourselves whether there might be a relationship whenever we make more than one diagnosis: in this example the patient may have developed a typical form of auditory hallucinosis after many years of heavy drinking (in which case we speak of **alcoholic hallucinosis**), or he may drink only because the voices tell him to (primary diagnosis therefore **schizophrenia**), or there may be no obvious relationship, in which case we simply make two diagnoses, putting the one highest on the hierarchy first.

Further examples of related diagnoses, where the second label gives information not implicit in the first, would be

1. *Agoraphobia,*
2. *Alcoholism,* or

1. *Anorexia nervosa,*
2. *Depressive illness.*

The second diagnosis is necessary since by no means all agoraphobics develop alcohol problems, and not all anorexics have depressive illness. In each case, the presence of the second diagnosis is likely to influence the treatment plan proposed for the patient. Note that the maladaptive behaviour has been put first in the latter example, implying that it may be causally implicated in the depression.

Diagnosis of a personality disorder may also be complementary to other diagnosis, and either help us to understand the aetiology or influence our management of the problem, for example:

1. *Paranoid psychosis,*
2. *Sensitive personality,* or

1. *Self-poisoning,*
2. *Histrionic personality.*

Having said this, it should be emphasized that two diagnoses should only be made if one will not do, so that one tries first to find a single diagnosis which will accommodate all the symptoms and signs. Only if this is not possible consider a second diagnosis.

Differential diagnosis is a quite separate process, which is concerned with alternative rather than complementary diagnoses, and is discussed in the chapter on formulation.

CLASSIFICATION SYSTEMS

The terminology used to label the different syndromes is embodied in various systems of classification. The ninth revision of the International Classification of Disease includes a classification of mental disorders. The World Health Organisation also provides a glossary describing the diagnostic criteria for each condition in this classification. This is the system that has been most widely used, both in the United Kingdom and abroad. It has been shown that different psychiatrists working in different hospitals, and in different countries, reach a high level of agreement in making diagnoses for the same patients when applying this classification.

The Diagnostic and Statistical Manual of the American Psychiatric Association (now in its third edition, and revised, thus 'DSM-IIIR') provides another classification which has recently aroused much interest. It differs from the International Classification of Disease in some important respects, notably in that it tends to give more emphasis to clear operational rules in making diagnoses.

FURTHER READING

American Psychiatric Association (1980) *Diagnostic and Statistical Manual.* Washington, DC.

Kendell, R.E. (1975) *The Role of Diagnosis in Psychiatry.* Oxford: Blackwell Scientific.

World Health Organisation (1978) *Mental Disorders: Glossary and Guide to their Classification in Accordance with the Ninth Revision of the International Classification of Diseases.* Geneva: World Health Organisation.

5 / AETIOLOGY

In this chapter we will look at the general principles that underlie the causes of mental disorders and the way in which these can be used to form hypotheses about the aetiology of an individual patient's illness. An accurate assessment of aetiology is important but should be based on well-observed data rather than wild speculation. It then serves as a logical basis for the plan of management (Chapter 7). The particular causes of each syndrome will be considered in Part 2.

AETIOLOGICAL FACTORS

When we look for the aetiological factors of a patient's illness we are in effect trying to answer the following questions:

Why this disorder?
Why this particular time?

In more chronic disorders we must also ask:

Why no recovery?

Aetiological factors can contribute at different stages: first by predisposing to illness, then as precipitants, and finally as maintaining factors. The first of these questions deals with predisposition, the second with precipitation, and the third with maintaining factors.

Predisposing factors

Predisposing factors are those which increase an individual's vulnerability to develop an illness at any time in the future. They address the *'Why this disorder?'* question. The predisposition may operate in a general way (for example **personality traits** of anxiety) so that the patient is at increased risk of developing different illnesses at a later stage in his life; or it may operate in a highly specific way (for example a **genetic predisposition** to Huntington's chorea) to increase the risk of one particular disease. Some kinds of **abnormal personality** are at higher risk of particular illnesses, and these will be described at the end of this chapter.

Precipitating factors

Precipitating factors determine when the illness starts (*'Why at this particular time?'*). Some people are vulnerable to mental illness but may go for many years without becoming ill, so we have to determine the factors that bring about this change from health to illness. Usually precipitating factors act in a non-specific way, that is they determine when the illness starts but not the type of illness: for example **life events** (see p. 56) which involve loss can help to precipitate almost any disorder to which the patient has a predetermined vulnerability.

Maintaining factors

In addition we have to consider whether there may be additional maintaining factors which prolong a disorder, if it continues for longer than would usually be expected (*'Why no recovery?'*). For example, the majority of affective disorders lead to recovery within weeks or months so, if the condition persists for longer, is there any evidence of causes which continue to affect the patient and prevent recovery?

A systematic approach

We should use the available data to answer these questions for each patient that we assess. *Table 2* provides a guide to a systematic approach and each stage needs to be considered in turn. At each stage the aetiological factors may be divided into biological, social, and psychological. Consider whether you have discovered anything about your patient which might fit into these categories, in turn, but you are likely to use only a few of these for each patient.

Aim to write a systematic account of the possible aetiological factors that you have discovered after you have taken the history and completed the examination of the mental state. This will form part of the formulation (see Chapter 9). This initial hypothesis will have to be tested, and perhaps modified, when you attempt to support it by investigations (see Chapter 6).

In the past there was some controversy about whether the origins of mental illnesses are mainly genetic or acquired: nowadays it is more appropriate to consider the extent to which each makes a contribution.

Table 2   *Examples of aetiological factors*

---

1 predisposing

A biological: genetic; intra-uterine disadvantage; birth trauma; or disorders of later onset resulting in cerebral disease or physical handicap. Some forms of personality disorder.

B social: physical or emotional deprivation during childhood due to family discord, bereavement, or separation. Chronic difficulties in work, marriage, housing, or finance. Lack of supportive relationships.

C psychological: inappropriate parental models, e.g. agoraphobic mother or violent father; constitutional predisposition to neurotic traits (may be partly biological), low self-esteem. Some forms of personality disorder. Habitual use of particular defence mechanisms.

2 precipitating

A biological: recent physical disease, e.g. infections, injury resulting in disability, malignant disease with threat of disfiguring surgery or death.

B social: recent life events, particularly those involving threat and loss, such as redundancy, child leaving home, separation, or divorce, loss of a supportive relationship.

C psychological: subject's responses to biological or social factors, e.g. following bereavement or mutilating surgery; feelings of loss of self-esteem; helplessness; hopelessness.

3 maintaining

A biological: physical handicaps; pain from physical disease; failure to take medication or unwanted effects of medication.

B social: adverse social circumstances; no intimate relationships; negative interactions at home; no support from key relative.

C psychological: hopelessness (no expectation of recovery); low self-esteem; marked adverse personality traits, e.g. long-standing dysphoric symptoms; no satisfaction of dependency needs.

THE GENETIC CONTRIBUTION

Evidence for the inheritance of a mental illness is based on the following:

1. Higher prevalence rates in first-degree relatives than the risk for the general population.
2. Higher prevalence rates in the children of probands who are adopted by healthy parents.
3. Higher concordance rates in monozygotic than dizygotic twins.
4. The persistence of this increased concordance, even when monozygotic twins have been separated in infancy and reared apart.

There is a considerable variation in the extent to which different diagnostic categories have a genetic contribution. For example, the concordance rates for first-degree relatives of schizophrenics is between 5 and 15 per cent compared with a lifetime prevalence of about 1 per cent in the general population. The concordance rates for monozygotic twins is between 40 and 60 per cent and this remains almost as high in twins that are raised separately by adoptive parents. The picture for manic-depressive (bipolar affective) disorder follows a similar pattern.

From these figures there can be no doubt that there is an important genetic contribution to the aetiology of these illnesses. However, the nature of this contribution is in doubt. It cannot be determined either by a simple dominant or recessive gene because concordance rates are too low. It has therefore been suggested that inheritance is likely to be due either to polygenic interactions (that is a number of different minor genes acting to complement or modify each other) or to a single gene with incomplete penetrance. The fact that the concordance rates in monozygotic twins are considerably less than 100 per cent demonstrates the importance of the contribution from environmental factors.

There are few mental disorders in which the genetic contribution is substantially greater than this and these are due to single gene transmission following the recognized Mendelian patterns. Examples are

Huntington's chorea (autosomal dominant inheritance)

and some of the uncommon causes of severe mental handicap such as

tuberose sclerosis (autosomal dominant), and
phenylketonuria (autosomal recessive).

The genetic contribution to most of the common psychiatric disorders – the non-psychotic forms of affective disorder – is probably small and based on the inheritance of a general neurotic tendency rather than a predisposition to specific diseases. It is greater for anxiety states and obsessive compulsive disorders than for depressive disorder. It has been suggested that individuals who score high on 'neuroticism' may readily form conditioned responses when anxious.

Some mental illnesses are **familial** in the sense that they tend to aggregate in particular families, even though the evidence for a specific genetic contribution is not very good. Depressive illness is an example of this, but it is not known in what way members of a family 'communicate' depression to each other.

ENVIRONMENTAL FACTORS

Many different factors in the environment that play a part in the aetiology of mental illness have already been mentioned. Some specific events – like bereavement in childhood – can have a long-term effect which may not be evident until much later in life. Others are more chronic difficulties, such as an unhappy marriage or an unrewarding job, which may have a cumulative effect over many years.

LIFE EVENTS

Life events refer to discrete changes in a person's environment that may cause some form of threat or stress to the individual. Some studies have been concerned with specific types of stressful event, while others have dealt with the effects of any kind of stressful event. In the former type of study, groups of subjects who have all had a similar experience – such as death of their spouse – have been followed up prospectively to find out how many develop mental illness during the following year compared with control subjects who have not been bereaved.

In the latter type of study, a group of patients suffering from the same illness – for example, depression – are studied to see whether they have experienced more stressful events than controls in the months prior to the onset of illness. Careful research has excluded those events which might have been the effect rather than the cause of the illness, and demonstrated which types of events are important in the aetiology of various psychiatric illnesses. Events which can precipitate an episode of schizophrenia are any that involve change and include such 'desirable' events as promotion, getting a new job, and moving house in addition to undesirable events. In the three weeks prior to an episode of schizophrenia there is a threefold increase in life events of all types compared with controls. The brevity of this increased period of risk indicates that the event is merely concerned with the exact *timing* of an episode of illness – we must look elsewhere for factors which cause the illness.

By contrast, research into life events prior to the onset of depressive disorders shows a fivefold excess of undesirable events, and these may occur throughout at least the six-month period preceding the onset of illness. 'Loss events' such as bereavement, divorce, severe illness in a close relative, or redundancy have been shown to be particularly important. This means that the contribution of life events to the precipitation of a particular episode of depression is relatively greater than in schizophrenia. Of course many people experience such events without developing schizophrenia, depressive disorders, or any other mental illness, and this demonstrates the essential interaction between life events and predisposition. In the case of depression a stressful life event is much more likely to be followed by an episode of depressive illness in a woman who lacks an intimate confidant (a social predisposing factor) and who has low self-esteem (a personality factor).

PSYCHOLOGICAL DEFENCE MECHANISMS

The description of psychological defence mechanisms stems from the psychoanalytic work of Sigmund Freud (1856 to 1939). These are *unconscious* processes used to *protect the individual from anxiety* arising from inner impulses or environmental threat. The subject is consciously unaware of painful experiences and of the unpleasant feelings attached to them. Individuals tend to have particular mechanisms which they acquire in childhood and use habitually, although sometimes they may emerge for the first time in the face of an unusual crisis. However, if a particular mechanism is used habitually it sometimes helps us to answer the *'Why this disorder?'* question, since different mechanisms tend to be used in different illnesses.

Repression and denial

Defence mechanisms are a part of the healthy repertoire of all people, since we all need to ward off anxiety. **Repression**, for example, refers to the exclusion from our awareness of impulses or emotions which would otherwise cause us distress. It would be difficult to remain healthy if we were unable to suppress unpleasant material, but it is easy to see that the process could go too far. Sometimes the defence against anxiety may prevent the subject from being aware that there are problems in his life which require constructive action. At other times the defence mechanism used may lead the subject to act in inappropriate ways which are maladaptive.

Thus defence mechanisms play an important part in the aetiology of mental illness: sometimes helping to protect against them, at other times contributing to their predisposition or precipitation. We shall be concerned only with those mechanisms which are of particular importance to an understanding of illness.

Denial is a mechanism by which experiences or feelings that might cause anxiety are *denied*, or prevented from entering conscious awareness.

> *A widow may keep all her late husband's personal possessions intact, cook meals for him, and anxiously await his return: she is said to be denying his death.*

Patients who have been told by their doctors that they have malignant disease may afterwards not remember that they have been told and behave as though they are going to recover: they have *denied* the information.

Projection

Projection is a process by which your own feelings or impulses are attributed to others.

> *For example, a patient does not accept his doctor's reassurance, and complains that no one will be able to help him. He is projecting his own feelings of helplessness into his doctor.*

Projection is an important mechanism in paranoid psychoses, which are illnesses in which the patient is convinced that others are persecuting him: his own self-critical feelings are being attributed to others.

Introjection

Introjection is the reverse process by which aspects of another person may be incorporated into the subject's perception of himself.

> *A patient may constantly criticize himself for being a failure in life, even though objectively he has done well. His criticism of himself stems from his father's critical*

attitude towards him which he has now introjected: it has become part of his perception of himself.

Idealization

Idealization is a means by which ambivalent feelings towards another person may be split, so that the bad feelings are denied, or sometimes introjected, and the other person is then regarded as perfect. It is thus a feature of being in love. However, it is also a common feature of morbid grief.

> *For example, Mrs Woods (see p. 15) had an extremely ambivalent relationship with her mother, being very dependent on her but was never able to please her. Following her mother's death Mrs Woods responded by unconsciously using idealization so that she remembered only her mother's good qualities and her own feelings of affection towards her mother. Her more negative feelings of anger and resentment were introjected and took the form of ideas of guilt and self blame: it was no longer her mother whom she regarded as at fault, but herself. (A further example of introjection was the way in which she developed chest pain similar to that suffered by her mother, a process also involving 'identification'.)*

Somatization and conversion

The term **'somatization'** can be used in a descriptive sense to indicate a psychological disorder presenting primarily with physical symptoms (see p. 125) but can also be used to describe a defence mechanism by which the focus on physical complaints serves to divert the subject from awareness of anxiety-provoking conflicts. Closely associated with this is the concept of **conversion**. This refers to the process by which the affect caused by a conflict is replaced by (or 'converted' into) a physical symptom. Idealization is also commonly associated with conversion: in extreme cases the patient claims that he has no problem of any kind in his life other than physical illness and if this is cured his life will be perfect in all respects (a truly remarkable state).

> *An example was a man who had been severely disabled due to headache for three years. He insisted that he could not remember any distressing event that occurred in the year prior to the onset of his symptoms. The history from his wife revealed that during that year he had experienced the bereavement of his father, a brother, and his closest friend, and had been so distressed that he could not attend the funerals.*

Dissociation

Dissociation is a defence mechanism which involves the splitting of two (or more) mental processes which would otherwise be integrated, one part then becoming unconscious. The splitting of conscious awareness is thought to result in such phenomena as **hysterical amnesia** or **fugue states** in which highly organized behaviours are carried out despite gross disturbance of memory or grasp of the environment. Dissociation and conversion are the defence mechanisms thought to predominate in **hysteria** (see p. 221), and the resulting symptoms are described as 'dissociative' and 'conversion' symptoms, respectively.

PERSONALITY DISORDERS

A person's personality refers to long-standing ways of behaving in a wide variety of situations. The characteristic ways of behaving are called **traits**, and particular constellations of traits are said to constitute **personality types**. Thus normal populations may be described in terms of 'extraversion–introversion', of 'stable–neurotic', or of other dimensions of personality derived by multivariate analysis of responses to questionnaires. We shall not give a full account of normal personality here but there is a wide range of information available in post-graduate textbooks.

We shall be concerned with those aspects of personality that are of especial importance to doctors: either because they *increase an individual's vulnerability* to a particular disease, or because they help us to understand *how an individual is likely to behave when he is ill.*

Personality disorders refer to characteristics of individuals that cause them to suffer or which cause others in society to suffer: they have been described by the International Classification of Disease as:

> *deeply ingrained maladaptive patterns of behaviour generally recognizable by the time of adolescence or earlier and continuing throughout most of adult life, although often becoming less obvious in middle or old age.*

Two points must be emphasized from the outset. First, a personality disorder is not an illness, so concepts of 'treatment' and 'recovery' are simply irrelevant. It is sometimes possible to modify habitual patterns of behaviour to some extent, although typically such modification takes a great deal of time and effort if it succeeds at all. Second, by their very nature, personality disorders are dimensional rather than categorical. That is to say, there are infinitely graded steps between normality and any of the 'disorders' described below. The distinction between having, and not having, such a disorder is arbitrary: individuals present such traits to a greater or lesser extent, and it is possible to have some traits but not others under each heading.

Possession of some of the traits can be quite adaptive: for example, mildly obsessional people make good doctors, accountants, or lawyers; mildly histrionic people are good public speakers and fun to be with; and a cyclothymic personality can be very creative during upswings of mood.

It is better to get into the habit of describing which traits best describe your particular patient rather than forcing them into one of the descriptions given below.

Schizoid personality

DESCRIPTION

A withdrawal from social and interpersonal contacts with emotional coldness and a preference for fantasy and introspection. The patient will have had few friends outside his immediate family and is often indifferent to praise or criticism from others. He tends to be aloof and cold, has little enjoyment in close personal relationships, and no desire for sexual experience.

AETIOLOGY

Uncertain; probably genetically related to schizophrenia. Increased incidence of schizoid personalities in the first-degree relatives of schizophrenic probands.

MEDICAL RELEVANCE

Schizoid personalities are at somewhat greater risk for developing an episode of schizophrenia and, having developed such an illness, the prognosis will be worse. However, it must be emphasized that only a minority of schizoid personalities develop schizophrenia; many schizophrenics have normal personalities before they become ill.

Cyclothymic personality

DESCRIPTION

A lifelong tendency to experience periods of pronounced mood disorder. During periods of elation there is an unshakeable optimism and an enhanced zest for life and activity; while periods of depression are marked by worry, pessimism, low output of energy, and a sense of futility.

AETIOLOGY

Imperfectly understood: probably genetically determined. Cyclothymic personalities occur more frequently in families with manic-depressive probands, although not in families with (unipolar) depressive psychosis.

CLINICAL RELEVANCE

Individuals with pronounced cyclothymic traits are at increased risk for the development of both manic and manic-depressive illnesses. The majority (75 per cent in one study) of patients with manic-depressive psychosis will describe cyclothymic traits in their pre-morbid personality.

Sensitive personality
(also known as 'paranoid personality')

DESCRIPTION

The patient has displayed excessive sensitivity to humiliations and rebuffs; a tendency to misconstrue neutral or friendly actions of others as hostile and contemptuous, and a combative and tenacious sense of personal rights. There may be proneness to jealousy or excessive self-importance. Such people feel easily humiliated and put-upon, and there is excessive self-reference.

AETIOLOGY

Unknown. There is a high incidence of this disorder in first-degree relatives of patients with paranoid psychoses.

MEDICAL RELEVANCE

Those with pronounced sensitive traits are especially likely to develop ideas of reference when depressed; some will even progress to frank persecutory symptoms during illnesses which respond to treatment with antidepressants.

In the general wards of the hospital such patients readily misinterpret medical advice, and may be hostile and critical about treatment given to themselves or to their relatives.

Depressive personality

There is no single personality type that is at greater risk for depressive illness. Personality tests measuring general **neuroticism** have been shown in some studies to increase the risk for depressive illness, and several recent epidemiological studies have identified **low self-esteem** as a personality characteristic that greatly increases the risk of a depressive illness following a stressful life event. Subjects tend to regard themselves in a critical and disparaging way and have a low opinion of themselves. Negative views about oneself, one's future, and one's surroundings are said to constitute the **'cognitive triad'** which render people vulnerable to depressive illness. It is likely that the concept of 'passive dependent personality', which will be described next, has considerable overlap with 'low self-esteem'. The two have been kept separate in this account since it is quite possible to have the latter without the former.

AETIOLOGY

This is imperfectly understood. However, recent surveys have shown early loss of mother during childhood to correlate with low self-esteem in adults, and have also identified some features in people's adult lives which relate to low self-esteem, such as women having an unemployed spouse, or more than three children living at home.

Among children, those with low self-esteem have been shown to be associated with authoritarian styles of parenting as well as with indifferent and neglectful parenting.

MEDICAL RELEVANCE

Patients who have a low self-esteem will be at greater risk than others of developing states of anxiety and depression when stressed: it must be remembered that new episodes of physical disease are psychological stressors, while many other sources of stress exist in the patient's social world outside hospital, and will be discovered only by clinicians who are prepared to get to know the patient as a person.

Passive dependent personality

DESCRIPTION

The patient has always let others make decisions for him, and has few resources of his own. He will agree with people with whom he really disagrees to avoid disturbing a relationship, and will remain in a relationship in which he is mistreated for fear of being left alone. When a close relationship ends he is devastated and helpless, as he is often preoccupied with a fear of being abandoned. He constantly seeks reassurance and approval from others, and is easily hurt by disapproval.

AETIOLOGY

No systematic studies have been reported. Authoritarian parents, who enforce rules and edicts without discussion, have been shown to produce children who are miserable, socially withdrawn, and have low self-esteem. It is possible that this might form the basis of the adult disorder, marked as it is by resourcelessness and a desire to please dominant people.

MEDICAL RELEVANCE

These people are at high risk for depressive illness when they lose the dominant person by death or separation. Left to themselves, they may drift down the social scale and become unemployed or homeless.

Obsessional personality

DESCRIPTION

Feelings of personal insecurity, doubt, and incompleteness lead to excessive con-scientiousness, checking, stubbornness, and caution. There is perfectionism and meticulous accuracy and the need to check repeatedly in an attempt to secure this.

Rigidity and excessive doubt may be conspicuous, and there may be insistent and unwelcome thoughts.

AETIOLOGY

Twin studies have shown that genetic factors are important in determining obsessional traits, and that there is an association between such traits and 'neuroticism' – which together may manifest as obsessional symptoms.

Ritualistic behaviour and excessive orderliness appears to be a normal developmental stage in childhood. There is no association between such traits and coercive toilet training, although there is some association between such traits in mothers and children. One study showed that parenting practices characterized as 'restrictive warmth' were associated with children who were submissive, dependent, polite, neat, and obedient: but that is about as near as the various studies of child development seem to get to 'obsessional personality'.

MEDICAL RELEVANCE

People with obsessional traits are especially likely to develop obsessional symptoms during episodes of depressive illness: in such patients special treatment for the obsessional symptoms is not required since they will respond to antidepressants. Obsessional traits are commonly observed in the pre-morbid personalities of those with obsessional states (p. 215).

Histrionic personality
(originally, and confusingly, called 'hysterical personality')

DESCRIPTION

The patient – who is usually female – behaves in a histrionic way, tending to exaggerate and dramatize her descriptions of both symptoms and circumstances. Aspects of her own behaviour which are inconsistent with the romanticized version she relates are either ignored or denied. Displays of emotion (both weeping and angry tantrums) commonly accompany the history – but they strike the observer as being too easily aroused, and they disappear as quickly. She tends to be egocentric in personal relationships, showing too little attention to other people's feeling to form any very deep relationships. Indeed, although she is often sexually provocative her own sexual relationships are unsatisfactory, as she tends to be both frigid and sexually naive. She is often an attractive girl, who has learned to be flirtatious as a way of gaining her own ends rather than as a way of initiating a sexual relationship.

DIAGNOSTIC CRITERIA

The label tends to be fixed on to any female patient who succeeds in irritating the (male) medical staff, by giving an exaggerated account of her symptoms, or who behaves in a manipulative way. This is a pity, since *if the term is used in this way it becomes meaningless*. In this one case we will therefore give diagnostic criteria.

All three of the following should be present:

1. Attention-seeking or histrionic behaviour.
2. Demanding interpersonal behaviour.
3. Displays of emotion which are easily aroused, or more intense than the circumstances require.

AETIOLOGY

Unknown. When measured as a personality trait there appears to be no genetic component. It can probably best be thought of as a set of behaviours that are learned by some immature girls who have been starved of parental affection. It is difficult to escape the impression that these patients use their behaviour to gain attention and admiration from older men: but there have been no systematic studies on this point.

MEDICAL RELEVANCE

The concept came about as a way of describing those thought to be at high risk for hysteria: thus the original name. Although these girls are at higher risk for conversion phenomena than those without such traits, it is now recognized that the majority of those with hysterical illnesses do not have such personalities.

You are far more likely to meet these patients in the accident room than in the neurological wards. They are certainly at very high risk for manipulative and attention-seeking interpersonal behaviours, and they will arrive in hospital having poisoned themselves with drugs, or having made superficial cuts on their forearms.

You should be on your guard when someone begins to behave in this way for the first time in adult life: the diagnosis is much more likely to be an affective illness than a personality disorder!

Antisocial personality
(originally called 'psychopathic personality')

DESCRIPTION

A lifelong tendency to disregard social obligations, and lack of real feeling for other people which may show itself either in impetuous violence or by callous unconcern. The patient may be abnormally aggressive, and tends to be affectively cold and irresponsible. They tolerate frustration poorly and tend to be impulsive. They tend to blame others or offer plausible rationalizations for the behaviour which brings them in conflict with society.

The assessment is made from the personal history, which will show many of the following features:

1. An *unstable work record*, with significant periods of unemployment at times when work was available, repeated episodes of absence from work, or repeated episodes of walking out of jobs without good cause.

2. Failure to conform to social norms indicated by admitting to offences that have not been detected, or a *forensic history* showing episodes of larceny, destroying property, assault, and so on.

3. Irritability and aggressiveness indicated by fights, assaults, wife-beating, or child-abuse.

4. A repeated failure to honour financial obligations.

5. A failure to sustain a monogamous *sexual relationship* for a prolonged period of time.

6. Recklessness, impulsiveness, disregard for truth, and lack of remorse for offences.

AETIOLOGY

Perhaps because of its enormous social importance, much work has been done on the aetiology of sociopathic personality. Both genetic and environmental factors are undoubtedly important. There is a very much higher concordance for criminality in monozygotic than dizygotic twins. Adoption studies show that adopted offspring of criminal parents have a much higher expectancy of sociopathic personality than adopted children whose biological parents were not offenders. In one Danish study the expectancy of criminality in adopted children whose biological parents were not known to the police was not affected by criminality in the father of the adopting family. However since the MZ concordance rate for criminality in twins is only about 50 per cent, it is evident that environmental factors must also be important.

Criminality and social deviance in parents have repeatedly been shown in surveys of antisocial behaviour; as has conflict-ridden and 'broken' homes, lack of early training, and lack of caring supervision. Parents have repeatedly been shown to use poor disciplinary techniques: thus mothers have little control over their (delinquent) children and don't enforce obedience, while fathers are either too lax or too strict.

MEDICAL RELEVANCE

Many of the injured patients you see in an accident room on a Saturday night will either have been injured by sociopaths, or be sociopaths who have managed to injure themselves in fights.

Sociopathic personalities are at higher risk than others for alcoholism and drug dependence.

EXAMPLE OF AETIOLOGY

Now let's return to Mrs Woods – whom we last met in Chapter 3 – for an example of how to write an account of aetiological factors.

> *Mrs Woods appears to be predisposed to the development of depressive illness due to the* **family history** *of depressive disorder in her mother and her own* **bereavement in childhood** *(death of her father when she was aged eight). She has marked* **obsessional personality traits** *(has always been a perfectionist, checked excessively and was house proud to a fault) and appears to have had* **difficulty in adapting to change or loss**, *e.g. when her daughter left home to go to university. She had a close and* **over-dependent relationship with her mother**, *whom she phoned daily throughout her life but could never please, and this has made her particularly vulnerable to the loss of her mother. The present illness has been precipitated by the discovery of her mother's* **terminal illness six months ago and death** *three weeks ago. Mrs Woods felt unable to express her anger or grief whilst nursing her mother through this illness, or to express her ambivalent feelings since the bereavement: this has resulted in the process of* **introjection** *(giving rise to her perception of chest pains) and subsequent* **idealization** *of the mother.*

Notice that these factors are not independent. Although Mrs Woods has always been of impeccable character, and a dutiful daughter, her early experience of bereavement has left her vulnerable to loss, and her relationship with her mother has made her particularly vulnerable to the loss of her mother.

Notice that although she describes both obsessional *traits* and dependent *traits*, that she does not have enough features to satisfy the requirements for either type of personality *disorder*. However, she adapts poorly to change due to her obsessional traits and her dependent relationship with her mother will make her especially vulnerable to loss. Thus the gun is primed and waiting to go off. It only needs the mother's terminal illness to pull the trigger.

Her inability consciously to accept the negative aspects of her ambivalent feelings towards her mother results in *denial* of such feelings.

This example demonstrates another feature in the aetiology of mental illness: the interaction of **nature** and **nurture**. To some extent Mrs Woods's predisposition to depressive disorder may be genetically determined (suggested by the family history) although social and psychological factors have also played their part.

6 / INVESTIGATIONS

So far we have seen in the earlier chapters that the data collected from the history and mental state examination are used to formulate hypotheses about the differential diagnosis and aetiology. The next logical step is to start to test these hypotheses by planning the investigations. These provide additional data which will either support or fail to support our initial hypotheses.

The **purpose** of investigations can be summarized as follows:
1. To support the preferred **diagnosis** if possible and rule out the alternatives.
2. To confirm the identified **aetiological factors** if possible or, if this is obscure, collect new data which will lead to new hypotheses about aetiology.
3. To assess **change**, e.g. to monitor progress in response to treatment.
4. To assess likely **response** to treatment.

The investigations are therefore planned for each patient according to their particular needs. There are no 'routine' investigations (a blunderbuss approach for the unthinking doctor)! In this chapter we will consider how to plan investigations and then go on to describe a few special procedures which the houseman should know about. Investigations that are particularly relevant to individual diagnostic categories are noted in Part 2.

Although in many branches of medicine it is customary to think of investigations mainly as those sources of data derived from laboratory or radiological procedures, in psychiatry we also include all additional sources of information that are required after the initial history and mental state examination. For example, these will include interviews with other informants, examination of past medical records, in-patient observations of mood, sleep pattern, and weight chart, or a home assessment.

You will already be familiar with most of the physical investigations that may be needed but a number of procedures mentioned above will almost certainly be new. However, the following procedures require further explanation.

THE FAMILY TREE

When there is a possibility that a patient is suffering from a familial disorder (genetic or otherwise), it is often helpful to draw up a family tree. The data is gathered from interviews with the patient and relatives. It can be supplemented, if thought necessary, from hospital and general practice health records and from death certificates. It should include all consanguinous relatives for whom accurate data are available.

Figure 3 is an example for a patient, Jane Smith, aged 43, who has been referred on account of memory difficulties and involuntary movements. It illustrates the spread of a disorder through a family in a manner consistent with autosomal dominant inheritance.

The following conventions are used:

The **patient**, Jane Smith, is indicated with an arrow.
Marriages are joined by horizontal lines, e.g. Simon Smith and Ellen.
A **marriage ended by death** can be indicated by a double sloping line, e.g. John Smith and Mary.
A **marriage ended by divorce** can be indicated by a double cross, e.g. William Morris and Elizabeth.
Children are shown joined to parents by vertical lines and siblings to each other (in chronological order) by horizontal lines.
Abortions and still births are included, as shown for Mary Smith's first two pregnancies
Twins are indicated by a vertical line which branches at an acute angle, e.g. Keith and Lawrence Morris.
For each person the year of birth (and death) is shown.
Death is also indicated by a sloping line through the idiogram, e.g. Simon Smith, Fred Jones, and the cause of death is given.
Important illnesses are also shown for living relatives.
Those with illnesses (possibly) related to that of the patient are shown by a shaded idiogram, e.g. Fred Jones, Mary, Jane, and Philip.
Any other information that might be useful can be added such as place and date of birth or occupation.

PSYCHOMETRIC TESTING

Psychologists have devised standardized tests to measure virtually every conceivable aspect of human thought and behaviour. Although many, such as personality tests, have no place in clinical psychiatry, others make a valuable contribution to the process of assessment: particularly in differentiating patients with organic brain disease from those with affective disorders or without mental illness.

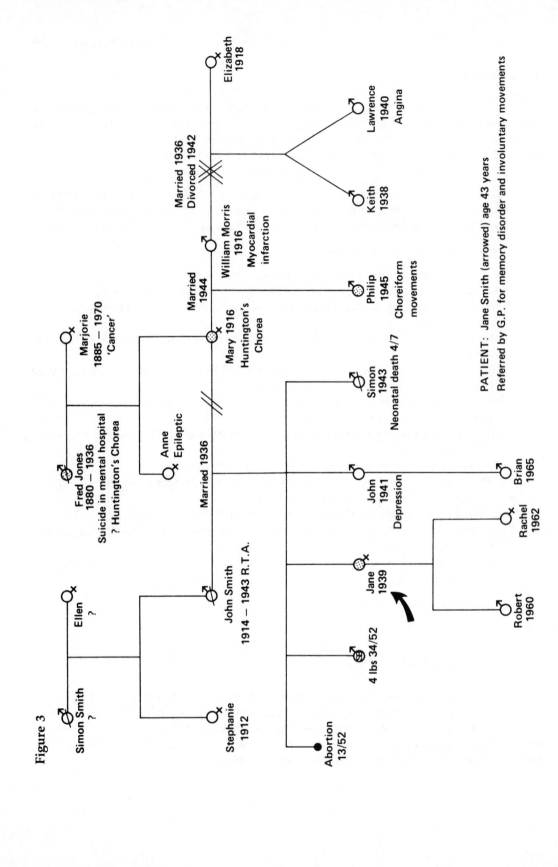

Figure 3

PATIENT: Jane Smith (arrowed) age 43 years
Referred by G.P. for memory disorder and involuntary movements

Assessment of cerebral organic disease

Many standardized tests are available to detect deterioration in brain functions that occur in the presence of organic disorders. Some of these are designed to assess specific functions, for example the visual–spatial functions of the parietal lobe or visual memory function of the non-dominant temporal lobe. Others are more general and include tests of a range of aptitudes such as those found in intelligence tests. While you are doing your psychiatry clerkship try to arrange to watch a clinical psychologist carrying out some of these tests.

INTELLIGENCE TESTS

The most widely used intelligence tests are the **Mill Hill Vocabulary test**, **Raven's Progressive Matrices**, and the **Wechsler Adult Intelligence Scale**. These provide an intelligence quotient (IQ), in which the scores obtained by the subject are expressed as a percentage of the mean scores obtained by the samples on which the tests are standardized. It is usual to subdivide the test score results and express these as two separate IQs, one for verbal tests and the other for 'performance' (that is non-verbal) tests.

Intelligence tests can contribute to the identification of organic brain disease in the following ways:

1. Testing on one occasion may reveal an IQ which is well below the past level of attainment as suggested by the history of educational and professional achievement. For example an overall IQ of 100 would be definitely suggestive of possible organic damage for a physicist but not for a shop assistant.

2. A gross disparity between a higher verbal IQ and a lower performance IQ (in the order of 20 or more) is suggestive of organic deterioration because verbal functions tend to be preserved longer than non-verbal functions. The reverse discrepancy is not usually of significance in this respect. Tests of vocabulary are particularly well preserved in early organic damage, and are therefore sometimes used to estimate premorbid ability.

3. Repetition of intelligence tests over a period of months or years may show a deterioration which usually provides a much better guide to the effects of organic cerebral disease than tests on a single occasion.

TESTS OF MEMORY

These are used to assess the ability to register, retain, and recall new material. They include tests of verbal learning, which are affected particularly by dominant hemisphere disease, and visual memory, which is mainly a non-dominant hemisphere function.

An example of a verbal learning test is the **Synonym Learning Test**. The subject is given definitions of ten words previously unknown to him, but related to his vocabulary level, and then asked to recall their meanings. The definitions are repeated and the subject retested. Scoring is based on the number of trials required. This test has proved moderately successful in differentiating between patients with dementia and those who have affective disorders or are not mentally ill.

In the **Benton Visual Retention Test** the subject is shown a card with a design for ten seconds and then asked to draw the design. The procedure is repeated with other cards. Scores are based on the number of cards correctly reproduced and the number of errors made. The perceptual and constructional skills involved can be separated from the effects of memory deficit by getting the subject to copy the cards while they are in front of him. This too has proved to be a useful test in discriminating between brain-damaged and non-brain-damaged subjects although there is some overlap in the scores obtained.

This is of course only a very brief account of a few of the many tests that are used in the assessment of organic brain disease. The important point is that abnormal findings help to increase the probability of an organic disorder, and the pattern of test findings may help to localize it. These tests are carried out only if there is already some other evidence suggestive of a possible organic disorder.

The findings have to be interpreted in the light of other data, both from the history and examination and from other special investigations.

Mood assessments

Mood assessments are based on standardized self-rating questionnaires or interviews, but the latter require special training in their use as well as postgraduate knowledge of psychiatry. Questionnaires, such as the Beck Depression Inventory (BDI) or the State-Trait Anxiety Inventory (STAI), can be easily administered and scored. However, they are not diagnostic instruments, for example the BDI can provide a measure of the severity of depressive symptoms but cannot differentiate between the affective symptoms that may occur in the setting of a depressive illness, dementia, or schizophrenia. It does not take into account objective signs of illness but is based on the patient's subjective experience. It does not differentiate between mood 'state' and 'trait', although the STAI does attempt to do this. Despite these limitations they provide a useful measure, particularly if administered repeatedly in order to assess change, for example to monitor the response to treatment. Mood scales are also available for both depression and mania based on observations by the nurses looking after the patient.

THE ELECTROENCEPHALOGRAM (EEG)

This is essentially a voltmeter which measures changes in potential transmitted from the brain to the scalp. Electrodes (usually eight or sixteen) are placed bilaterally on the scalp in standard positions and simultaneous tracings are made on a polygraph. The healthy adult, relaxed, awake, and with eyes closed, shows a characteristic **alpha rhythm** of about ten cycles per second and low frequency. On opening the eyes, or with increased mental activity, the tracing flattens. The records of young children normally show **delta waves** which are much slower (fewer than four cycles per second) and of greater amplitude. During adolescence these are replaced by **theta waves** (four to seven cycles per second). These slow waves are not usually present in the adult except during sleep.

The most valuable contribution of the EEG is in the diagnosis of **epilepsy**. 'Spikes' (brief high amplitude discharges) or 'sharp waves' (more prolonged but also high amplitude) are characteristic. Alternating spikes and delta waves at three cycles per second are a classic feature of petit mal epilepsy.

The EEG may be a valuable adjunct in identifying the presence of organic brain disease. In delirium there is usually an irregular slow wave pattern. In dementia the most useful findings are the loss of normal alpha activity and the emergence of delta activity in the waking state. These changes also tend to occur gradually in the normally ageing brain so they have to be interpreted with care. Negative findings do not exclude the possibility of organic disease but a grossly abnormal record is very highly suggestive. It can therefore be valuable in helping to differentiate between dementia and depressive pseudo-dementia, particularly as it is relatively cheap, non-invasive, and painless. The EEG can also be useful in helping to localize a lesion because the abnormal findings may then be limited to tracings from a few leads rather than appearing as a generalized abnormality. A major limitation is the non-specific nature of the abnormal findings, which tend to be similar regardless of the underlying pathology.

HOW TO PLAN INVESTIGATIONS

It is best to plan the investigations methodically. First consider whether it is necessary to get further information about the history and then remember the familiar categories of **biological**, **psychological**, and **social** factors. *Table 3* shows some examples of the commoner investigations that are needed together with some of their indications. As usual, this is only a guide: it is not intended to provide an exhaustive list of all possible investigations. Now let's find out how to apply this procedure: back to Mrs Woods.

*First consider the **history**. We already have an independent account from the husband which is consistent with that of the patient so we probably don't need to see other informants. However it would probably be helpful to find out more from the general practitioner about the episode when he prescribed medication for her 'nerves', and we must certainly send for her mother's psychiatric case records.*

*Next we have to sort out the **differential diagnosis**. In this case the possibilities are limited as she seems to have a wide range of depressive symptoms and some features of a morbid grief reaction. However, she has been complaining of chest pain.*

***Biological** investigation will certainly have to include physical examination and an ECG, if only to provide an informed basis for reassuring her (and ourselves) that she does not have heart disease. As we examine Mrs Woods we note faded bruising on her left*

Table 3   *Examples of investigations*

---

1. history
Always at least one additional **informant**, but sometimes others.
Include employers or teachers if likely to be useful (*with patient's consent*).
Patient's past **general medical and psychiatric records**, and information from general practitioner.
Relative's medical records, if there is positive family history of mental illness.

2. biological
Includes any necessary assessment of physical disease (whether or not related to the mental state) including:
Physical examination: (if not yet done).
Haematology: e.g. ESR, white cell count in infections.
Biochemistry: liver function tests – alcoholism; thyroid function tests – hyperthyroidism; electrolytes – delirium or anorexia nervosa.
Bacteriology, virology, serology: for urinary tract infection, herpes zoster, neurosyphilis.
Electroencephalogram: epilepsy, delirium, dementia.
Radiology: CAT scan – dementia or space-occupying lesion.

3. social
Assessment of family members: by interview (alone or with patient) to see what they are like and how they relate to each other.
Home assessment: (*if necessary*) by psychiatric social worker or others to determine adequacy of accommodation and services and home atmosphere.
Financial assessment: (*if appropriate*) balance of family income from all sources, expenses, and debts.
Occupational: by occupational therapist, to determine nature and severity of disablement, in self-care or employment.

4. psychological
Exploratory psychotherapy (see p. 105)
Standardized psychometric tests: organic psychosyndromes, mood disorders.
Behavioural assessment: to identify maladaptive behaviours and their environmental reinforcers, e.g. in agoraphobia or obsessive compulsive disorder.

---

upper arm and left thorax. She reminds us that she fell downstairs three weeks ago, after taking the sedative prescribed by her GP.

*At this stage **social investigations** do not seem to be indicated.*

*Psychological investigations will certainly include serial observations of her mood and other aspects of the mental state, and if she is an in-patient we will want to ask the nurses to observe the daily pattern of her mood, sleep, and appetite and to keep a weight chart. This will help to confirm the presence of depressive illness as the preferred diagnosis. Later on these will also provide a base line for assessment of change in response to treatment. Further interviews with Mrs Woods in order to explore her relationship with her mother and her reaction to the mother's illness and death may help to confirm their central importance as **aetiological factors** (and may also be therapeutic).*

THE CONTRIBUTION OF OTHER PARAMEDICAL WORKERS

Psychiatric social workers

PSWs have special training in the management of the mentally ill and their families. They contribute to the social aspects of assessment and treatment with regard to material welfare such as financial status and living conditions; the impact of the mentally ill and their families on each other; and the patient's social interactions, sources of support, and satisfaction. In addition some social workers have **approved social worker** status which carries particular responsibilities with regard to the Mental Health Act (1983) (see p. 305).

PSWs may contribute to assessment, for example by interviewing family members to collect additional histories or to assess the attitudes of the relatives to the patient; or by carrying out a home assessment to determine the adequacy of material resources and to observe the nature of family relationships within the home environment.

Psychiatric nurses

Psychiatric nurses have received a special training in mental nursing and play a major part in the care of severely ill patients. It is unwise to judge patients entirely on what you observe at interview: the nurses observe the patient closely for long periods of time in a variety of settings, and regularly provide invaluable additional information about patients. They are responsible for administering medications and they participate in group therapy on the ward as well as providing intensive care for individual patients. **Community psychiatric nurses** are trained to provide nursing care in people's homes.

Occupational therapists

OTs have special skills in the management of disability in the mentally ill. They help those with acute illnesses regain their self-confidence and to interact with others. They discover a patient's assets and exploit them, as well as helping patients to cope with disabilities. They may be involved in the assessment of 'activities of daily living' which include the essentials of self-care such as washing, dressing, cooking, and the use of public services; in the assessment of work, leisure, and recreational activities; and in the assessment of psychological problems through the use of 'projective techniques' such as art and drama.

The contribution of OTs is particularly valuable in the rehabilitation of those with chronic disorders.

7 / TREATMENT

In the chapter that follows we shall give *far more information than you need to pass* your Finals Examination. For Finals, you merely need to know the indications and side-effects of the more important psychotropic drugs, the indications, contra-indications, and side-effects of ECT, and some idea of the principal varieties of psychotherapy. However, we make no apology for giving you more information than you are going to need before you qualify, since we are sure that you will return again and again to this chapter when you have patients under your care.

Treatment in psychiatry should always be considered under the headings **physical**, **psychological**, and **social**. This may seem different from treatments in general medicine but the example of epilepsy will serve to illustrate the model:

Physical – anticonvulsants, and folic acid if necessary.

Psychological – supportive psychotherapy and reassurance about the diagnosis and its implications; advice about avoiding stressful situations and alcohol if these precipitate fits; appropriate treatment for depression or anxiety if these occur.

Social – counselling the patient about employment, driving, marriage, and having children, helping the family coping with the epileptic fits. The person may require being registered as disabled.

Doctors vary in their inclination to regard the psychological and social aspects of treatment as important. For example, anxiety, depression, and sexual problems frequently follow mastectomy and can respond to appropriate treatment. However, some surgeons are more likely than others to detect and treat these symptoms among patients who have undergone the operation. We give separate accounts of physical treatments and psychological treatments. Some forms of social help are included in the latter section, while other forms depend upon local resources and on the needs of the individual patient: you should always seek advice from the **medical social worker**.

PHYSICAL TREATMENTS: DRUGS

Although it has been known since time immemorial that chemical agents can induce perceptual, cognitive, and affective changes, and can grossly modify human behaviour, it is only for the past thirty years that the use of drugs has become generally established in the treatment of psychiatric disorders. Thus **psychiatric toxicology** (that is the production of mental disturbance by drugs) has been complemented by **psychiatric therapeutics** (that is the alleviation of the symptoms of mental illness or the modification of the course of mental illness by drugs). Often the boundary is blurred between these two major areas: the same drug can be toxic or therapeutic under different circumstances!

Drugs used therapeutically fall into two major categories:
1. Drugs that have primarily a direct action on the central nervous system (CNS).
2. Drugs that have an indirect action on the CNS due to their influence on other organ systems of the body.

In this latter group we find drugs which act primarily on the cardiovascular, respiratory, alimentary, or endocrine systems, and thereby can correct a hypoxic or metabolic disturbance of the brain (e.g. the beneficial effect of diuretics in a toxic confusional state caused by cardiac failure).

However, we shall restrict ourselves to the drugs that have a primary action on the central nervous system. The discipline dealing with these drugs is called **neuropharmacology**; **psychopharmacology** is the branch of neuropharmacology concerned with the effects of drugs on behaviour. Drugs that have a primary action on the central nervous system (neuropharmacological agents or centrally acting drugs) are summarized in *Table 4*.

The two major classes are **non-selective** and **selective** drugs. Non-selective drugs have an action on every neurone in the brain and spinal cord: they either decrease ('CNS depressants') or increase ('CNS stimulants') neuronal excitability. Selective drugs, on the other hand, affect only certain groups of neurones or only some aspect of nervous function.

It is obvious that all neuropharmacological agents have to be able to pass through the blood–brain barrier. An important consequence of this feature of these drugs is that they can pass through other lipid membranes, such as the placenta: all centrally acting drugs have a ready access to the foetus. Therefore the general rule is that all these drugs should be avoided during the first trimester of pregnancy, and should be used with great caution during the rest of the pregnancy (see pp. 267–68).

In this chapter we shall concentrate on the discussion of centrally acting drugs which have important roles in the treatment of psychiatric disorders.

Table 4 *Classification of neuropharmacological agents*

I. non-selective agents
    A. general CNS depressants
        1. anaesthetic gases and vapours (nitrous oxide, ether, halothane)
        2. aliphatic alcohols (ethanol)
        3. barbiturates

    B. general CNS stimulants
        1. convulsants (strychnine, picrotoxin)
        2. xanthines (caffeine)

II. selective drugs
        1. anticonvulsants (phenytoin, carbamazepine)
        2. centrally acting muscle relaxants (mephenesin)
        3. centrally acting antihypertensives (clonidine)
        4. narcotic analgesics (opiates)
        5. analgesic antipyretics (aspirin)
        6. anti-Parkinsonian drugs (L-DOPA, central anti-cholinergics)
        7. psychopharmacological drugs ('psychotropics')
            a. neuroleptics (chlorpromazine, haloperidol)
            b. anxiolytics (benzodiazepines)
            c. antidepressants (imipramine, phenelzine)
            d. psychostimulants (amphetamine, cocaine)
            e. hallucinogens (LSD, psilocybin)
            f. other drugs (lithium, tryptophan)

Barbiturates

Barbiturates are general, non-selective depressants of central nervous system activity. These drugs were the most important therapeutically used psychoactive agents during the first half of this century; however, their use has become very limited over the past fifteen years or so. In small doses, they cause a degree of psycho-stimulation and euphoria; in higher doses, however, they cause sedation, and eventually coma. Tolerance readily develops to all barbiturates. Tolerance means that, on repeated medication, the same dose becomes gradually less and less effective (or that increasing doses are needed to evoke the same effect). The tolerance is partly **pharmacokinetic** (*drug disposition tolerance*: the metabolic removal of the barbiturate becomes more effective due to the induction of microsomal enzymes in the liver) and partly **pharmacodynamic** (adaptation of the nervous tissue to the presence of the drug). It is important that while tolerance can develop to the hypnotic effect of the drug, this is not accompanied by an increase in the lethal dose. Both psychological and physical dependence can develop in patients taking these drugs: withdrawal is accompanied by a rebound hyperexcitability of the brain, leading to convulsions. Therefore the use of barbiturates should be avoided for the treatment of insomnia and anxiety; for these indications the benzodiazepines are safer drugs (see below). Barbiturates are often abused by drug addicts, especially in combination with amphetamine since a barbiturate can reduce the unpleasant excitement produced by amphetamine and also enhance the euphoria. **Phenobarbitone** is still used therapeutically as an effective anticonvulsant in generalized epilepsy, and lipid soluble barbiturates (for example, thiopentone) are used as intravenous anaesthetics. Barbiturates, especially **amylobarbitone**, still have some limited use in psychiatry:

1. For *abreaction* (induction of a state of clouded consciousness in which a skilled interviewer can induce the patient to reveal suppressed psychological material).

2. For *activation of the EEG* (a small dose of barbiturate increases the amplitude of high frequency waves and can provoke the appearance of seizure activity).

Anticonvulsants

Epilepsy is a common disorder with psychiatric complications; therefore patients suffering from epilepsy are often referred to psychiatrists. The psychiatrist has to be familiar with the pharmacological management of epilepsy, the side-effects of the drugs, and also with possible interactions between anti-epileptic drugs and other psychoactive medication.

Although general depressants of the central nervous system have anticonvulsant properties (for example, barbiturates), their clinical use is seriously hampered by their sedative properties. Thus only phenobarbitone has survived as a useful drug, but even with this barbiturate daytime sedation and impairment of psychomotor performance can be a problem. The ideal anticonvulsant has a selective effect on the seizure focus without affecting other parts of the CNS. None of the existing anticonvulsants satisfies completely this requirement: apart from an effect on the focus, they also influence other neurones, usually preventing the spread of epileptic discharge through the brain.

PHENYTOIN

Phenytoin (diphenyl-hydantoin) is chemically related to barbiturates. It is a broad-spectrum anticonvulsant with effectiveness in all types of epilepsy with the exception of absence seizures. There are great inter-individual variations in plasma levels on the same dosage, and the determination of plasma concentration is important in selecting a clinically effective non-toxic dosage regimen. Although the drug does not cause sedation, there are some other adverse effects which have been described in patients on chronic medication:

1. Cerebellar-vestibular effects (ataxia, nystagmus).
2. Psychiatric symptoms (a toxic delirium).
3. Gastrointestinal symptoms (nausea, vomiting, diarrhoea, gingival hyperplasia).
4. Impaired calcium metabolism resulting in osteomalacia.
5. Megaloblastic anaemia.

6. Hirsutism.

7. Swollen gums.

Other drugs can influence the plasma concentration of phenytoin:

1. Phenobarbitone and carbamazepine reduce phenytoin plasma levels due to the induction of microsomal enzymes in the liver.

2. Ethanol increases plasma levels due to reduction of phenytoin inactivation.

CARBAMAZEPINE

Carbamazepine is chemically related to the tricyclic antidepressants. This drug has become increasingly popular, over the past decade, for the management of both generalized and partial seizures. Plasma level assessments help in selecting the appropriate oral dosage. The drug is generally well tolerated; toxic effects include *diplopia, blurred vision, drowsiness, dizziness, ataxia, nausea.* The most severe, albeit rare, side-effect is *aplastic anaemia;* patients on this drug require regular haematological monitoring. A recently discovered effect of carbamazepine is it possible effectiveness in the prophylaxis of recurrent manic-depressive episodes, especially in patients who do not respond to lithium (see p. 92).

VALPROIC ACID

Valproic acid (sodium valproate) is a branched chain carboxylic acid with well-documented efficacy in generalized grand mal, myoclonic-atonic and absence seizures; it is less effective in partial seizures (for example, temporal lobe epilepsy). It is believed that the drug acts by *enhancing GABA-mediated inhibition* in the CNS.

BENZODIAZEPINES

Although most **benzodiazepines** have anticonvulsant properties, *clonazepam* and *diazepam* are the two most frequently used drugs in the management of epilepsy. These are broad-spectrum anticonvulsants with effectiveness in most types of epilepsy. Both diazepam and clonazepam, in the form of intravenous injection, are the first line of treatment in major status epilepticus; clonazepam is used to treat absence and myoclonic seizures in children; diazepam can be used in alcoholic withdrawal states for sedation and prevention of fits.

ETHOSUXIMIDE

Ethosuximide is the primary drug for the treatment of absence seizures.

The modern treatment of epilepsy involves clinical and electroencephalographic identification of the type of seizure involved, selection of an appropriate drug, and continuous monitoring of the clinical response, side-effects and plasma concentration of the anticonvulsant.

It is especially important to monitor serum levels of phenytoin. The aim is *'monotherapy'*, that is the control of seizures with one anti-epileptic drug. Drug combinations should be avoided because of complex pharmacokinetic interactions between anti-epileptic drugs and difficulties in identifying adverse effects attributable to a particular medication.

Anti-Parkinsonian drugs

Parkinsonism is an extrapyramidal syndrome consisting of the triad of *hypokinesia*, *rigidity*, and *tremor*. Parkinsonism can be defined neurochemically as a **striatal dopamine-deficiency syndrome**. The syndrome can be brought about by a reduction in the dopaminergic input to the striatum in the following ways:

1. Destruction of the nigro-striatal pathway: Parkinson's disease, postencephalitic Parkinsonism, manganese poisoning.
2. Depletion of nigro-striatal neurones of dopamine by reserpine, tetrabenazine.
3. Blockade of striatal dopamine receptors by neuroleptics.

It follows from this model that **dopaminergic drugs** restoring the functional integrity of dopaminergic neurotransmission in the striatum will be beneficial in treatment. It has been found that **anti-cholinergic drugs** can also alleviate the symptoms of Parkinsonism, suggesting that there may be a functional antagonism between dopaminergic and cholinergic influences in the striatum. Thus anti-Parkinsonian drugs fall into two major categories:

1. Dopaminergic drugs.
2. Centrally acting anti-cholinergics.

The dopaminergic drugs comprise

1. *Dopamine dispensers* (precursor: L-DOPA; releaser: amantadine)
2. *Dopamine mimetics* (e.g. apomorphine, bromocriptine)
3. *Dopamine conservers* (e.g. selegiline – a centrally acting monoamine oxidase-B inhibitor which prevents the degradation of dopamine).

Of these drugs, **L-DOPA** is the primary agent in the treatment of Parkinsonism due to the degeneration of the nigro-striatal system; the other dopaminergic drugs are useful adjuncts in management. L-DOPA is usually administered together with a peripheral aromatic-L-amino-acid decarboxylase inhibitor: the use of the enzyme inhibitor prevents the conversion of L-DOPA to dopamine in the periphery thereby reducing peripheral side-effects and enabling a reduction in the dosage of L-DOPA. The use of L-DOPA, and to some extent of the other dopaminergic drugs, is associated with important psychiatric side-effects:

Mild side-effects (anxiety, insomnia, daytime sedation) are very common but subside with time.

Severe side-effects occur in about 15 per cent of patients treated with L-DOPA and comprise

1. Acute brain syndrome
2. Affective psychosis (depression leading to suicide, hypomania).
3. Paranoid psychosis.

The centrally acting anti-cholinergics readily pass through the blood–brain barrier and can produce effective central muscarinic receptor blockade with relatively little effect on peripheral muscarinic receptors. These drugs have only a limited use in the management of Parkinsonism resulting from the degeneration of the nigro-striatal system, but they are the treatment of choice in managing neuroleptic-induced Parkinsonism. In neuroleptic-induced Parkinsonism the symptoms are due to the blockade of striatal dopamine receptors by the neuroleptic drug, and thus dopaminergic drugs, whose action relies on the activation of these receptors, are ineffective. The most commonly used *centrally acting anti-cholinergics* are **benzhexol**, **benztropine**, **procyclidine**, and **orphanedrine**. These drugs can be useful in alleviating the symptoms of neuroleptic-induced Parkinsonism, and procyclidine in injection form can relieve the symptoms of neuroleptic-induced *acute dystonic reactions*.

The routine use of these drugs should be avoided since they can reduce the effective concentration of the neuroleptic in the body and may also promote the development of tardive dyskinesia. The *side-effects* are the same as those of atropine: dry mouth, cycloplegia, constipation, urinary retention. In susceptible individuals or on high doses an *'atropine psychosis'* (a toxic delirium) may develop.

Anti-cholinergic drugs can produce *euphoria* in some individuals, and thus these drugs have some abuse potential.

Neuroleptics

These drugs are also called 'ataractics', 'major tranquillizers', and 'anti-psychotics'. The term **neuroleptic** was coined by Delay and Deniker in 1952 to describe the characteristic pattern of sedation ('neuroleptic syndrome') caused by these drugs: *psychomotor slowing, emotional quieting, and affective indifference without any clouding of consciousness and/or ataxia.* The terms 'ataractic' and 'major tranquillizer' are alternatives to describe this pattern of sedation. The term 'antipsychotic' refers to the ability of these drugs to affect some 'target symptoms' of psychotic states, such as hallucinations, delusions, and thought disorder. The sedative and anti-psychotic effects can be separated: while tolerance develops to the sedative effect, this is not the case with the anti-psychotic effect. The classification of neuroleptic drugs is shown in *Table 5*.

Neuroleptics of different classes have a common mode of action: they *block transmission through dopaminergic synapses*. Most neuroleptics achieve this by their ability to block post-synaptic dopamine receptors, whereas rauwolfia alkaloids, together with some synthetic drugs such as tetrabenazine, impair dopaminergic transmission due to their ability to deplete presynatpic stores of dopamine (and also of noradrenaline and 5-hydroxytryptamine). Thus the central effects of the neuroleptics are related to the four areas of the brain where dopaminergic synapses, and thus dopamine receptors, are located:

1. **Limbic system and neocortex**. Dopamine-containing neurones in the midbrain project to the limbic system ('mesolimbic pathway') and to some areas of the prefrontal cortex ('mesocortical pathway'). It is believed that the blockade of dopamine receptors at these sites is the basis of the anti-psychotic effect of the neuroleptics.

2. **Striatum**. Dopamine-containing neurones in the pars compacta of the substantia nigra project to the striatum ('nigro-striatal pathway'). The blockade of striatal dopamine receptors is thought to be the basis of neuroleptic-induced Parkinsonism.

Table 5 *Classification of neuroleptics*

I. tricyclic neuroleptics
  A. phenothiazines
      1. with aliphatic side-chain (e.g. chlorpromazine)
      2. with piperidine side-chain (e.g. thioridazine)
      3. with piperazine side-chain (e.g. trifluoperazine)
  B. thioxanthines
      e.g. flupenthixol, clopenthixol
  C. azepines
      1. dibenzoxapines (e.g. loaxapine)
      2. dibenzodiazepines (e.g. clozapine)

II. butylperidines
  A. 'butyrophenones' (phenylbutylperidines)
      e.g. haloperidol, droperidol, spiroperidol
  B. diphenylbutylperidines
      e.g. pimozide, fluspiriline

III. other heterocyclic compounds
  A. indoles
      e.g. oxypertine
  B. substituted benzamines
      e.g. sulpiride

IV. rauwolfia alkaloids
      e.g. reserpine

---

3. **Hypothalamus**. Dopamine-containing neurones in the arcuate nucleus project to the infundibulum of third ventricle ('tubero-infundibular pathway'). The blockade of infundibular dopamine receptors is thought to be the basis of neuroleptic-induced hyperprolactinaemia.

4. **Brain stem**. Dopamine receptors have been identified in an area of the lower brain stem which lies outside the blood brain barrier ('chemoreceptor trigger zone'). Neurones in this area project to the dorsal nucleus of the vagus, and their stimulation can result in vomiting. It is believed that the anti-emetic effect of neuroleptics is based on the blockade of dopamine receptors in the chemoreceptor trigger zone.

There are three major uses for neuroleptics in psychiatric treatment:

1. **Acute calming of agitated patients**. An injection of a potent short-acting neuroleptic (e.g. droperidol) can be very effective.

2. **Treatment of acute psychotic states**. Both organic psychoses (including most drug-induced states) and functional psychoses (acute schizophrenia, mania, psychotic depression) can respond to treatment with neuroleptics. Apart from a psychomotor calming effect, the drugs help to abolish specific 'psychotic' symptoms (hallucinations, delusions, thought disorder). As the psychosis subsides, the patient becomes more responsive to the environment, and amenable to other forms of treatment (for example, occupational and social therapy).

3. **Maintenance treatment** in chronic and recurrent psychotic states. This form of treatment is especially important in schizophrenia where symptoms can persist or recur over many years. Maintenance treatment helps to control the psychotic symptoms and to maintain the patient's social functioning at its optimum level, and can prevent the recurrence of acute psychotic episodes.

The choice of drug and form of administration depends on the indication and on the clinical features of the individual patient. For the treatment of acute psychoses oral medication on the ward can be used; drugs can be administered in the form of syrup. **Chlorpromazine** is the oldest and best-known phenothiazine, and it is usually a safe choice in most cases. **Thioridazine** has more anti-cholinergic and anti-adrenergic side-effects, but is less likely to produce extrapyramidal side-effects probably due to its 'built-in' central anti-cholinergic anti-Parkinsonian property.

Trifluoperazine, haloperidol, and **pimozide** are potent neuroleptics: these drugs are not sedative, and are relatively free from autonomic side-effects, but can produce troublesome extrapyramidal syndromes. These drugs can be used in small doses on an out-patient basis in the management of **chronic paranoid states**. Although drugs in tablet form are suitable for long-term maintenance treatment, depot injections are usually preferred for this purpose since they help to ensure patient compliance. The depots are usually oily injections of esters (decanoates or enanthates) of drugs; the active drug is gradually released from the injection site into the blood stream. There are depot injections for **fluphenazine, flupenthixol, clopenthixol, haloperidol**, and **fluspiriline**.

Injections are administered every one to four weeks, usually at a 'depot clinic' or in the patient's home.

The neuroleptics are relatively safe drugs: they have a high therapeutic index (toxic dose/therapeutic dose), and as they have a shallow dose–response curve, they can be administered over a wide dosage range. The side-effects and drug interactions are shown in *Table 6*.

Anxiolytics

These drugs are also called 'minor tranquillizers'; they are effective in reducing pathological anxiety, tension, and agitation without general depression of the CNS (cf. barbiturates). These drugs are also devoid of any anti-psychotic activity (cf. neuroleptics). Of the diverse compounds included in this group only the **benzodiazepines** will be considered since they have almost completely replaced other anxiolytics (e.g. meprobamate, methaqualone).

BENZODIAZEPINES

The mode of action of benzodiazepines is closely related to GABA-mediated inhibition in the CNS. Specific binding sites for benzodiazepines ('benzodiazepine receptors') have been demonstrated in most parts of the neuraxis; the highest concentrations have been found in the neocortex, limbic system, and cerebellum. The benzodiazepine receptor is closely associated with the GABA-receptor ('GABA-benzodiazepine receptor complex'), and the activation of the benzodiazepine receptor results in potentiation of GABA-mediated responses. The anti-anxiety effect is thought to be mediated via the enhancement of GABA-mediated inhibition of 5-hydroxytryptamine – and noradrenaline-containing neurones; the integrity of the monoamine-containing neurones is believed to be essential in mediating the suppression of certain behaviours and increased arousal associated with fear responses. Similarly the enhancement of GABA-mediated neuronal inhibition in certain neuronal circuits has been related to the anticonvulsant and central muscular relaxant effects of benzodiazepines.

Each benzodiazepine possesses, to greater or lesser extent, five important pharmacological effects:

1. Anxiolytic.
2. Hypnotic.
3. Muscle relaxant.
4. Anticonvulsant.
5. Amnestic.

The **anxiolytic effect** is utilized in the management of anxiety states. While these drugs are effective and relatively harmless in the treatment of short-lived situational anxiety, their use in the management of anxiety neurosis is more controversial. The current recommended practice is to use these drugs for only a limited period (two to four

Table 6 *Side-effects of neuroleptics*

central side-effects extrapyramidal syndromes	Parkinsonism	hypokinesia, rigidity, and tremor (alleviated by centrally acting anti-cholinergic drugs)
	akathisia	'inability to sit still', inner restlessness, and compensatory foot-shuffling
	acute dystonic reactions; oculogyric crises	spastic contractions of the muscles of the neck and shoulders; relieved by an injection of procyclidine
	tardive dyskinesia (late onset)	orofacial dyskinesia whole body chorea
	neuroleptic malignant syndrome	rigidity, hyperpyrexia, and coma (extreme dopamine receptor blockade: potentially lethal) treat with bromocriptine (dopamine receptor stimulant) and dantrolene (muscle relaxant)
lowering of the seizure threshold	fits	
central autonomic side-effects	thermoregulatory failure	body cools in cold temperature → dangerous hypothermia in heat, → heat stroke
	orthostatic hypotension	partly central origin (see below!)
endocrine complications	hyperprolactinaemia	galactorrhea, gynaecomastia, impotence, and infertility
	reduction in gonado-trophins, oestrogens and progesterone	amenorrhoea and infertility
psychiatric complications	apathy, lassitude, lack of initiative	(like chronic schizophrenia!)
	disturbance of the sleep/wakefulness cycle	
	depression	
	acute brain syndrome ('atropine psychosis)	esp. potent anti-cholinergic drugs (like thioridazine)
peripheral autonomic side-effects (phenothiazines > butyrophenones)	blockade of muscarinic receptors	cycloplegia, dry mouth, constipation, urinary retention

Table 6   *Side-effects of neuroleptics (cont.)*

	blockade of α_1-adrenoceptors	miosis, orthostatic hypotension, nasal stuffiness, ejaculatory incompetence
hypersensitivity reactions		
	cholestatic jaundice	
	blood dyscrasias	agranulocytosis
	allergic skin reactions	urticaria, dermatitis
skin reactions		
	contact dermatitis	affects nurses handling phenothiazine solutions
	photosensitivity	problem in sunny climates
	patchy hyper-pigmentation (long-term medication)	
drug-interactions		
	blockade of uptake of drug into peripheral noradrenergic neurones	inhibition of the anti-hypertensive effect of guanethidine
		potentiation of the effects of sedative drugs (including ethanol and opiates)

weeks) during which the patient will become more amenable to other (e.g. behavioural, social) forms of treatment. The long-term use of these drugs should be avoided because of the possibility of development of *tolerance and dependence.* **Diazepam**, a long-acting drug, may be more suitable for the management of persistent high levels of anxiety, whereas shorter-acting drugs (e.g. **lorazepam, oxazepam**) can be used for the management of episodic or situational anxiety.

Several benzodiazepines are suitable **hypnotics**: triazolam and temazepam are short-acting drugs suitable to *induce sleep and relatively free from hangover effects during daytime,* whereas longer-acting drugs, such as diazepam, nitrazepam, and flurazepam can both *induce sleep and maintain sleep throughout the night.*

Diazepam is used as an effective **muscle relaxant** in the treatment of spasticity, and diazepam and clonazepam are established **anticonvulsants** (p. 80).

Some benzodiazepines (e.g. diazepam, lorazepam, midazolam) can produce **anterograde amnesia**; this property of the drugs is utilized in pre-anaesthetic medication and in performing minor surgical or diagnostic interventions (dentistry, endoscopy).

Almost all the **side-effects** of the benzodiazepines are related to their actions on the CNS. Daytime sedation, drowsiness, impairment of psychomotor performance can occur both in conjunction with anti-anxiety treatment and the use of long-acting hypnotics ('hangover effect'). Increased hostility and aggressive behaviour can occur as a rare but unpleasant complication. Physical dependence has been reported, especially in association with large-dose long-term medication.

Withdrawal symptoms are common; these are more severe following the use of short-acting potent drugs (e.g. lorazepam) than long-acting drugs (e.g. diazepam). Withdrawal symptoms include increased anxiety, rebound insomnia, dysphoria, anorexia; rarely more severe symptoms (severe agitation, panic, depression, delusions, hallucinations, convulsion) can occur. These withdrawal symptoms can take a few weeks to resolve, and patients must be encouraged to persevere if they are not to continue their dependence. The benzodiazepines are relatively safe drugs in overdosage; fatalities are usually due to the concomitant use of CNS depressants (ethanol, barbiturates).

Antidepressants

These drugs are effective in the treatment of pathological depressive states; they do not have any specific effects in non-depressed individuals. There are four major classes of antidepressant drugs:

1. Tricyclic antidepressants.
2. Novel, atypical, or second-generation antidepressants.
3. Monoamine oxidase inhibitors.
4. Tryptophan.

TRICYCLIC ANTIDEPRESSANTS

These drugs have been in clinical use for almost thirty years, and they are still the most important antidepressants. Chemically they are related to the phenothiazines. They have characteristic effects on a number of central and peripheral synapses and/or receptors:

1. **Noradrenaline**: These drugs block the (re-)uptake of noradrenaline into presynaptic terminals, and thereby potentiate the synaptic effects of noradrenaline. They also block post-junctional α_1-adrenoceptors, resulting in antagonism of the effect of noradrenaline. After chronic administration (one to three weeks), these drugs reduce the number of post-junctional β-adrenoceptors (*'down-regulation of β-receptors'*), and thereby attenuate β-adrenoceptor-mediated responses (for example activation of the enzyme adenylate cyclase).

2. **5-Hydroxytryptamine**: These drugs can both block the uptake of 5-hydroxytryptamine into presynaptic terminals, thereby potentiating the synaptic effect of the monoamine, and block postsynaptic 5-hydroxytryptamine receptors, thereby antagonizing the effect of the amine.

3. **Acetylcholine**: blockade of muscarinic receptors.

4. **Histamine**: blockade of histamine H_1-receptors.

According to the monoamine theory of affective disorders (p. 184), the anti-depressants relieve depression by correcting a deficiency in central monoaminergic neurotransmission; this is achieved by an increase in the synaptic concentrations of noradrenaline and/or 5-hydroxytryptamine via (re-)uptake blockade. More recently it has been proposed that a more relevant common mode of action of these drugs is the *down-regulation of central β-adrenoceptors*: the development of this effect has the same time-course as the development of the antidepressant effect, and antidepressants of other classes also share this effect. The blockade of central α_1-adrenoceptors, muscarinic, and histamine receptors is believed to be responsible for the sedative effects of tricyclic antidepressants; the blockade of these receptors in the periphery results in characteristic autonomic side-effects.

Indications: Tricyclic antidepressants can be effective in the treatment of different forms and severity of depression, both on the ward and on an out-patient basis. The therapeutic effect appears gradually, usually after one to three weeks on the drug; therefore in severe retarded or psychotic depression a faster-acting treatment, such as ECT, may be more appropriate. It is important to administer a therapeutically effective dose, and plasma level assays may be helpful in dosage selection. It has been recommended that the antidepressant medication should be continued after remission of the depressive symptomatology since there is an increased risk of relapse for the first six to twelve months following a depressive episode. There are a large number of tricyclic antidepressants available on the market. **Imipramine** is the prototype drug with established effectiveness. **Desipramine** is less sedative than impramine and has more marked sympathomimetic activity. **Amitriptyline** is a widely used and effective drug with marked sedative and peripheral antimuscarinic and adrenolytic properties. **Clomipramine** does not cause appreciable sedation, and it has been claimed to have beneficial effects in obsessional states. The side-effects are shown in *Table 7*.

The most important **drug interaction** involving these drugs is diminution of the effectiveness of some **antihypertensive agents** either due to uptake blockade in peripheral noradrenergic neurones (bethanidine, debrisoquine) or to a central effect (clonidine); β-adrenoceptor blockers are not affected.

NOVEL (ATYPICAL) ANTIDEPRESSANTS

These drugs differ structurally from the tricyclic antidepressants, and they also have varied pharmacological properties. The most important are:

1. **Mianserin** (blocks 5-hydroxytryptamine receptors and α_2-adrenoceptors).

2. **Maprotiline** (blocks noradrenaline uptake).

3. **Trazodone** (blocks α_1-adrenoceptors).

Since most of these drugs are relatively free from peripheral anti-cholinergic and

Table 7   *Side-effects of anti-depressants*

central neurological side-effects	fine static tremor
lowering of the seizure threshold	convulsions
peripheral autonomic side-effects antimuscarinic	cycloplegia, mydriasis, tachycardia, constipation, urinary retention
sympathomimetic (due to noradrenaline uptake blockade)	mydriasis, tachycardia
adrenolytic (alpha$_1$-adrenoceptor blockade)	miosis, orthostatic hypotension, nasal stuffiness, ejaculatory difficulties
cardiovascular side-effects	tachycardia
	orthostatic hypotension
	arrhythmias
reduction in cardiac contractility	reduced cardiac output
psychiatric side-effects	hypomania
	paranoid–hallucinatory states
potent anti-cholinergics like amitriptyline	acute brain syndrome ('atropine psychosis')
hypersensitivity reactions (relatively rare)	cholestatic jaundice
	blood dyscrasias
	allergic dermatitis

cardiotoxic side-effects, they have been especially recommended for the treatment of elderly patients and of those suffering from heart disease. It should be noted, however, that clinical experience with these drugs is still rather limited compared to the tricyclic antidepressants. Moreover, these drugs are not completely devoid of side-effects: maprotiline can cause convulsions, mianserin and nomifensine can produce potentially lethal blood dyscrasias, and trazodone can produce sedation, orthostatic hypotension, and impairment of male sexual functions (ejaculatory incompetence, priapism).

MONOAMINE OXIDASE INHIBITORS

This is an old-established class of antidepressants; the use of these drugs, however, is much more limited than that of the tricyclic antidepressants, because they are both less effective and more toxic. The antidepressant action of these drugs has been directly related to their main pharmacological action – the *inhibition of the enzyme monoamine oxidase*: enzyme inhibition results in an increased concentration of cerebral monoamines which would correct the neurochemical deficiency underlying depressive illness (see monamine theory of affective disorders, p. 184).

There are three monoamine oxidase inhibitors in clinical use:

1. Phenelzine.
2. Tranylcypromine.
3. Isocarboxazide.

The clinical uses of these drugs are:

1. As a *second line of treatment* in case of patients whose depression does not respond to treatment with tricyclic antidepressants.
2. They have been recommended for some *atypical forms of depression* characterized by features such as 'reversed diurnal variation', weight gain, or for the treatment of patients with histrionic or hypochondriacal features.
3. *Phobic anxiety states*, in which they are as effective as tricyclic antidepressants. Relapse is common on withdrawal of the drug.
4. *Narcolepsy.*

These are potentially toxic drugs, and **side-effects** are common and troublesome. These are:

1. *Excessive central stimulation* (agitation, hypomania, convulsions).
2. *Orthostatic hypotension* (probably due to sympathetic ganglion blockade).
3. *Hepatocellular jaundice* (as a rare but severe hypersensitivity reaction).

Drug-interactions are important and basically of two kinds:

1. Potentiation of the effects of **monoamine precursors** (e.g. L-DOPA) and indirectly acting sympathomimetic amines (e.g. tyramine, amphetamine). The potentiation of the effects of sympathomimetic amines can lead to a hypertensive crisis (as in the **cheese reaction** following the ingestion of tyramine-containing foodstuffs, such as cream cheese, broad beans, pickled herrings, avocado pears, Marmite, and Chianti).
2. **Inhibition of the detoxification** of a number of drugs (barbiturates, ethanol, centrally acting anti-cholinergics, tricyclic antidepressants).

TRYPTOPHAN

Tryptophan is the amino-acid precursor of 5-hydroxytryptamine. It is believed that the administration of tryptophan results in increased 5-hydroxytryptamine synthesis in the brain which in turn would lead to the replenishment of presynaptic stores. Tryptophan has only weak antidepressant properties, and is usually administered as an adjunct to enhance the effectiveness of tricyclic antidepressants or monoamine oxidase inhibitors in case of treatment-resistant depression.

Psychostimulants

These drugs increase the level of alertness, stimulate mental activity, and suppress fatigue in the normal person. The two major classes of psychostimulants are the **amphetamines** and **cocaine**; the **xanthines** (e.g. caffeine) are classified as non-selective CNS stimulants (see *Table 4*). Both the amphetamines and cocaine exert their alerting effects by increasing the central actions of monoamines: amphetamine releases both noradrenaline and dopamine (and at higher doses 5-hydroxytryptamine) from presynaptic stores; cocaine blocks the (re-)uptake of noradrenaline. These drugs also possess powerful sympathomimetic effects. Of these drugs only the amphetamines have therapeutic uses.

AMPHETAMINES

The most important amphetamines are:

1. Amphetamine.
2. Methamphetamine.
3. Methylphenidate.
4. Fenfluramine.

Apart from a psychostimulant/anti-fatigue effect, these drugs also have anorectic (appetite suppressant) properties. However, they have no place in the treatment of obesity, since they are not effective and produce dependence.

Before the advent of the tricyclic antidepressants, amphetamine was the most popular drug for the treatment of depression. The current clinical use of these drugs is limited, and it includes the treatment of the following:

1. **Narcolepsy** (alerting effect).
2. **Hyperkinetic children** (a paradoxical 'calming' effecting of amphetamine and methylphenidate).
3. **Nocturnal enuresis** (partly a central alerting effect, partly a direct effect on the bladder sphincter).

SIDE-EFFECTS

1. Excessive **central stimulation** (anxiety, over-activity, insomnia)
2. **Paranoid psychosis** (especially on larger doses). Since most of the amphetamines cause euphoria, they have an abuse potential; **psychological dependence**, rapidly develops on these drugs.

Lithium

Lithium cannot be classified with other psychoactive drugs: it is a unique drug which has no psychotropic effect in normal individuals. However, it has remarkable effectiveness in manic-depressive psychosis (acute 'anti-manic' effect and 'mood-stabilizing' effect on maintenance treatment). Lithium is a monovalent cation which is available for clinical use in the form of carbonate or citrate salts. The most important cellular effects are:

1. Competition with sodium ions for the *sodium pump*: interference with the maintenance of membrane potential and action potential generation in neurones.
2. Increase in the *uptake of catecholamines* into nerve terminals.
3. Reduced effectiveness of the *activation of central α_1-adrenoceptors and muscarinic receptors*.
4. Inhibition of the activation of *adenylate cyclase*
   - by antidiuretic hormone (ADH) in renal tubules;
   - thyroid stimulating hormone (TSH) in the thyroid gland.

The first three effects have been related to the anti-manic and mood-stabilizing properties of lithium, whereas the effect on adenylate cyclase activation seems to be the basis for some side-effects (nephrogenic diabetes insipidus; hypothyroidism).

The elimination of lithium from the body is almost entirely through the kidneys. In steady state, the serum lithium concentration is determined by the ratio of the *daily lithium intake* and the *renal lithium clearance*. Renal lithium clearance is the product of the fractional tubular excretion of lithium and the glomerular filtration rate. The elimination of lithium through the kidneys can be impaired if either of these components is reduced: fractional tubular excretion of lithium will be reduced if the serum sodium concentration declines (for example, as a result of thiazide diuretics, Addison's disease); glomerular filtration rate can be reduced as a result of dehydration, cardiac failure, kidney disease.

Lithium can be used clinically both in acute affective episodes and in prophylactic maintenance treatment. The oldest use of lithium is in the treatment of **mania**. The therapeutic (anti-manic) effect of lithium does not appear for about a week, therefore the additional use of neuroleptics is often required. The plasma concentration aimed at is higher (0.6–1.2mEq/1) than in maintenance treatment; thus there is an increased risk of lithium toxicity. In general, a neuroleptic is more effective and safer for the management of acute mania.

There is increasing evidence that lithium has an **antidepressant effect**, and its use has been recommended to treat depressive states unresponsive to tricyclic antidepressants. The most important use of lithium is the **prophylactic maintenance treatment of recurrent manic-depressive psychosis**. Patients with both bipolar (manic and depressive) and unipolar (only depressive) episodes can respond to maintenance treatment: relapses may be completely prevented or their frequency and/or intensity reduced. Patients with frequently alternating mood states ('*rapid cycling manic-depressive psychosis*') usually respond only poorly to lithium; such patients may benefit from maintenance treatment with **carbamazepine** (see 'Anticonvulsants' p. 79). Patients on lithium maintenance treatment are usually followed up at 'lithium clinics' where plasma concentration of lithium, therapeutic response, and side-effects can be monitored. This is done monthly until a steady state has been achieved; three-monthly thereafter. The recommended plasma level is 0.4–0.8 mEq/1 for maintenance treatment.

Lithium maintenance treatment is contra-indicated in the following conditions:
1. Renal and cardiac insufficiency.
2. Addison's disease.
3. Hypothyroidism.
4. Pregnancy.

It is usual to do a **blood urea** before starting lithium; other tests only if clinically indicated. Lithium has a low therapeutic index, and **toxicity** quickly appears as the plasma concentration rises above 1.2 mEq/1.

SIDE EFFECTS

Side-effects can occur even at 'therapeutic' plasma levels:

1. **Gastrointestinal side-effects** are common, especially early in treatment, and include nausea, vomiting, indigestion, metallic taste, diarrhoea.
2. Of the **neurological side-effects** a fine static tremor is the most common; the appearance of coarse tremor, ataxia, fasciculations are the signs of intoxication.
3. Of the **metabolic effects** a nephrogenic diabetes insipidus (polyuria, polydipsia), increased water retention leading to ankle oedema, and an increase in weight are the most important.
4. An important **endocrine side-effect** is the development of hypothyroidism.

Drug interactions involve:

1. **Thiazide diuretics** (these can lead to sodium loss and thus to lithium toxicity).
2. **Neuroleptics** (these can increase the neurotoxicity of lithium).

PHYSICAL TREATMENTS: ELECTROCONVULSIVE TREATMENT (ECT)

The use of electroconvulsive therapy has been the cause of much controversy both in psychiatry and among the general public. This is partly because the treatment has been used outside those situations where its use is appropriate and partly because there has been difficulty in performing accurate research. Several large studies have established that ECT is superior to antidepressant drugs, and far superior to placebo, in the treatment of depression. The necessity of the seizure has now been proven by studies comparing the effects of ECT with 'simulated' ECT (administration of the anaesthetic and muscle relaxant but without the electric shocks).

The relative effects of treatments for severe depressive illness were demonstrated in a study some years ago:

> *After four weeks over 70 per cent of those receiving ECT had few or no symptoms (they had received four to eight treatments during this time). Just over one-half of those receiving imipramine had made a similar response, to be compared with 39 per cent of the placebo group and only 30 per cent of the phenelzine group.*

Mode of action

It is a highly probable that grand mal seizure activity is necessary for the antidepressant effect, and there is some evidence that seizures elicited by higher currents have greater antidepressant activity than those elicited by lower currents. Thus attempting to minimize confusion and memory loss by minimizing the current may reduce the therapeutic efficacy. However, unilateral ECT to the non-dominant hemisphere evokes a bilateral seizure with much less confusion and, at most, marginally reduced efficacy.

ECT potentiates behaviour mediated by serotonin (5HT) and there is neurochemical evidence from work with experimental animals that this is due to an increase in post-synaptic 5HT receptor numbers. Behaviours mediated by dopamine are also enhanced by ECT, and there are also influences on nor-adrenergic functions similar to those described for antidepressant drugs (see pp. 88–9). In particular, it has been shown that ECT has an effect in down-regulating β receptors.

The neurochemical and behavioural effects of ECT parallel its antidepressant actions since the changes emerge after several treatments and sub-seizure currents are ineffective.

Clinical uses

The principal use of ECT is in **severe depressive illness**. Features of that illness that predict a good response to ECT are:

1. Severe weight loss.
2. Pronounced early morning wakening.
3. Psychomotor retardation.
4. Psychotic features – especially depressive delusions.

In clinical practice ECT is used:

1. When a **depressive illness with the appropriate features fails to respond** to antidepressant treatment.
2. In psychotic depression where suffering is severe, especially when **depressive delusions** are present.
3. In **depressive stupor**.
4. In **catatonic stupor**.

5. In **puerperal psychoses**, especially those with clouding, perplexity, and marked affective features.

More controversial indications include:

6. *Acute schizophrenia* with clouded consciousness and perplexity.
7. In *schizophrenia* where there are pronounced depressive features.
8. In *mania* when neuroleptic and lithium have failed to control persistent over-activity.

Administration of ECT

ECT requires a general anaesthetic and the usual precautions are observed. The treatment is usually given early in the morning so the patient is starved from midnight. Atropine is administered as pre-medication to dry up bronchial and salivary secretions and also to prevent an extreme bradycardia. A short-acting anaesthetic is administered together with a muscle relaxant to modify the fit. Following ventilation with oxygen (this has been shown to reduce amnesia afterwards), the electrodes – moistened to ensure good contact with the skin – are placed one on the temporal region and one near the vertex of the side of the non-dominant hemisphere for unilateral ECT. (For bilateral ECT the electrodes are placed on each temporal region.) Treatment is given twice a week with two clear days between treatments until a satisfactory response has been obtained: this is usually after six to eight treatments.

Unwanted effects

ECT is a safe treatment. The mortality rate is similar to that of a brief anaesthetic when used for dental or investigative procedures. The largest series demonstrate a mortality of 1 death per 20,000 treatments.

The treatment causes *alteration of pulse rate, a rise in blood pressure*, and *a great increase in cerebral blood flow*.

The **contraindications** are therefore illnesses affecting the cardiovascular and central nervous systems:

Cerebral and aortic aneurysms.
Recent cerebral haemorrhage.
Myocardial infarction.
Cardiac arrhythmias.
Raised intracranial pressure and brain tumour.
Acute respiratory infections form a contraindication to the anaesthetic and require treatment before ECT is given.

Physical side effects following ECT are rare. However, *physical problems following the anaesthetic* may include:

Myocardial infarction.
Cardiac arrhythmias.
Pulmonary embolism.
Pneumonia.

If the *muscle relaxant has not been properly given* the following may occur:

Dislocations.
Fractures (and consequent fat embolism).

Increased blood pressure during the fit itself may occur, causing:

Cerebral haemorrhage.
Bleeding from peptic ulcer.

PSYCHOLOGICAL SEQUELAE

Mania is precipitated by ECT in approximately 5 per cent of cases. This figure is similar to that found with tricyclic antidepressants and occurs in those patients known to have, or be vulnerable to, bipolar manic depressive illness.

A post-ECT **confusional state** usually lasts for about half an hour, a headache may also occur but is usually short-lived.

Memory loss is a more important side-effect. There is a short and rapidly dwindling amnesia for the time preceding each treatment (retrograde amnesia) and a longer post-ECT (anterograde) amnesia. Patients may also complain of *subjective difficulty in remembering* previously well-learned material, like telephone numbers or addresses. These problems are usually hard to demonstrate with objective tests of memory. However, the following factors will reduce the memory problems:

1. Unilateral shock to the non-dominant hemisphere.
2. Not giving too many treatments.
3. Not giving treatment too frequently.
4. Oxygenating the patient well before the shock.
5. Not using an unnecessarily big shock.

BEHAVIOURAL TREATMENTS

These treatments are environmental manipulations based on principles derived from experimental psychology in order to bring about changes in overt behaviour, thoughts ('cognitions'), or autonomic functions. Behaviour therapy is in no way antagonistic to physical approaches to treatment: rather the two approaches are complementary. Many patients derive benefit from a combination of the two types of treatment.

Theoretical foundations

The fundamental principles of behavioural change are:

1. **Classical (Pavlovian) conditioning**. This is the process by which a neutral stimulus (the 'conditioned' stimulus, or CS) acquires the ability to elicit an involuntary response (a CR) as a result of repeated association with a stimulus (the 'unconditioned' stimulus, or UCS) which normally evokes that response. Pavlov's famous experiments on gastric acid and salivary excretion in dogs exemplify this form of learning. Thus the sight of food (UCS) usually evokes salivation, and by initially pairing this with a bell (CS) Pavlov was subsequently able to make the dog salivate (CR) when the bell rang in the absence of food.

   A clinically relevant example of classical conditioning would be the hypothetical explanation of the origin of phobic anxiety, whereby the phobic object (for example, spiders) act as a CS eliciting a fear response because of earlier pairing with such responses.

2. **Operant (instrumental) conditioning**. This is the process whereby voluntary behaviours are strengthened ('reinforcement') or weakened ('punishment') because of their consequences. Skinner's experiments in which rats pressed levers for food reinforcement typify this type of learning in animals, while a clinically relevant example in humans would be the engendering of temper tantrums in a young child when he discovers that such behaviour is particularly effective in obtaining his parents' undivided attention.

Both classical and operant conditioning tend to be situationally specific (that is to say, the learned responses occur most readily in situations similar to those prevailing when the conditioning took place). Both types of conditioning are deemed to be reversible. Thus a classically conditioned fear of crowded places would be expected to **extinguish** as a result of repeated visits to busy shops, while tantrums cease when they no longer elicit the same parental attention.

Many pathological behaviours involve a complex interplay between classical and operant conditioning. For example, although phobic **anxiety** may arise from a classical learning experience, phobic **behaviour** is more likely to be maintained by operant conditioning – that is the reinforcement of avoidance behaviour by anxiety reduction.

General principles of behaviour therapy

All behaviour therapies start with **behavioural analysis**. The objective symptomatology is clearly defined, and details of the frequency, duration, and intensity of the symptoms are recorded together with events that occur at the time when symptoms are experienced. This is usually accomplished by asking the patient to keep a diary for a week or so before any formulation is attempted. Such a formulation must take account of:

A. The Antecedents – the environmental context in which the symptom occurs;

B. The Behaviour;

C. The Consequences – events which may contribute to the maintenance of the behaviour.

The formulation constitutes a **hypothesis** about the nature and origin of the symptom. The hypothesis will usually suggest appropriate treatment strategies: for example, the hypothesis that a patient's withdrawal from social contact is maintained by anxiety reduction might suggest a different type of intervention from the hypothesis that it stems from an inadequate repertoire of social skills. The treatment thus constitutes a test of the hypothesis, which itself may require modification in the light of success or failure of the treatment.

Behavioural treatment invariably involves a clear objective goal agreed upon by the patient. Most therapists also use **intermediate goals** or 'targets', the attainment of which provide an important source of reinforcement for the patient.

Specific techniques

RELAXATION

Since the conditioned response in so many of the above states is one of anxiety the patient must first be trained to produce the opposite response, relaxation. This is done initially well away from any anxiety-provoking stimulus. The patient is first taught to recognize the signs of tension in her body and how these can be altered by voluntary control. She is then given an audiotape which describes exercises to relax the body and the mind and takes this home to practise. The technique of relaxation must become sufficiently rehearsed so that it can be applied even in situations which have previously caused anxiety.

DESENSITIZATION

With the therapist's help, the patient constructs a **hierarchy** of anxiety-provoking stimuli. These stimuli are then presented to the patient, starting with the most innocuous. As each stimulus is mastered, the patient progresses to the next one. The stimuli may be presented in one of two ways.

Desensitization in imagination consists of the patient imagining anxiety-provoking scenes while in a relaxed state.

Graded exposure (or 'in vivo' desensitization). This treatment consists of the patient having to encounter anxiety-provoking stimuli in real life, starting with those which provoke least anxiety. This procedure is favoured by most therapists since confrontation with stressors in real life is always the eventual goal of treatment, and it is more effective.

Here is an example of graded exposure:

Mrs X presented with a moderately severe fear of wasps. On occasion this resulted in her running away leaving her baby and pram unattended in the street. A twelve-step hierarchy of increasingly anxiety-provoking wasp-related stimuli was constructed and this determined a programme of graded exposure, starting with reading about and looking at pictures of wasps in books, and ending with killing a wasp trapped against a window. Initial exposure to each item took place in the clinic, the patient then being encouraged to complete similar assignments at home without the therapist.

The duration of each exposure to an item was dependent on the rate of habituation of the anxiety response: exposure was discontinued when the patient described a significant reduction in anxiety. In practice this was rarely more than fifteen minutes per item. Usually more than one item was completed at the same appointment. After only five treatment sessions, the patient completed the hierarchy, and remained anxiety-free in the presence of wasps at a six-month follow-up point.

FLOODING

Whereas desensitization is a 'little-by-little' approach, flooding plunges in at the deep end. The patient is confronted with a situation at the top of her hierarchy (for example, shopping in a crowded department store, or travelling on a bus in the rush hour), and is required to remain in that situation until her anxiety has spontaneously dissipated ('habituation'). Although it is often difficult to persuade patients to undergo flooding, it is a rapid and a generally more effective treatment than desensitization.

Mrs Y had not ventured more than a quarter of a mile from her home and had completely avoided all shopping areas for more than a year, because of agoraphobic anxiety difficulties. The patient and therapist travelled by car into the city centre on a Saturday afternoon and spent two and a half hours in a crowded shopping mall. Initially the patient complained of extreme panic, the therapist both reassuring and prompting her to remain in spite of an intense desire to exit from the situation. These feelings began to subside after about thirty minutes, and by the end of the session the patient was euphoric. Two further sessions of the same took place, and these were characterized by even more rapid habituation of anxiety. Subsequently Mrs Y was encouraged to travel alone to the same shopping centre, and this was accompanied by a generalization of the treatment effect to other public situations. After only three weeks from the commencement of treatment she was able to travel to and shop in local supermarkets and city centre department stores.

BIOFEEDBACK

Many visceral and neuromuscular activities of which we are normally unaware can be brought into consciousness by providing an auditory or visual 'feedback' signal (for example, a tone whose pitch varies with frontalis muscle tension). This technique is often used as an adjunct to relaxation training, but can also be used in the treatment of specific symptoms such as tension headache, or in the treatment of hypertension.

RESPONSE PREVENTION

This is used in the treatment of compulsive rituals. The patient feels compelled to perform some act such as washing hands but is firmly persuaded from doing so. This must be maintained for prolonged periods to be effective. It is best performed while the person is repeatedly faced with a situation in which the compulsion occurs such as touching dirt. In this way it is similar to flooding – the patient is faced with intense anxiety which gradually wanes as it is not relieved by the habitual means of giving in to the compulsion.

> *Mr Z presented with an obsessional preoccupation with dog excrement. After returning home from walking in the street, he would be compelled to engage in a decontamination ritual beginning with scrubbing his shoes with disinfectant (these were not normally soiled to the objective observer). He would then take all his clothes off, and place them in the washing machine, then scrub his hands, and bath himself. The ritual took more than two hours to perform. Treatment involved the patient being encouraged to deliberately soil his shoes with dog excrement and return home, leaving his contaminated shoes on the door step. The therapist then spent an hour or more with the patient, preventing any cleaning ritual from occurring and distracting him with other activities. After two months of twice-weekly visits by the therapist the patient was able to venture out alone and return without performing the ritual, apart from washing his hands in a normal fashion.*

COGNITIVE-BEHAVIOURAL THERAPY

This treatment approach is of particular value in depressive states. It can be used in conjunction with pharmacological treatment, and is especially useful in milder or long-standing depressive conditions where antidepressant drugs are either ineffective or undesirable. It is based upon the observation that depressed patients often have erroneous and highly pessimistic beliefs about themselves, their circumstances, and their future (the 'negative triad').

Cognitive therapy aims to correct these gloomy thoughts, and at the same time to demonstrate to the patient that he is capable of surmounting problems which because of his pessimistic beliefs he would not normally undertake. Although the primary focus of this type of therapy is the patient's beliefs, it can be included with behaviour therapies because of the emphasis on practical goals, and because thoughts appear to be subject to the same laws of reinforcement as acts.

> *Mr A who six months previously had failed to obtain an important job promotion, was diagnosed as suffering from a moderately severe depressive illness. He was preoccupied with thoughts of incompetence at work and in the home, worries that nobody liked him, and ideas of low self-esteem. He was asked to keep a diary in which he recorded recurrent negative thoughts and their underlying assumptions. Treatment sessions focused on reality-testing these assumptions. For example, one recurrent thought suggested that he had been passed over for promotion because he was incompetent in his current position.*

Underlying assumptions included:

1. *His manager paid particular attention to every error that he had made over the years, no matter how insignificant.*
2. *Because of (1), the manager believed Mr A to be the most incompetent person in the firm.*
3. *It was because of (2) that Mr A had not been promoted.*
4. *Mr A would not be promoted at any future date.*

As a result of treatment sessions and reality-testing assignments, the patient began to realize that most of these assumptions were incorrect. This led to adjustments in his attitude towards his work and career, and after three months of treatment the depression was ameliorated.

SOCIAL SKILLS TRAINING

Sophisticated social behaviour is largely acquired by learning. Many people cope poorly with social situations because they have never acquired a full repertoire of appropriate social responses. Social skills training is usually undertaken with groups of patients, and aims to provide explicit training of such social responses. Mock social situations are set up, and the patients practise by **role-playing**, after the therapist has provided a **model** of the appropriate behaviour ('modelling'). The patient's performance may be videotaped, so that particular problems can be discussed and corrected in debriefing sessions.

BELL AND PAD TRAINING

This is a behavioural treatment for nocturnal enuresis. A pad containing electrical contacts is placed under a sheet on the patient's bed. If the patient urinates in the bed a circuit is completed, setting off an alarm bell which wakes the patient. This is one of the most effective treatments for enuresis, although the underlying psychological processes remain obscure. Simple classical conditioning cannot provide a full explanation for the treatment's efficacy, because the alarm bell (CS) occurs after the unconditioned reflex of micturition. It seems likely that as a result of extensive practice the patient learns to become more aware of stimuli associated with bladder distension.

INDICATIONS

It can be seen that behavioural treatments are helpful in a very wide range of psychological disorders. In **affective disorders** like anxiety, phobias, or depression; in **maladaptive behaviours** such as obsessional states and sexual problems; in **abnormal illness behaviours**; and in deficient social skills and nocturnal enuresis.

PSYCHOTHERAPY

The doctor–patient relationship is one in which the patient places great trust in the doctor. The patient discusses personal problems which he would otherwise keep private, and he may be prepared to comply with whatever treatment and advice that the doctor prescribes. Some knowledge of how this relationship operates is essential to be a good doctor. However, it is important to realize that this relationship can be used in a therapeutic way. This is formalized in psychotherapy, in which the doctor aims to help the patient by recognizing his needs and helping him with them through the medium of the therapeutic relationship.

Types of psychotherapy

Psychotherapy may be divided according to the type of recipient: thus **individual, marital, family, and group psychotherapy**; or it may be divided according to the kind of technique used. We will now consider first, the kinds of psychotherapeutic techniques that should be possessed by every doctor; and second, techniques which are better left to those with greater experience.

Ingredients of psychotherapy relevant to general medical practice

There are many different forms of psychotherapy, but even in a crowded general practitioner's surgery or a busy out-patient clinic there are a number of techniques that a doctor will find helpful. Taken together, they are sometimes described as '**supportive psychotherapy**'.

ACTIVE LISTENING

Students are often surprised to find that taking a full history in the psychiatric out-patient clinic leads to the patient saying that he feels much better! The patient will probably have never before had such an opportunity to review all aspects of his life and to express emotions associated with events in his life. In addition the student's intense interest in what the patient is saying demonstrates a concern which the patient appreciates.

Active listening is an important part of the therapeutic process. There is no need for such listening to be a time-consuming business – in fact it can save time. The patient with a sexual problem, for example, can spend many fruitless consultations with the doctor who is not skilled in gaining her confidence and listening for clues as to the nature of the underlying worry.

VENTILATION OF FEELINGS

Allowing expression of feeling is an important aspect of the therapeutic relationship. It is especially useful to be able to express anger, frustration, or grief that has previously been suppressed.

REASSURANCE

The patient who correctly suspects that he has cancer may ask the doctor about the diagnosis. He may well be asking for reassurance rather than for information. Even if there is nothing in the prognosis about which the doctor can reassure, if he listens carefully to the patient he may understand his particular fears, such as unrelieved pain, incontinence, or the effect on his relatives. On these matters he can reassure and in doing so relieve some of the patient's suffering.

It is important to realize that a properly conducted **physical examination** may be a vital ingredient in the ability to provide reassurance, and that the doctor's own behaviour during a physical examination can serve either to increase or to decrease the patient's anxiety.

A doctor frequently has to reassure a patient (especially an anxious one) that he does not have a serious disease. In spite of his efforts he may later discover that his attempts at reassurance have failed and the patient has sought further tests elsewhere. This is because the doctor has either not fully understood the patient's underlying worries or not explained adequately the cause of the symptoms.

EXPLANATION

The patient who fears that his headaches indicate an underlying brain tumour is less reassured by the doctor's statement *'All the tests show that nothing is wrong'* than:

> *Your headaches are due to the muscles of your scalp tightening; this is why they also affect the back of your neck and occur when you get tense.*

Thus an explanation by the doctor can be very therapeutic, although it uses neither technological investigations nor drugs.

You may observe a patient in the out-patient clinic look greatly relieved by the consultant's authoritative statement that he recognizes the patient's illness and can prescribe appropriate treatment. The 'explanation' may just be a name for a disease whose aetiology is not understood; the 'treatment' something that is known to work, although no one is quite sure why. Yet until this time the patient has been perplexed as to what has been happening to him, and the *doctor's explanation is reassuring.*

ADVICE/GUIDANCE

Patients often turn to the doctor for advice. These may be matters about which the doctor can be precise (such as giving up smoking, or stopping benzodiazepines), or they may be related to problems such as leaving a job, or getting a divorce. The doctor must avoid telling people what they should do, although it is legitimate to tell them what effect a particular change might be expected to have upon their health.

Thus the doctor might advise that if the patient took time off from caring for a sick parent it would help in the treatment of her own depressive illness: but whether the patient does so or not must be her own choice.

SPECIAL INTERVIEW TECHNIQUES

1. Instead of asking questions, use statements to encourage the patient to talk.
2. Be prepared to try to understand what the patient is feeling (using empathy) and then to make intelligent guesses to prompt her to go on.
3. Allow the patient to show her emotions to you, whether they be crying, anger, distress. You can respond with a supportive comment, such as 'I can see you've been through a difficult time'; but remember that silence can also be supportive.
4. The doctor is not always right. Give the patient the chance to correct your ideas about her feelings.
5. Don't reassure too soon.

It is easier to get an idea of such techniques by looking at what might actually be said during a consultation. They are often used in an attempt to reconstruct possible original causes and look for continuing causes of the patient's problems, and are then described as **insight-oriented psychotherapy**. We will return to Mrs Woods, and first see how a doctor who has no knowledge of psychotherapeutic techniques might interview her, using a traditional 'question-and-answer' format:

Doctor:	**Mrs Woods**
What is the matter?	*Nothing.*
Then why are you looking so depressed?	*Wouldn't you if your mother had just died?* (awkward silence)
Have you been taking the antidepressant tablets?	*Yes.*
Is your sleeping improving?	*A bit.*
Why aren't you talking much?	*Nobody understands how I feel.* (eyes fill with tears)
I do, it's normal to feel like this after a death; don't distress yourself.	

A more experienced doctor might say:

Doctor	**Mrs Woods**
You look very down, Mrs Woods.	*Yes.*
You look as though you are about to cry.	*I can't cry, they won't let me.*
They?	*My relatives. They say how well I've taken it; I don't want to let them see me cry.*

Doctor	Mrs Woods
Perhaps your husband doesn't like you crying. . . or perhaps it's your own wish not to cry.	*It's not my husband, it's my sister.*
(Silence)	*She was always mother's favourite and it upsets her too much to see me cry, it's always been my job to comfort her.*
You sound cross about that.	*Well, wouldn't you be? All those years I did far more for my mother than my sister – but my mum thanked her, never me.* (bursts into tears)
Yet you always felt that you had to do more for her.	

Distress is bound to follow a bereavement, but the doctor's comments in the second extract have led to a much fuller understanding of the patient's distress. It is this understanding, combined with his or her familiarity with the normal grief reaction, that puts the doctor in a position to help Mrs Woods. It has become clear that she cannot cry in front of her sister, and her guilt is perhaps becoming easier to understand.

Formal exploratory psychotherapy

This type of psychotherapy is more intensive and is usually given by those who have received some special training. It aims to help the person modify long-standing aspects of their feelings and behaviour, often by modifying defence mechanisms. It is more formal in the sense that the doctor spends a specified time with the patient each week, the therapy may last for some time, and in the longer forms of treatment there is much greater emphasis on analysis of the doctor–patient relationship.

TECHNIQUES USED

Getting the patient to express his or her most intimate feelings and to react spontaneously within the therapy requires:

1. Careful selection of suitable patients.
2. A fixed time each week for the therapeutic session which is held in a quiet and private office where interruptions are prevented.
3. A trusting relationship in which the doctor facilitates the patient's spontaneous expression of emotion and yet makes the patient feel that it is safe for this to occur.
4. Treatment takes place in the framework of a **therapeutic contract** which makes clear to the patient how much treatment is being offered, and what should be achieved during these sessions. The doctor must be very careful not to break his side of the contract so that if the patient breaks his side the doctor can interpret this behaviour.

INDICATIONS

This type of psychotherapy may be used as an adjunct to other treatments in anxiety disorders, depressive illness, and anorexia nervosa. It is occasionally used alone in any of these conditions and in the management of maladaptive behaviours such as self-poisoning and bulimia. Patients are selected who are well motivated to engage in this form of treatment and who can understand it. They must be able and willing to make some important changes in their lives.

CONTRA-INDICATIONS

This treatment is generally not recommended for patients who:

1. Are psychotic.
2. Show marked paranoid traits.
3. Are seriously dependent on drugs or alcohol.
4. Are unable to tolerate personal discomfort.
5. Are involved with an impossible life situation which cannot be expected to change.
6. Have an antisocial personality.

HAZARDS

The principal hazard is **excessive dependency**, so that the patient relies so completely on the doctor that he needs to consult him on every aspect of his life and termination of treatment is impossible. This should be avoided by careful selection of patients for this form of treatment, by not allowing treatment to be prolonged unnecessarily, and by recognizing the early signs of dependency and dealing with them appropriately.

CONTENT OF TREATMENT SESSIONS

Psychotherapy often starts with the patient asking *'What do I talk about?'* There is usually a presenting problem to initiate the discussion but the doctor is deliberately non-directive. This is partly to ensure that the patient does the work of exploring his own feelings and partly so that the patient, not the doctor, leads the discussion.

It is assumed at the outset that the doctor and patient can together make sense of the patient's symptoms and life situation. This requires a theoretical model around which the material brought up during psychotherapy may be arranged. Any such model must enable the doctor to identify key problems, provide explanations for the present problems, and prescribe a means of change.

A case treated by formal exploratory psychotherapy will now be used to illustrate several general principles:

THE PROBLEM

A forty-year-old man presented to the neurologist with a marked tremor at times of stress. This had been present for twenty years, but was becoming more of a problem as the patient was promoted at work. Previous treatment with propranolol and tranquillizers had been ineffective and he increasingly used alcohol to suppress the tremor.

INDICATIONS FOR PSYCHOTHERAPY

He was treated with psychotherapy in view of the failure to respond to other treatments, and the evidence that the tremor was related to interpersonal conflicts. The patient also showed considerable determination to find a psychological cause for his tremor.

THE CONTRACT

It was agreed that the patient would attend six sessions of forty minutes each and progress would then be reviewed. During these sessions the patient's emotions would be explored to try and understand why he reacted to particular situations.

THE TREATMENT

When tackled directly no progress was made: the patient simply went over his habitual thoughts on the matter – saying that his marriage was happy, his friendships normal, and others become nervous in front of a crowd; it was inexplicable that his anxiety was so marked.

Once the patient began to trust the doctor, however, it became appropriate to point out that the patient repeated this description as though he was trying to hide his true feelings ('denial'). It eventually transpired that he felt a failure in his own eyes and that he felt he had let his parents down. This emotional arousal was accompanied by tears. Rather than try to ignore these, he was encouraged to dwell on the feeling of failure. This sense of failure was profound and extended to another problem which had only been hinted at previously, namely premature ejaculation.

The doctor suggested that the patient normally kept such feelings well hidden, which meant that the patient lived in terror of being exposed. But the true fear of exposure did not become apparent until later when, with great anxiety, he admitted to **dreams** of a homosexual nature. He felt enormous relief that his bisexual feelings could be accepted by the doctor as a normal part of his personality.

The whole set of problems then began to make sense. The tremor had begun soon after he had left a boys' boarding school (where homosexual activity had been common) and at a time when he was beginning to experience a sense of rejection in his heterosexual relationships. His aspirations to be a great success both socially and in his career were proving unrealistic, and those situations where he felt he was under scrutiny were those in which he developed anxiety.

He then felt able, for the first time, to tackle the sexual problem which had previously seemed insuperable. The anxiety symptoms did not at this stage disappear but he also felt able to tackle these and a course of behavioural therapy utilizing relaxation and desensitization was successful.

PARTICULAR TECHNIQUES USED DURING PSYCHOTHERAPY ARE ILLUSTRATED IN THE ABOVE CASE HISTORY

Analysis of the **patient's reaction to the doctor**: the patient habitually promoted a self-confident image. When the doctor persistently suggested that this facade hid anxiety and doubt the patient became annoyed. It was analysis of this annoyance that led to exposure of the feelings of failure.

The **emotional arousal** that occurs during treatment may lead to the patient expressing strong feelings (love or hate) towards the doctor. The origin of such feelings may be in the patient's past experience and this must be pointed out. It emerged that sitting with the doctor aroused feelings of being with his father; this elicited feelings of dislike and frustration that were initially directed to the doctor.

Such **linking of the present with the past** is often helpful in psychotherapy but is most efficacious if the present is actually within the psychotherapy treatment session.

The **doctor's reaction to the patient**. In the above case the doctor felt irritated that the patient repeatedly asserted that he was really no different from anyone else. He noted that the patient was using denial too forcefully and this prevented the treatment progressing. The patient initially refuted the doctor's suggestion that he was using denial, but later said that if he had allowed himself fully to accept the need for treatment he would have crumbled into a nervous wreck.

Interpretation of dreams. This technique is simply a way of gaining access to unconscious material which is usually blocked by defence mechanisms. In the above example there had been little or no hint of the patient's homosexual feelings – he was so ashamed they had been well hidden – and it cost the patient an enormous effort to describe them to the doctor. Yet having described the dreams the patient felt enormous relief. The fact that the doctor could accept these as part of the patient's make-up without expressing the revulsion that the patient himself felt was the starting-point of improvement.

Group therapy

Some patients benefit from discussing their problems in a group. Groups are especially sensible for those who have difficulty relating to other people, or for people sharing a

Table 8 *The treatment plan*

---

acute illness

1. *Where will treatment take place and who will provide it?*
   Consider the extent to which supervision and physical care are required:
   Psychiatric unit as in-patient, day-patient, out-patient; or domiciliary care; general practitioner; social services; clinical psychologist.

2. *What should be done if the patient refuses treatment?*
   Is compulsory admission clinically necessary and legally justifiable? What is the risk to the patient or to others?

3. *Is urgent intervention required to relieve distressing or life-threatening symptoms?*
   For example, change of environment by hospital admission; sedation.

4. *Treatment aimed at relieving mental illness or its symptoms*
   Physical: neuroleptics, minor tranquillizers, antidepressants, hypnotics, electroplexy.

   Psychological: psychotherapy – insight, supportive, individual, or group;
   behaviour therapy – desensitization, flooding, response prevention, operant conditioning.

   Social: Environmental manipulation, marital or family therapy or support; use of social agencies or legal advice.

   Occupational: Diversionary, creative, expressive; maintenance of or training in skills or social behaviour.

5. *The treatment of associated physical disorders*
   Specific treatments for organic brain syndromes, e.g. thyroxin, vitamins, antibiotics. Correction of fluid and electrolyte balance, vitamin depletion due to malnutrition, treatment of intercurrent infection.

6. *The correction of handicaps*
   Vision, hearing, speech.

chronic illness

1. *Rehabilitation and resettlement*
   To what extent does the patient need help with accommodation, work, social interactions which may affect the long-term outcome?

   For example, psychiatric after-care or other hostel; referral to disablement resettlement officer, occupational retraining or sheltered work shop; domiciliary social services such as home help, family-aid, meals-on-wheels; community services such as luncheon club.

2. *Other prophylactic measures for those vulnerable to relapse*
   Physical: Long-term depot phenothiazines, tricyclic antidepressants, lithium.
   Psychological: Supervision, support, social casework.

3. *Liaison between psychiatrist, general practitioner, community psychiatric nurse, psychiatric social worker*
   What information do they need? Who will prescribe?

---

common problem. Large numbers of specialized groups exist for helping patients with particular problems: for example, groups exist for patients who have had operations such as mastectomy or colostomy; for recovered alcoholics, and for those who have recently been bereaved. Support comes from the knowledge that others are experiencing similar problems, and learning ways of coping from other group members.

PLANNING TREATMENT

Treatment should follow logically from the specific aetiology of the illness as well as from the diagnosis. A plan of treatment should be drawn up and recorded for each patient, and an outline of factors to be considered is shown in *Table 8*.

In addition to the usual categories of physical, psychological and social aspects of treatment, it is important to consider the order in which they are appropriate. This can be divided for convenience into the earlier stages, which are concerned with arrangements for treatment, symptomatic relief and the treatment of the underlying causes; and the later stages which include rehabilitation, prophylaxis, and arrangements for after-care.

FURTHER READING

Beech, H. and Vaughan, M. (1978) *Behavioural Treatment of Obsessional States.* Chichester: John Wiley and Sons.

Bloch, S. and Crown, S. (1979) *An Introduction to the Psychotherapies.* Oxford: Oxford University Press.

Lader, M. (1975) *The Psychophysiology of Mental Illness.* London: Routledge & Kegan Paul.

Meyer, V. and Chesser, E. (1970) *Behaviour Therapy in Clinical Psychiatry.* Harmondsworth: Penguin Books.

Shaw, D., Kellam, A., and Mottram, R. (1982) *Brain Sciences in Psychiatry.* London: Butterworth Scientific.

8 / PROGNOSIS

The outlook for a psychiatric illness depends partly on the particular condition under consideration, but partly on factors that cut across diagnoses, and will be considered in this short chapter. If you are trying to predict the future course of a particular patient's illness, read the section on prognosis in the appropriate section and then take the following factors into account as well.

GENETIC FACTORS

A patient with a strong family history of an illness known to be partly determined by genetic factors – such as schizophrenia or manic-depressive illness – can be expected to have a worse outlook than one with a slight or no family history. However, do not put much reliance on this factor, because there are exceptions in each direction: those with a strong family history can have a good prognosis, and vice versa.

EARLY CHILDHOOD FACTORS

Severe deprivation in early childhood often leaves scars for the rest of a lifetime. If your patient will need to settle down in some stable relationship in order to improve, ask yourself what experience life has so far offered your patient of such relationships. A person who has been bereaved in early childhood will always carry a greater vulnerability to losses in later life.

PRE-MORBID PERSONALITY

Don't forget that personality characteristics are by definition relatively constant, so you must not expect your patient to improve much in these respects. For example, a person who has always had depressive traits in their personality is unlikely suddenly to cheer up in middle age: in real life, Scrooge would have been found to have had a manic illness or a temporal lobe lesion!

Similarly, the damage done to antisocial personalities has been inflicted in childhood, and cannot be undone. If your patient is aged over thirty, the best level of their pre-morbid adjustment indicates the probable limits of what can be expected of them in the future.

MATURITY AND IMMATURITY

If your patient is under thirty, ask yourself to what extent they can still be expected to mature. Emotionally healthy people in our society, who have not experienced deprivation and upheaval in childhood, can be expected to have completed the greater part of maturation before the age of twenty; in developing countries, it is much earlier than that.

However, those who have had disrupted childhoods and who have had no good parental role-models, may take much longer to grow up. Thus a young woman from a miserable home, who has endured divorce of her parents, and has been poorly parented may present in her twenties with episodes of wrist-cutting and self-poisoning. With sympathetic and patient handling such patients may settle down in life later on, so that the demands they have made on medical services during the time of their repeated episodes of self-injury appear, in retrospect, to have been a phase in growing up.

Try to assess your young patient's maturity by asking yourself these questions about them:

1. How physically mature do they look?
2. Are they emotionally independent of their parents yet?
3. Are they financially independent of their parents and, if they are, are they earning their own living?
4. Have they succeeded in having a lasting sexual relationship with another adult?

To the extent that your patient is still immature, there is scope for further improvement. With help, maybe he or she can learn to adapt more successfully.

LEVEL OF PRE-MORBID ACHIEVEMENT

Ask yourself what your patient has been able to achieve in their life before they became ill. Those who have achieved much – emotionally and occupationally – have a much sounder basis to build on after an episode of psychotic illness or head injury. Try to identify any ways in which your patient was disadvantaged **before** he became ill: these are his **pre-morbid handicaps**, and it may be very important to help him with them during rehabilitation. But to the extent that they may be severe and irremediable, the prognosis is poor.

PREVIOUS PSYCHIATRIC HISTORY

This is critically important. As any actuary can tell you, if you want to know about the future, look at the past. One saying has it that in psychiatry 'the diagnosis is from the mental state, but the prognosis is from the history'.

If your patient has never been ill before, there is a much better chance that he will recover completely. If a patient tells you that she has been depressed off and on for the past twenty years, the chances are that she will continue to have episodes of depression in the future.

PRECIPITATING FACTORS

To what extent can your patient's illness be understood as a reaction to a stressful environment? To the extent that it can, and provided that the patient has a good record of pre-morbid adjustment, the future is likely to be good.

CURRENT LIFE ADJUSTMENT

What sort of social environment has your patient got to go back to in the community? Has the patient someone in whom he or she can confide, and how much support does this confidant provide at times of crisis? What are the living conditions like? And is there financial hardship?

These factors seem especially important in determining the course of non-psychotic affective illness.

MODE OF ONSET

How did the illness begin? Generally speaking, psychological illnesses that begin suddenly have a much better outlook than those with a gradual onset. The best combination is to have a severe stress followed by an illness with an acute illness, while the worst is to have an unprovoked illness of insidious onset.

LENGTH OF PRESENT ILLNESS

Once more, on actuarial considerations: the longer, the worse.

COMPLIANCE WITH TREATMENT

Is the patient likely to comply with treatment? Some people with eccentric personalities, and many of those with sociopathic personalities, are less likely to accept any treatment which requires prolonged cooperation.

If they have had previous episodes of illness, to what extent have they complied with treatment in the past?

THE NATURE OF THE DISORDER ITSELF

Generally speaking, the majority of patients with psychiatric illnesses will recover, and a substantial proportion may never have another episode of illness. Even major psychoses like schizophrenia and psychotic depression can have wide variability in their course, with some patients getting completely well, some having only a partial recovery, some having a fluctuating course, and others having a progressive course.

Remember that disorders like manic-depressive psychosis are known to be remittent, so that although you can assure your patient that they will get well, they are actually very likely to have further episodes of illness.

Other disorders – like Alzheimer's disease and Huntington's chorea – are progressive and incurable: details will be found in the appropriate sections.

When considering an individual patient's prognosis, avoid such uninformative terms as 'guarded'. Weigh up the different factors which suggest a good or bad outcome for that particular patient. Remember that the expected outcome may vary according to which aspects of the case we are considering: for example, we might predict:

> *Complete recovery from florid symptoms, but will probably fail to return to work and there is a high probability of further episodes.*

9 / FORMULATION

THE PURPOSE OF THE FORMULATION

The formulation is the method used to integrate all the clinical data that are required in order to treat the patient and evaluate the outcome: *it is not a case summary*. It follows a logical sequence which we have dealt with in turn in the preceding chapters. The purpose of this chapter is to show how these are integrated, and why.

No doubt you will by now be in the habit of making and using diagnoses and may wonder why that isn't good enough for psychiatry, but we have already noted in Chapter 4 that diagnoses have important limitations. A diagnosis involves a 'nomothetic' (literally 'law-giving') process. This means that all cases included within the identified category have one or more properties in common. For example, all those with a diagnosis of pulmonary tuberculosis will have an infectious disease of the lungs caused by the tubercle bacillus. While this is useful information it is quite inadequate as a basis for management. It tells us little about the clinical state, which might range from a chance radiological finding in an apparently healthy person to a fulminating pneumonia, and it certainly won't help us to decide which are the appropriate drugs to use.

By contrast the formulation is an 'ideographic' process (literally 'picture of the individual'). This means that it includes the unique characteristics of each patient's case which are needed for the process of management. So, while nomothetic processes are the only way we can advance knowledge about *diseases*, we use ideographic methods to understand and study the *individual*.

To pursue the example of pulmonary tuberculosis, the additional information that is taken into account might include the subject's previous state of immunity, nutrition, and the state of health of those with whom he lives. It would also take into account the varieties of clinical presentation, sensitivities of the tubercle bacillus, the extent to which he is likely to be compliant with medication, and the risk of relapse through cross-infection.

THE FORMAT OF THE FORMULATION

Demographic data

Begin with the name, age, occupation, and marital status.

Descriptive formulation

Describe the nature of onset, for example acute or insidious; the total duration of the present illness; and the course, for example cyclic or deteriorating. Then list the main phenomena (that is symptoms and signs) that characterize the disorder. As you become more experienced you should try to be selective by emphasising the phenomena that are most important, either because of their greater diagnostic specificity or because of their predominance in severity or duration. *Avoid long lists of minor or transient symptoms and negative findings*. These basic data are chiefly derived from the history of the present illness, the mental state, and physical examinations and are used to determine the syndrome diagnosis in the next section. Note that this is not the place to bring in other aspects of the history: that comes later.

Now let's return to Mrs Woods for an example. We have already seen most of the history and examination findings in earlier chapters, but this is how it would be used in the formulation.

> *Mrs Woods is a forty-five-year-old married housewife. Three weeks ago, following the death of her mother, she experienced an acute onset of an illness characterized by depressed mood, anhedonia, poor sleep, early morning waking, poor appetite and weight loss, poor libido, and constipation. She has had intermittent left chest pain. On examination she shows mild retardation of movement and speech, weeps frequently, and appears depressed. Her thought content is focused on the death of her mother and she has the delusion that she is responsible for her mother's death. Physical examination reveals recent and older bruising.*

Differential diagnosis

List in order of probability all diagnoses that should be considered and include any disorders that you will wish to investigate. These will usually be syndrome diagnoses based on the descriptive formulation above. Give the evidence for and against each diagnosis that you consider. Include any current physical illness which may account for some or all of the phenomena. A common error is to include, for example, thyroid function studies in the investigations without including thyroid disease in the differential diagnosis. If you think a condition is worth investigating then you are obviously including it in your differential diagnosis; if it's not worth mentioning don't bother to investigate it.

Remember that in addition to the primary diagnosis you may need to consider a supplementary diagnosis, for example alcoholism in a patient presenting with delirium, or a personality disorder in a patient with an anxiety state. Regarding Mrs Woods:

1. **Depressive illness: Morbid grief reaction** (preferred diagnosis). *The symptoms and signs are essentially those of a depressive illness, with depressed mood, depressive thought content; and neuro-vegetative features. This has developed in the setting of bereavement and the content of abnormal beliefs and perceptions is limited to the bereavement.*

2. **Manic depressive disorder:** *in view of the psychotic symptoms it is necessary to consider the possibility that this is a depressive episode in a bipolar affective disorder. However there is no evidence of manic episodes in the past.*

3. **Angina pectoris:** *the distribution of chest pain is more characteristic of anxiety than of myocardial insufficiency, but this possibility will have to be investigated before it can be excluded.*

Aetiology

The various factors that have contributed should be evident mainly from the family and personal histories, the history of previous illness, and the pre-morbid personality. Remember you should aim to answer these questions: why has this particular patient developed this particular illness at this particular time? If necessary look back to *Table 2* for the systematic method used to identify the relevant factors. We have already considered the aetiology of Mrs Woods's case in some detail (p. 67) but this is how it might be presented in the formulation:

> **Predisposing factors** *include a family history of depressive illness in her mother, the death of her father during her childhood, and marked pre-morbid obsessional and dependent traits. The illness has been **precipitated** by the illness and subsequent death of her mother and her inability to face the ambivalent nature of that relationship.*

Investigations

List all investigations that are required to support your preferred diagnosis and to rule out the alternatives, and also any that you think are required to improve your understanding of the aetiology. Give reasons for investigations if they are not self-evident. Include all sources of additional information. Have another look at *Table 3* to remind yourself about how to plan investigations systematically.

> *Investigations should include contacting her general practitioner to find out more about her past history of mental illness and review of her mother's hospital records. She also*

requires physical examination, chest X-ray, and an ECG. It will be important to observe her mood state through the day, sleep, and appetite, and to keep a weight chart. Insight-oriented psychotherapy may help to determine the aspects of her bereavement that have determined morbid grief.

Treatment

Outline the treatment plan that you wish to follow. This should stem logically from your discussion of the aetiology as well as from the diagnosis. Consider each stage of management in turn as described in Chapter 7, starting with the preliminary arrangements and finishing with the possible need for prophylaxis.

> **Treatment:** *It is preferable initially to provide treatment on an in-patient basis in view of the severity of Mrs Woods's depression and self-neglect, and this should be on a voluntary basis. If the physical investigations confirm that there is no evidence of cardiac disease she should be told of this and the ways in which psychological factors can give rise to chest symptoms should be explained. If the depressive symptoms persist in hospital following a few days' observation she should then be started on a tricyclic **antidepressant drug** with sedating properties, e.g. Amitryptyline, increasing to a full dose of 150 mgm at night after a few days. If no improvement occurs within two to three weeks it may then be necessary to consider **ECT**. She should be encouraged to attend occupational therapy in order to maintain social and occupational skills. **Psychotherapy** should initially be supportive and, although some insights may be obtained, it should not be interpretive – at least until her depressive symptoms are much improved. It is too early to predict how much help she will need to adjust to her mother's death in the longer term.*

Prognosis

Describe the expected outcome of management of this illness episode, both with regard to the symptoms and also subsequent function, e.g. self-care and return to the community. Consider the risk of subsequent relapse. Give your reasons for these predictions based on the principles described in Chapter 8.

> **Prognosis:** *Mrs Woods is likely to make a complete recovery from her present illness because it is an affective disorder (and these generally result in recovery); it had an acute onset and a specific precipitant; she has a supportive husband and no material hardship. The prominence of neuro-vegetative symptoms suggests a good response to tricyclic antidepressant drugs. However, she is likely to have some continuing difficulty in adjusting to her mother's death. She is constitutionally predisposed to suffer from depressive illness and is likely to suffer further episodes in the future, particularly when she experiences bereavement or other loss.*

HOW TO USE THE FORMULATION

Aim to write up formulations for each patient you clerk during the psychiatric attachment and discuss them with the medical staff. The formulation should be written up as soon as you have clerked the patient and written up the record of the history and mental state examination. Of course you will probably want to modify your formulation later on when you have additional information.

We have referred in earlier chapters to the hypotheses that are an intrinsic part of the clinical approach and this requires explanation. In the formulation the clinical data are used to set up hypotheses concerning the diagnosis and aetiology of the case. The investigations, and even more important the response of the illness to the treatment, provide the method for testing them. By observing the outcome of investigations and management we are able to discover whether our initial hypotheses were correct, but we can do so only if we recorded them in the formulation.

If our hypotheses are not supported, for example the patient has failed to improve with the planned treatment, then we have to review the accuracy of the original data. This will require reappraisal of the history and mental state and possibly further investigations.

FURTHER READING

Greenberg, M., Szmukler, G., and Tantam, D. (1986) *Making Sense of Psychiatric Cases.* Oxford: Oxford Medical.

PART 2
THE SYNDROMES
OF PSYCHIATRIC
DISORDER

10 / PSYCHIATRIC ASPECTS OF PHYSICAL DISEASE

This chapter will first consider the kinds of relationships which can exist between psychological and physical ill-health, and will give an extended account of the phenomenon of 'somatization'. We will then consider the psychological manifestations of various physical illnesses, and we will include psychiatric aspects of epilepsy. A final section will deal with acute and chronic pain.

Numerous studies have shown that there is a strong relationship between physical and psychological illness, which cannot be accounted for by chance association. All too often, doctors in hospital practice consider the possibility that there is something psychologically wrong only when they have failed to find a physical cause for their patient's symptoms. This is a very bad policy, since most psychologically disturbed patients on the medical wards *have a physical disorder as well*. Nor is it true that patients in whom we have failed to make a physical diagnosis necessarily have psychological disorders! *Psychiatric diagnoses should be made on positive evidence of disorder, and not by exclusion.*

At one time it was usual to divide physical diseases into those in which psychological factors were thought to be relatively unimportant, and others called 'psychosomatic diseases' which were thought to be partly caused by psychological factors. Eczema, asthma, coronary heart disease, diabetes, and ulcerative colitis were thought to be examples of such diseases. However, the term is no longer used since no one now supposes that diseases can be divided up in this way. It is impossible to think of a disease which is not affected in some way by psychological factors, and to the extent that the word 'psychosomatic' is still used it refers to the systematic study of psychological factors in physical disease processes.

RELATIONSHIPS BETWEEN PHYSICAL DISEASE
AND PSYCHIATRIC ILLNESS

There are in fact five kinds of relationships between psychiatric disorders and physical symptoms which account for the high rates of psychiatric illness seen on surveys in general medical settings.

1. **Psychiatric disorder may provoke or release physical disease**. Depression is the illness most likely to do this. In surveys of psychiatric illness in medical in-patients, a proportion of cases will be found where the sequence is:

   stressful life event → episode of depression → physical ill-health

   It is possible that these apparently causal sequences are just part of the tendency for illnesses to come in clusters in people's lives, rather than at random time points. There is no doubt that 'functional' illnesses like asthma and migraine are more likely to occur when patients are psychologically unwell, and there is some evidence that the same is true for conditions such as eczema and carcinoma of the cervix.

2. The **psychiatric symptoms may be the presenting symptoms of a physical disease**. This is not all that common, but it happens. Thyrotoxicosis may present as an anxiety state, myxoedema and pernicious anaemia may present as depression, myasthenia gravis may be mistaken for a minor mood disorder. A full account of such disorders is given later in this chapter (p. 128).

3. **Psychiatric illness may be the direct consequence of a physical disease**. If the physical disease had not occurred, the psychiatric illness would not have done so – at least, not at that particular time in the patient's life. This is a common relationship, and is perhaps the easiest one to understand. A patient who has noticed a potentially serious symptom like a breast lump or an episode of rectal bleeding may become anxious about the possible cause; a patient who knows he has cancer may become depressed. It is important to recognize these illnesses, since they cause much suffering and respond well to treatment.

4. **Psychiatric disorder may exacerbate the pain of a physical disease**. Patients who are depressed experience pains and discomforts more severely than when they are well, and the experience of anxiety has been shown to lower the pain threshold. This general relationship holds for any chronic pain, from sciatica to malignant disease. When a patient who is known to have some chronic disease complains of an exacerbation of their pains it is tempting to conclude that the underlying disease has deteriorated, but it is often not true.

5. **Psychiatric illness may present to doctors with physical symptoms which have no organic basis**. This phenomenon is called the 'somatization' of psychological distress, and its existence explains why some clinicians consider psychological causes only when they have failed to make a physical diagnosis. However, as we shall see, somatization can be expanded to cover cases where there is

undoubted physical disease, but this disease does not really account for the patient's physical symptoms.

SOMATIZATION

Somatization can be defined as **the expression of personal and social distress in an idiom of bodily complaints with medical help-seeking**. The majority of such patients are also experiencing symptoms of depression and anxiety, but they do not complain about these symptoms unless the doctor asks about them. Instead, they complain of pains and other somatic symptoms, and they do not consider themselves psychiatrically unwell. They may have physical disease as well (in which case the psychological disorder is exacerbating their symptoms, as in '4' above); or it may not be possible to demonstrate any physical disease (as in '5').

Epidemiology

Most surveys have shown that between 20 and 40 per cent of patients admitted to medical wards can also be diagnosed as having a psychiatric illness. Only a small minority of these see themselves as psychiatrically ill: most will satisfy criteria for somatization.

In primary care almost 20 per cent of patients presenting to their doctors with new episodes of illness can be shown to satisfy criteria for somatization, because in addition to the features described above, a research diagnosis of a depressive illness or an anxiety state can be made, treatment of which would ameliorate the patient's presenting somatic symptoms. A physical disease will be demonstrable in about 70 per cent of such somatizing patients, but it will not by itself account for the patient's symptoms.

Clinical features

1. The commonest kind of patient with psychiatric illness on the medical wards will have symptoms of a **depressive illness accompanied by anxiety symptoms** (see p. 183), but the patients will have been admitted for investigation of an undoubted physical illness. In most cases their psychiatric disorder is making a material contribution to their physical symptoms: most usually by making their pains or discomfort more intense. Another, much smaller group, are 'somatizing' without demonstrable physical disease.

2. The next commonest group of patients are complaining of mild **anxiety states** (see p. 177) in addition to their physical symptoms.

3. A third group turn out to have **alcohol-related problems**, often with affective symptoms as well. The remaining patients are a mixed bag and include those with acute and chronic brain syndromes (see p. 140) and others with abnormal illness behaviour (see p. 218).

Aetiology of somatization

We have seen that there are a number of reasons why such patients may be experiencing pains. We must now understand why they choose to focus upon somatic symptoms to the relative neglect of their affective symptoms.

1. The patient does not connect his affective symptoms with his pain, and concentrates on the pain **because it hurts**.
2. The patient is afraid that the pain may indicate some **serious physical disease**.
3. The patient may feel that his emotional problems are his own affair, but excluding physical causes for pains is very much his doctor's job. Some doctors share this view, and may respond with greater interest to physical symptoms than they do to psychological symptoms. This is called '**differential reinforcement**' by the doctor.
4. Key people in the patient's family may be more sympathetic to physical symptoms than they are to psychological problems: this is **differential reinforcement** by relatives.
5. The patient may feel that there is some **social stigma** attaching to emotional illness: societies vary in the extent to which they stigmatize such illnesses, but even in our own it is more acceptable to be thought to have a physical illness.
6. The last reason is a development of the same point: failing to recognize that one has an emotional illness means that one doesn't have to ask oneself awkward questions about one's own personal responsibility for the life predicament that one is in. To have a physical illness is a misfortune, but in most cases one need not feel responsible for it. A somatizing patient **need not blame himself**, nor need he examine the life problem in which he is enmeshed.

Course

In both primary care and psychiatric settings it has been shown that the presence of somatic symptoms as part of a mood disorder is associated with a longer course and a less favourable outcome than can be expected for mood disorders that are unaccompanied by somatic symptoms.

Nevertheless, it must be emphasized that the majority will remit with symptomatic treatment. Two studies have shown that detection and treatment of such disorders will shorten their course.

TREATMENT OF PSYCHIATRIC ILLNESS ASSOCIATED WITH PHYSICAL DISEASE

Psychiatric symptoms as presenting symptoms of a physical disease

Treatment will of course be directed at the underlying disease. However, do not forget to explain to your patient that their disease has been responsible for the psychiatric symptoms described to you, and ask the patient to let you know if these symptoms do not remit.

Psychiatric disorder secondary to physical disease

Allow the patient to ventilate his anxieties, and be sure to correct any fears that are unrealistic or just wrong. If it is not possible to reassure the patient, give information about the investigations that are to be carried out, and promise to keep the patient informed. Only use benzodiazepines for short periods where anxiety has not responded to discussion, and the patient is clearly distressed and agrees to have some medicine to calm himself down. If the patient has a depressive illness an antidepressant should be prescribed. Tetracyclic antidepressants such as mianserin, trazodone, or maprotiline are better tolerated by patients with physical illnesses, since they have fewer side-effects than tricyclic antidepressants.

Psychiatric illness exacerbating symptoms of an undoubted physical disease

Treatment of such affective illness is an extremely important part of your general management plans for the patient's illness. However, the principles are the same as those described already: see p. 181 for anxiety states, and p. 188 for depressive illnesses with anxiety.

Somatic presentations of psychiatric disorder

In cases where either no physical disease is demonstrable, or the physical disease which is present does not account for the patient's symptoms, it is essential to help the patient to see his symptoms in a different way. The **worst thing you can do** is to indicate by your words or actions that

> Our investigations are normal, so there's nothing wrong with you

The patient knows that isn't correct since his pain is real enough. The patient will usually be complaining of numerous other psychiatric symptoms, but he will not have connected them with the pain.

Let us suppose that a patient with severe epigastric pain has reported numerous symptoms of a depressive illness, and you have been asked to tell him that the results of all investigations, including a gastroscopy, are quite normal:

> I'm glad to be able to tell you that you haven't got an ulcer or a tumour causing this pain, and all our investigations have been completely normal. Nevertheless, you have had a lot of pain, haven't you, and it has gone well beyond your usual indigestion pain? . . .
> (Having acknowledged the reality of the pain, pause for agreement.)
>
> . . . When you came into hospital you told me how depressed you have been feeling since

you didn't manage to get promoted at work. You mentioned that you have lost over a stone in weight and tended to wake early in the morning brooding about the things that you feel you've made a mess of in your life . . .

(Mention about three of the more striking symptoms, always including the mood disorder. Be prepared to remind your patient about the others if necessary.)

. . . We think that you are undoubtedly depressed, and that your depression has made your pain very much worse than it would have been otherwise. It's one of the things that depression does, I'm afraid . . .

(Pause for patient's response. Be prepared to repeat that you know that the pain is real, but depression can cause real pain.)

. . . We think that it is very important to give you some treatment for your depression, and I would now like to discuss some of the ways we might help you . . .

(If you have got this far, you have done well. From now on the management is the same as that for any other depressive illness – see p. 188 – but with one advantage. The patient's pain will act as a key symptom to indicate your success – or lack of it – in dealing with the problem.)

OTHER USEFUL STRATEGIES

1. Asking the medical social worker to help by carrying out a home visit, by seeing a relative on your behalf, or by providing some tangible social help for the family.

2. Arranging to see a key relative yourself in order to explain the nature of the patient's symptoms and treatment, since the family will probably share the patient's views that he has an undiagnosed physical illness.

PSYCHIATRIC PRESENTATIONS OF PHYSICAL DISEASE

Many physical diseases have psychological symptoms as part of their presentation. This is true of most endocrine disorders, many metabolic disorders, and some neurological diseases.

ENDOCRINE DISORDERS

Hypothyroidism

Mental symptoms are as prominent as physical symptoms in myxoedema, and take the form of memory loss, somnolence, and depressed mood. The cognitive changes may be so severe that the patient is thought to have a **chronic brain syndrome**: since the condition is reversible in its early stages, **thyroid function tests** should be done in all cases of **pre-senile dementia** (see p. 148). The patients complain of lethargy: they feel slowed up, are disinclined to undertake even familiar tasks, and are unable to concentrate. Patients are often diagnosed as depressed, and the hypothyroidism is missed. Major psychotic illness may also occur.

Hyperthyroidism

Patients are over-aroused, distractible, and anxious. The presentation may be irritable, show easy startle responses, and be intolerant of frustration. They can therefore closely resemble **anxiety states**, but the additional feature of hyperthyroidism should allow the correct aetiology of the anxiety to be diagnosed. There may be histrionic disturbed behaviour, and sometimes excitement is such that the patient satisfies the criteria for a **manic illness**. As with myxoedema, other psychotic illnesses, including agitated depression and schizophreniform illnesses, have also been reported. The thyroid disease is presumably releasing psychosis in vulnerable people.

Cushing's syndrome

Depression is easily the commonest psychosyndrome seen, ranging in severity from mild to severe with paranoid features. Well over 50 per cent of patients with Cushing's syndrome may be expected to have depressive symptoms. These symptoms are directly due to the increased level of corticosteroids, since treatment of the hormonal disorder causes the depressive symptoms to disappear, yet they reappear if the Cushing's syndrome relapses. In theory one might expect manic syndromes since exogenously administered steroids produce euphoria: but such syndromes are rare.

Hypopituitarism and hypoadrenalism

The psychosyndrome consists of weakness, lack of energy, tiredness with defective memory, and poor concentration. The patient may be somnolent and self-neglectful, so the condition can be misdiagnosed either as depression or as dementia.

Sheehan's syndrome

This is a postpartum necrosis of the pituitary. There is chronic ill-health with lack of energy, depression, and sensitivity to cold: think of it if lactation did not occur and menstruation did not resume after the postpartum haemorrhage; confirm by the absent pubic and axillary hair, followed by appropriate biochemical investigations.

Acromegaly

Earliest symptoms often include apathy and loss of initiative. Some patients become depressed and irritable, while others show lability of mood.

Parathyroid disease

The commonest psychological disorder is **depression**, which tends to be both marked and early. It occurs in both hypo- and hyper-parathyroidism, and appears related to calcium rather than to parathormone levels.

Diabetes mellitus

Listlessness, irritability, and confusion may usher in diabetic coma. Later complications include some degree of chronic brain syndrome if there have been cerebrovascular accidents, or if there has been damage secondary to prolonged hypoglycaemia.

Hypoglycaemia

This may occur with diabetes mellitus, with an insulinoma ('spontaneous hypoglycaemia'), or it may be provoked by alcohol. Early psychological symptoms are anxiety or panic, weakness, and sometimes depersonalization. This may be followed by ataxia or clouding of consciousness, or by peculiar and uncharacteristic behaviour. The patient may be aggressive and noisy, and there is usually some degree of motor incoordination. If treatment is delayed, irreversible brain damage will result. When hypoglycaemia is provoked by alcohol a malnourished person takes a large quantity of alcohol and lapses first into stupor, then coma. Surrounding drinkers assume he is 'dead drunk'. Unless the true diagnosis is made, death is indeed a possibility.

METABOLIC DISORDERS

Electrolyte imbalance

These are best set out as a table:

Alkalosis	dulling of perception, confusion and tetany
Acidosis (includes hypercapnia)	dulling of mental functions, drowsiness, impaired consciousness, eventual papilloedema
Hyponatraemia	lassitude, weakness, irritability, confusion
Hypokalaemia	apathy, lethargy, confusion
Hypomagnesaemia	depression, disorientation, delirium

Renal failure

Mental clouding, poor concentration, and listlessness lead to drowsiness and disorientation. 'Uraemia' may thus present as **delirium**, or it may aggravate a mild dementing illness in an elderly patient. Depression can be marked and require treatment. Symptoms are not due to urea itself, but to electrolyte imbalance and toxic levels of drugs.

RENAL DIALYSIS

This is associated with three psychological problems: patients often complain of *anxiety and depression*; rapid reduction of urea may lead to *headache, muscular twitches, fits, and confusion* – perhaps because of cerebral oedema; and a *progressive dementia* has been described associated with high brain aluminium concentration ('dialysis encephalopathy').

Hepatic failure

The features of hepatic pre-coma are psychological and motor, and are due to nitrogenous substances derived from food. The patient may be noted to have a fixed, staring appearance with a reduction of spontaneous movements.

There are periods of clouded consciousness with perplexity, forgetfulness, dysarthria, and ataxia. Hypersomnia occurs, and the characteristic flapping tremor can be elicited. There is sometimes a fatuous personality change similar to a frontal lobe disorder (see p. 160).

Acute intermittent porphyria

This is a rare disorder, but psychotic symptoms may be prominent, in association with unexplained abdominal pain. Histrionic behaviour and emotional lability are common. It is beginning to look as though George III did not suffer from it.

TOXIC STATES AND DEFICIENCIES

Carbon monoxide poisoning

This is a cause of a severe amnestic syndrome. Extrapyramidal damage may also occur: personality changes include impulsiveness, moodiness, and aggression.

Thiamine

Depression, irritability, lassitude, and anorexia occur in those deprived of dietary thiamine. Vague somatic complaints and forgetfulness occur as deficiency becomes more severe; finally Korsakow's syndrome (see p. 157). Acute depletion will cause Wernicke's encephalopathy (see p. 157).

Nicotinic acid

Pellagra has prominent psychiatric abnormalities, of which the most dramatic is a *paranoid hallucinatory psychosis*. However, other psychological manifestations include disorientation and confusion, excitement with outbursts of violent behaviour, and depression.

Vitamin B$_{12}$ and folic acid

Amnestic syndrome, subacute delirium, and chronic brain syndrome may either antedate or accompany the megaloblastic anaemia, and are reversible with treatment. *Vitamin B$_{12}$ deficiency* has been said to lead to depressive symptoms, but the evidence is unclear. *Folic acid deficiency* is associated with depressive symptoms accompanied by low drive and anergia, and also with chronic brain syndrome in the elderly (see p. 275).

NEUROLOGICAL DISEASE

We deal with cerebral tumours and dementia in Chapter 12. Two neurological illnesses are strongly linked with *affective illness*:

Parkinson's disease

There is an important association with *depression*, which often follows the onset of Parkinsonian symptoms. Treatment of the depression may dramatically alleviate the motor symptoms.

Multiple sclerosis

At one time students were taught that patients tended to develop euphoria. This can happen when there is general cerebral impairment, but it is not common. Most patients will describe symptoms of *anxiety and depression*, and such symptoms can greatly add to the burden which their disease imposes.

EPILEPSY

Most of those prone to epilepsy are psychiatrically normal, and are not at particular risk for chronic brain syndromes, for major mental illness, or for personality disorder. However, there is an increased risk for such disorders in those whose epilepsy is symptomatic of some organic cerebral disorder, and pathology in the temporal lobe seems especially important in this respect.

Nevertheless, most epileptic patients experience prejudice from others, and this may cause both social handicaps and depressive symptoms which are more disabling than the fits.

Epidemiology

The prevalence of epilepsy in the general population has been estimated to be between four and six per thousand at risk, with an equal sex incidence. Of these, about 30 per cent will have psychiatric difficulties. Among children, psychiatric disorders occur among 7 per cent of those without epilepsy, in 30 per cent of those with uncomplicated epilepsy, and among 60 per cent of those with epilepsy complicated with brain damage.

Clinical features and classification

The principal distinction to be made is between *partial seizures* which start focally and those which are *generalized* from the beginning. Partial seizures may or may not become generalized, so it can be seen that a clear description of the *beginning* of an attack is of the greatest importance diagnostically.

PARTIAL SEIZURES

These may be elementary or complex. An *elementary partial seizure* may include motor or sensory phenomena, and there will usually be no impairment of consciousness. There may be a 'Jacksonian march', as ictal activity spreads in the motor cortex to involve adjacent areas.

A *complex partial seizure* is a term which replaces what used to be referred to as 'psychomotor epilepsy' and 'temporal lobe epilepsy'. The ictus has a focal origin – so there may be an *aura* – but the subject will fall to the ground and become unconscious only if the complex partial seizure becomes generalized. Otherwise, he will appear to be out of touch with his surroundings during the attack and a fixed stare with circumoral pallor may be seen. Voiding of urine or faeces may occur.

The auras usually last only a few seconds, and take the form of hallucinations of hearing, vision, smell, taste, or various bodily sensations. An example of the latter would be the 'epigastric aura', which is usually experienced as a central abdominal churning feeling that spreads upwards through the chest – but many others can occur, including feelings of flushing, tachycardia, fear, and dizziness. Particularly memorable are sudden feelings that unfamiliar surroundings are familiar – the *'déjà-vu'* experience – or the reverse, called *'jamais-vu'*. (However, it should be pointed out that many people report such experiences who have no evidence of temporal lobe epilepsy!)

Psychomotor seizures are examples of complex partial seizures in which automatic behaviours may occur in states of clouded consciousness. They may take the form of grimacing or changes in respiration, or there may be more complex stereotyped behaviour, for example, button-fiddling, lip-smacking, mouthing, including **fugues** (see *p. 311) and **automatisms** (see *p. 310). These usually last only a few minutes, although they may last longer if this form of seizure goes into *psychomotor status*.

GENERALIZED SEIZURES ('GRAND MAL')

This is the familiar major epileptic seizure – classically seen in barbiturate withdrawal or hypoglycaemia – with sudden onset; *tonic then clonic generalized convulsions*; and profound unconsciousness for at least several minutes. If the patient is examined during an attack the corneal reflexes will be lost and the plantar responses extensor. The patient may bite his tongue or be incontinent of urine. Immediately on coming round the patient will be disoriented, and will usually report a severe headache.

In contrast, a 'hysterical' or psychogenic 'seizure' will show none of these features. Patients will tend to fight the examining doctor during the attack, which tends to take place only before an audience. However, they appear to be unconscious during the attack and they thrash their limbs about in ways which can be quite convincing if they have seen others with genuine seizures, or if they have experienced them themselves on other occasions. They tend to be in a bad temper on 'coming round' – but they share this characteristic with those emerging from genuine attacks.

Myoclonic and akinetic seizures refer to other patterns of generalized seizure; the former characterized by widespread myoclonic jerks and the latter by sudden diminution of motor tone – so that the seizure begins without warning by the patient collapsing unconscious. Needless to say, such patients are at high risk of injury during the attack.

Epilepsy in childhood

Epilepsy presents in distinctive ways.

1. **Neonatal seizures** are often the presenting symptoms of serious congenital abnormalities or meningitis. Unless they are due to hypocalcaemia, the prognosis is grave.

2. **Febrile fits** are the commonest form of epilepsy, affecting 3 per cent of children at some time. They accompany fevers and are generally bilateral; brief and benign. If they take their onset in the first year of life, last for more than half an hour, or are lateralized the prognosis is more serious.

3. **Infantile spasms** take the form of recurrent forward flexion of the trunk ('Salaam epilepsy') coming perhaps three times a day. The onset is between four and eighteen months, there is an association with early infantile autism (see p. 236), and there may be failure of normal intellectual development.

4. **The Lennox–Gastaut syndrome**, or 'atypical petit mal', is associated with four kinds of attack: generalized seizures, drop attacks, tonic attacks, and atypical absences. The EEG shows atypical 'notched' spike and wave discharges.

5. **Petit mal** occurs in childhood: the child maintains posture, but is unconscious during attacks (which may be referred to as '*absences*'). The EEG shows three per second spike and wave during an absence, and the child may have generalized seizures at other times.

6. **Petit mal status** ('status of minor epilepsy') is commoner in childhood and old age than in adult life: it can persist for prolonged periods (several months!) and although the child is conscious there is clouding accompanied by inability to concentrate and motor incoordination: school work usually suffers, and the EEG shows continuous three per second spike and wave.

7. **Generalized epilepsy** (grand mal') is sporadic throughout childhood.

Aetiology

In about 66 per cent of cases no cause can be found for epilepsy even after full investigation ('idiopathic'); in such cases genetic factors appear to have some importance. In the remainder the epilepsy can be shown to be secondary to some known cerebral disease: birth injury, congenital malformations, exanthemata, and metabolic disorders in children; cerebrovascular disease, head injury, and degenerative disorders in the elderly.

Drugs may cause epilepsy in two ways: sudden withdrawal of agents known to have anticonvulsant properties such as benzodiazepines or barbiturates; or administration of agents known to lower the convulsive threshold, such as phenothiazines and, to a lesser extent, tricyclic antidepressants.

Withdrawal from large doses of alcohol also causes generalized seizures (see p. 197). Alcohol or drug abuse should therefore always be considered in a patient with no previous history of epilepsy who has a fit following admission to hospital.

Differential diagnosis

Organic conditions which must be distinguished from epilepsy include: syncope, spontaneous hypoglycaemia, and transient ischaemic attacks.

Psychiatric and behavioural disorders include: temper tantrums, breath-holding attacks, and night terrors in children; hyperventilation, panic attacks, and aggressive outbursts in unstable personalities, and hysterical 'loss of consciousness' in adults. The differentiation between generalized seizures and hysterical seizures has been given in detail above.

Psychiatric aspects of epilepsy

PERSONALITY CHANGES

Attitudes of dependency and insecurity may be engendered by over-protection during childhood or by the social and occupational problems which must be faced. These may increase vulnerability to depressive illness.

Patients with temporal lobe epilepsy can exhibit explosive irritability and aggressiveness, and also may report sexual problems: either hyposexuality or deviant practices such as fetishism or transvestism.

DEPRESSIVE ILLNESS

Depression, anxiety, and low self-esteem are common, perhaps because of the social handicaps experienced by most epileptics.

ICTAL

Increasing irritability, tension, and depression are sometimes reported as *prodromata* for several days before an ictus: they are usually relieved afterwards.

The types of complex partial seizures with psychological symptoms have been described above. Sometimes an ictus is followed by restless and combative behaviour. Very occasionally an ictus is followed by schizophrenia-like symptoms, the *paranoid hallucinatory state* accompanied by some clouding of consciousness ('epileptic twilight state').

THE SYMPTOMATIC SCHIZOPHRENIA OF TEMPORAL LOBE EPILEPSY

This is usually a chronic paranoid schizophrenia, taking its onset a decade or more after the onset of the temporal lobe epilepsy. It has been suggested that the dominant temporal lobe is more likely to be affected. The first-degree relatives of such patients have an expectation of schizophrenia no higher than chance, nor is there increased expectancy of schizoid personality, suggesting that the psychosis is indeed secondary to the epilepsy.

EPILEPSY AND CHRONIC BRAIN SYNDROME

There are two possible relationships: a dementing illness may present as epilepsy; or hypoxia associated with long-standing epilepsy may cause a chronic brain syndrome. In old age *petit mal status* may present as an apparent dementing illness of sudden onset. Diagnosis is on the EEG.

Treatment

Whenever possible use anticonvulsant drugs singly, starting with drugs of first choice. If combinations are tried choose those that work by different mechanisms. It is better to have occasional fits than to have a patient drowsy or muddled with side-effects of treatment. The drugs are described on pp. 79–81.

PAIN

Pain is a perception and as such is a part of the mental state. It is commonly associated with tissue damage, and peripheral nerves then play an important part in its transmission. However, central neural mechanisms play a predominant part in pain perception: pain can be caused by CNS lesions, and is also modified by CNS activity, serving both to exacerbate it (as in depressive illnesses) and to relieve it (as exemplified by the use of hypnosis for dental analgesia).

Frequency and diagnosis

Pain is the commonest symptom of which patients complain, accounting for between 50 per cent and 95 per cent of presentations in medical out-patient clinics. Frequently it remains undiagnosed: approximately half of all patients presenting with pain to neurologists, cardiologists, and gastroenterologists show no evidence of relevant organic pathology after intensive investigation and long-term follow-up. Of patients with diagnosed mental illness in general practice and psychiatric out-patient settings, about 60 per cent complain of pain. It seems likely that pain is associated as much with mental as with physical illnesses and occurs particularly in the setting of affective disorders. However, it has little diagnostic specificity and can occur as a symptom of any mental illness. As usual, diagnosis is based on the nature of associated symptoms.

Pain mechanisms

1. The physiological effects of anxiety are widespread. Increased muscle tension is believed to result in 'tension headache'; increased intestinal motility may be experienced as abdominal pain; palpitations may lead to chest pain.
2. Pain is often experienced at a site where there is, or has been, some minor organic pathology, which has not previously caused the patient distress, but serves as a focus once the patient becomes anxious or depressed.
3. Depression and anxiety result in reduced tolerance of pain, whatever its origins.
4. Somatization frequently presents as pain and may result from the use of other defence mechanisms, such as introjection. It is a common feature of anxiety states, depressive disorders, and morbid grief reactions.
5. The awareness of pain becomes more intense and the associated illness behaviours (see *Table 9*) become more frequent as a consequence of reinforcement by others who respond to the patient more positively when he shows such behaviours.

Acute pain

The intensity of pain associated with organic disease and trauma, including post-surgical pain, is related particularly to anxiety. Patients in hospital may experience anxiety for many reasons but much is often due to lack of familiarity with investigation and treatment procedures and the extent to which pain should be anticipated. Pre-surgical preparation which includes careful explanation of the procedures that the patient will experience and the availability of post-surgical analgesia have been shown to reduce both the post-surgical pain experienced and the need for analgesia.

Women patients and those with higher scores on measures of neuroticism tend to complain more about post-surgical pain and receive more analgesics from ward staff; others suffer pain of similar intensity but complain less and consequently suffer more

Table 9 *Aspects of illness behaviour*

1. symptom perception – quality and intensity

2. evaluation of significance of symptoms (morbid risk)

3. verbal communication – complaint behaviour

4. non-verbal communication – posture, gait, use of aids

5. consultation behaviour – the numbers of medical and non-medical people consulted and the number of consultations

6. self-treatment – e.g. number and frequency of medications

7. treatment compliance

8. maintenance of customary activities and roles

9. mood states – including denial of negative affects

because staff are unaware of their pain and fail to give analgesics. It is important to ask patients routinely about pain in order to determine the appropriate management.

Chronic pain patients

Patients with chronic pain (usually defined as of more than six months' duration) may suffer from a wide range of physical and mental disorders. It is a common error to suppose that such patients can be divided into those with 'real' or 'organic' pain and those with 'imaginary' or 'psychogenic' pain: first because both organic and psychological factors often play a part in the same patient, and second because pain is primarily a subjective experience and, if perceived, is always 'real', whatever its origins. Any combination of the mechanisms described above may play a part, and many aspects of illness behaviour (see *Table 9*) associated with the pain may appear inappropriate. Drug abuse is often an important secondary problem which may be iatrogenic.

Surveys of patients attending pain relief clinics show that at least half are suffering from mental illness, diagnosed using standardized methods, but few of these disorders are recognized by the anaesthetists who run the clinics and few are referred to psychiatrists. About two-thirds of those with mental illness have depressive disorders, most of the remainder having primary hypochondriasis.

FURTHER READING

Eastwood, M. (1975) *The Relationship between Physical and Mental Illness*. Toronto: University of Toronto Press.

Ford, C. (1983) *The Somatising disorders: Illness as a Way of Life*. Amsterdam: Elsevier Biomedical.

Kleinman, A. (1980) *Patients and Healers in the Context of Culture*. London: UCLA Press.

Williams, P. and Clare, A. (1979) *Psychosocial Disorders in General Practice*. London: Academic Press.

11 / ORGANIC BRAIN SYNDROMES

Organic brain syndromes may either involve the entire cortical canopy, in which case they are said to be **generalized**; or they may involve only a specific part of the cortex, in which case they are said to be **focal**. Generalized brain syndromes are further subdivided by their course, into **acute brain syndrome** and **chronic brain syndrome**. Even this distinction cannot always be made in a hard-and-fast way, and intermediate disorders can be referred to as **subacute brain syndromes**.

These are all syndromal diagnoses, and they will always require further investigations to establish the cause in a particular case.

ACUTE BRAIN SYNDROME
(also known as **DELIRIUM**)

Terminology

You may be confused by a variety of terms for an acute brain syndrome, all meaning almost the same thing. Old people are often said to present with an *'acute confusional state'*, and this term is further discussed on p. 273. A *toxic confusional state* refers to an acute brain syndrome secondary to toxic causes such as those listed in *Table 10*. Many clinicians use the word *delirium* to mean an acute brain syndrome with pronounced psychomotor agitation often accompanied by hallucinations and illusions, but others do not make this distinction.

Epidemiology

This a common condition occurring in 5–10 per cent of general medical and surgical in-patients. It is common in the elderly and up to 30 per cent of the population have been estimated to suffer from this syndrome at some time of their lives. It is the most common cause of a psychotic state that occurs in the general wards. The syndrome occurs when normal brain functioning is disturbed by any one of the many causes listed in *Table 10*.

Table 10   *Causes of acute brain syndrome*

	systemic	intracranial
trauma		head injury
degenerative		dementia with acute illness
epileptic		post-ictal states petit mal status
vascular	myocardial infarction anaemia heart failure internal haemorrhage	cerebral thrombosis or embolism subarachnoid haemorrhage transient ischaemic episode hypertensive encephalopathy
infections	exanthemata septicaemia pneumonia influenza typhoid typhus cerebral malaria trypanosomiasis	encephalitis meningitis rheumatic chorea cerebral abscess
metabolic	uraemia liver failure, alkalosis, acid-base disorders acidosis, hypercapnia electrolyte disturbances remote effects of carcinoma anoxia CVS, chest disease, and anaemia	
endocrine disorders	hyperthyroid crisis myxoedema Addisonian crisis diabetic pre-coma, hypoglycaemia parathyroid disease	
toxic	drugs: see text, pp. 143–44 alcohol: delirium tremens Wernicke's encephalopathy heavy metals: lead, arsenic, mercury	

Clinical features

Despite the plethora of aetiologies shown in *Table 10* the clinical picture is relatively constant. It is characterized by:

1. **Clouding of consciousness** (see p. 35) which has an acute onset and a fluctuating course – being worse at night, better during the day, and improving as the underlying pathological process resolves. Minor degrees of clouding of consciousness may be difficult to detect unless the patient is examined at night or when he is fatigued. Poor attention and impaired thinking may only be evident with persistent cognitive testing. In severe cases it may be impossible to gain the patient's attention at all as he is responding only to hallucinatory experiences, and his speech is an incoherent rambling, totally incomprehensible to the observer.

2. **Disorientation in time** (see p. 34) occurs first, followed by that of **space and person**. The disorientation fluctuates with level of consciousness and the person may be oriented by day and disoriented by night.

3. **Impaired thinking** ('confusion') occurs in conjunction with clouding of consciousness. Thinking may be slowed initially but progressively reasoning becomes less clear and incoherent.

4. **Disturbance of registration, retention, and recall** occur.

5. **Perceptual abnormalities** often make the staff first aware of the patient's abnormal mental state. *Illusions and misinterpretations* may dominate the picture. Unfamiliar objects and people are at greatest risk of being misinterpreted. Members of staff may be regarded by the patient as enemies or involved in a plot. Drugs may be misinterpreted as poison and these will be refused. *Visual hallucinations* are common, though *auditory and tactile hallucinations* also occur. The hallucinations may form complex scenes in which the patient feels he is involved and by which he may be terrified.

6. **Emotional changes**. Anxiety, irritability, depression, and apathy occur first but frank fear may occur with or without the hallucinatory or persecutory phenomena described above. The patient may attempt to leave the ward in order to escape the frightening scenes he is experiencing.

7. **Psychomotor changes**. Either change may occur: *psychomotor retardation* may be evident with apathy and withdrawal from the patient's surroundings; but in the more severe forms *restless over-activity* is more common, with the patient plucking at the bedclothes or attempting to get out of bed. The latter pattern is seen in *delirium tremens* (see p. 146).

The failure to learn new material is usually evident on recovery when a dense amnesia for the duration of the delirium is evident. Occasionally there have been lucid intervals when the patient's conscious level returns to normal, and there may be fragmented but vivid memories of emotionally charged scenes.

Diagnostic criteria

The following criteria may be used for research purposes.

Clouding of consciousness of acute onset, accompanied by *reduced capacity for attention,*

AND two or more of the following:

1. **Disorientation** or **memory impairment**.
2. **Perceptual disturbance** (misinterpretations, illusions, or hallucinations).
3. **Incoherent speech**.
4. Disturbed **sleep–wakefulness cycle** with insomnia and daytime sleeping.
5. Increased or decreased **psychomotor activity**.

Aetiology

The syndrome is produced by any cause that disrupts total brain functioning, and is the same irrespective of whether the exciting cause is intra-cranial (such as encephalitis or subdural haematoma) or systemic (such as pneumonia or uraemia). More than one factor may be present, and factors may contribute to the aetiology that have not been listed as 'main causes'. For example, following an operation *residual anaesthetic, pain, mild respiratory problems, toxins from blood transfusion, opiate analgesic drugs, dehydration, anxiety, and unfamiliar surroundings* may each be insufficient in themselves, but together account for delirium.

Examination of the time of onset of the condition may provide a clue to the principal factor; this may coincide with the onset of a pyrexia, the changing of a drug, or development of dehydration.

TOXIC EFFECTS OF DRUGS

A wide range of drugs are capable of causing an acute brain syndrome, particularly:

1. Dopamine agonists (especially in combination):
   Benzhexol
   L-DOPA
   Amantadine.
2. Antidepressants, notably Amitryptyline (especially when used in patients with severe physical illness or in large doses).
3. Tranquillizers and hypnotics:
   Barbiturates
   Benzodiazepines
   Phenothiazines.

4. Anti-cholinergic drugs:
   Atropine
   Hyoscine.

5. Antituberculous drugs:
   Isoniazid
   Cycloserine.

6. Cytotoxic drugs.

7. Anticonvulsants (especially in high dose).

Alcohol and barbiturates can cause toxic symptoms either by acute intoxication or by withdrawal. Thus an acute brain syndrome developing twenty-four to seventy-two hours after admission may result from the sudden cessation of regular alcohol intake or a drug upon which the patient is dependent.

Differential diagnosis

CHRONIC BRAIN SYNDROME

A previously undetected chronic brain syndrome can present for the first time as an acute brain syndrome if the patient develops some intercurrent infection which produces a state of acute cerebral decompensation. As the infection resolves, the chronic brain syndrome becomes apparent. The same can happen if there is some sudden change in the patient's environment, such as death of a spouse or moving to a new house. In either case, such a transient acute brain syndrome is sometimes referred to as a 'decompensated dementia'.

FUNCTIONAL ILLNESS

Depression in the elderly (see p. 278) may present with clouding of consciousness and impaired ability to concentrate. The acute onset of *mania* or *schizophrenia* may be accompanied by perplexity, clouding, and impaired ability to think in addition to more typical schizophrenic phenomena.

In these functional conditions clouding, disorientation, and impaired concentration will generally be less pronounced than other features of the mental state. Thus in severe depressive illness depressed mood and psychomotor retardation will predominate over the cognitive changes, and in schizophrenia the psychotic features will become clear with time.

Investigations

These will be ordered according to the abnormal physical findings present, unless a likely cause is evident from your physical examination.

A useful first round of investigations would be:

Full blood count
ESR

Urea and electrolytes
Liver function tests
Thyroid function tests
Blood sugar
Serology for neurosyphilis

Urine for microscopy and culture
Urine for drugs or porphyrins

Chest X-ray

To distinguish between delirium and functional illness:

EEG – shows slow waves in delirium

The following may be necessary:

Serum B_{12} and folate
Lumbar puncture
CAT scan

Treatment

The patient must be investigated in hospital.

TREATMENT OF THE UNDERLYING CAUSE.

Correction of the underlying physical abnormality is the primary goal of treatment. It may be necessary to correct a number of factors. Any abnormalities of fluid or electrolyte balance, or haematological and nutritional factors should be corrected. *Any drugs that are not essential should be stopped.*

SYMPTOMATIC AND SUPPORTIVE MEASURES

Tranquillizers may be necessary if the patient is otherwise unmanageable. Since such medication can itself cause delirium it should be kept to a minimum and used only if the nursing procedures described below are unsuccessful.

Haloperidol is preferable to chlorpromazine as it tranquillizes without sedating, is less hypotensive, and has fewer adverse effects on the liver. It does not accumulate in the body like diazepam, nor is it likely to release clouding and disturbed behaviour in the same way as benzodiazepines.

Chlormethiazole is useful in delirium from any cause in which epileptic fits might occur, such as delirium tremens.

These drugs are particularly useful at night, as sleep deprivation can exacerbate the delirium.

In order to minimize misinterpretations the patient should be nursed in a room that is *well-lit during the night* and by a small number of staff whom the patient can easily recognize. The patient will require *frequent reassurance* because of his fear, and *repeated explanation* by calm members of staff can reduce the need for sedation.

Early detection of acute brain syndrome may avoid the necessity for sedation, so any reports by the night staff of mild degrees of clouding or disturbed thinking in seriously ill patients should be investigated fully.

It is essential that a patient with an acute brain syndrome be kept in hospital for treatment. Occasionally this requires use of Section 5(2) of the Mental Health Act (see p. 307).

Course and prognosis

Following resolution of the underlying disorder, the delirious state may linger for days. In one study of delirium the majority of patients had either cancer or serious heart disease and the mortality rate during the index admission was 20 per cent and by one year nearly 50 per cent. However, the prognosis in cases due to drug intoxication or withdrawal is much better than for those in whom an underlying potentially fatal illness causes the delirium.

SUBACUTE BRAIN SYNDROME
(also known as SUBACUTE DELIRIOUS STATE)

This is a state intermediate between an acute and a chronic brain syndrome: the onset will have been less sudden than is usual in delirium, there will be a combination of features of the two, and the course is also intermediate. Wernicke's encephalopathy (p. 157) often presents in this way.

DELIRIUM TREMENS

About 5 per cent of patients admitted to hospital with physical complications of alcoholism will display delirium tremens. Typically it occurs in middle-aged men who have been drinking heavily for some years, but it can also occur after only a few months of heavy drinking.

The first twelve hours:

Mild withdrawal phenomena such as tremor and agitation occur;

Twelve to forty-eight hours after withdrawal:

Generalized epileptic seizures may occur;

Three to four days after withdrawal:

The clinical picture in delirium tremens occurs –

and is similar to that in acute brain syndromes of other aetiologies but the following features are marked:

1. Dramatic, sudden onset with restlessness, insomnia, and fear.
2. Clouded consciousness and disorientation.
3. Startle reactions, nightmares, and panic.
4. Face terror-stricken.
5. Ataxia and tremor present.
6. Perspiration, tachycardia, low pyrexia; flushing or pallor.

Later:

1. Profuse visual and tactile illusions and hallucinations (pink elephants rare; rats, snakes, and nameless small animals common, vivid, and terrifying).
2. Auditory hallucinations may be threatening or persecutory.
3. Disorientation and confusion

Treatment

This is an urgent matter; the patient is admitted to hospital and:

1. **Sedation** is essential with chlormethiazole or diazepam which have **anticonvulsant properties** in addition to being tranquillizers. These can be given four-hourly and intravenously if necessary. They should be given on a reducing regime and stopped after, at most, fourteen days.
2. Parenteral administration of **B vitamins** can prevent Wernicke's encephalopathy if instituted early.
3. **Fluid replacement** may be necessary as dehydration can be severe. Electrolyte balance must be obtained: hypokalaemia and hypomagnesaemia are common.
4. **Hypoglycaemia** is common and can cause serious cerebral damage. The infusion fluid should therefore include **dextrose**.
5. Concurrent **infection or head injury** often accompanies the delirium and treatment is instituted as necessary.
6. Once the acute phase is over the patient will require continuing **sedation at night** when vivid nightmares result from REM rebound. To avoid dependence on the sedative drug a *reducing regime lasting for approximately ten days* is used.

7. Upon recovery, the patient must be examined for all the **effects of alcohol** including evidence of chronic alcoholic brain damage (see p. 152). Assess motivation for treatment of alcoholism.

Course

Delirium tremens usually resolves in three days but continuing high levels of anxiety may continue for weeks or months afterwards. These require treatment as they contribute to the risk of the patient rapidly returning to alcohol.

Mortality of DTs has been 10–15 per cent with death due to epileptic fits, heart failure, infection, or self-injury during the most disturbed phase.

CHRONIC BRAIN SYNDROME
(also known as **DEMENTIA**)

Terminology

This syndrome, like the acute one, requires further investigation to establish its cause. All are agreed that some chronic brain syndromes are reversible. Although some clinicians use the above terms interchangeably, others reserve the term 'dementia' for those chronic brain syndromes which are irreversible.

Epidemiology

It is estimated that 10 per cent of the population over sixty-five years are affected by dementia. This figure rises to 22 per cent in the over eighty-year-olds (see p. 275). The majority remain in the community and fewer than one-fifth of the severe cases are admitted to hospital or live in an old people's home.

'Senile dementia' applies to chronic brain syndrome occurring over the age of sixty-five years. Senile dementia of Alzheimer's type (SDAT) and multi-infarct dementia are the commonest forms. Pick's disease is less common and Huntington's chorea and Creutzfeld–Jacob disease are least common. Those dementias presenting before the age of sixty-five years are known as the **pre-senile dementias**.

Clinical features

PRESENTATION

Failure of memory may be so insidious that it does not attract medical attention until it is very pronounced. There may be progressive failure to cope with social situations, or matters may come to a head when normal routines are disturbed, and the patient is unable to cope.

FEATURES

1. **Memory impairment** without clouding of consciousness is the hallmark of the syndrome. This may first be noticed by relatives and workmates rather than the patient himself, who may even deny the impairment. It may be so gradual that it is difficult to date the onset. Minor forgetfulness, failure to remember names and appointments, lead on to more definite evidence of amnesia. The patient may lose his way in familiar territory, a decline in performance at work may become evident and the patient may become hopelessly mixed up with complex tasks at home such as cooking from a recipe. Leaving the gas on, wandering at night, and forgetting the day are common ways in which the memory loss is brought to the attention of others. The impairment of memory is global, but loss of short-term memory is a conspicuous early sign with relative preservation of long-term memory initially. Recall is affected and the person may need prompts even for previously well-established memory traces. Some patients conceal their memory loss by using lists and sticking to a strict daily routine. A spouse or other close relative may have tolerated and helped to compensate for the patient's memory loss, in which case the death or move of the relative will bring the dementia to light.

2. **Personality deterioration** reflects both intellectual deterioration and changes in social awareness. The earliest change may be an exacerbation of personality traits producing obsessional or hypochondriacal symptoms. Loss of manners may occur, the person ignores the feelings of others, and becomes increasingly stubborn and withdrawn. In later stages personal care and hygiene deteriorate with food stains on clothing and chaotic living conditions resulting. Eventually urinary and faecal incontinence occur but the patient may have become so apathetic that he appears unconcerned by this.

3. **Thinking** becomes slowed and restricted with a tendency to brood on a few themes from the past. Perseveration occurs. The dementing person cannot cope with new ideas and abstract thinking is lost. Concentration is impaired and the person becomes easily fatigued. Judgement is impaired, and ideas of reference or even delusions develop because the power to reason is lost. Thus an item which is lost through forgetfulness and later found is regarded by the person as evidence that an intruder has been in the house. In later stages thinking is confined to very few themes and may become incoherent. These abnormalities of thinking are reflected in the **speech** of the dementing person, which is slow, impoverished, and may eventually become a series of incomprehensible words and phrases.

4. **Emotional changes** may be the presenting feature. These are initially a response to the intellectual deterioration and will therefore depend on the degree of insight and the previous personality. Anxiety, irritability, and depression are common reactions and suicide attempts occasionally reflect this. Affective responses later become blunted but are interspersed with apparently unprovoked outbursts of anger, distress, or laughter. Such emotional lability may be demonstrated during

cognitive testing when the patient becomes frustrated, bursts into tears, and gives up: a **catastrophe reaction**.

5. Sometimes the illness presents with **persecutory delusions** or **auditory hallucinations**.

Diagnostic criteria

Chronic brain syndrome may be defined as an acquired global impairment of intellect, memory, and personality without impairment of consciousness.

For research purposes it can be diagnosed when there is **loss of intellectual abilities** sufficiently severe to interfere with social or occupational functioning, **memory impairment**, and at least ONE of the following, in the absence of clouding of consciousness:

1. Impairment of **abstract thinking**.
2. Impaired **judgement**.
3. **Aphasia, apraxia, agnosia**, or **constructional difficulty**.
4. **Personality change**,

Aetiology

Senile dementia will be discussed in Chapter 19 (see p. 275); we shall here consider *chronic brain syndromes occurring before the age of sixty-five*.

The degenerative causes of such chronic brain syndromes (sometimes called '**pre-senile dementias**') are sufficiently important to be discussed separately.

ALZHEIMER'S DISEASE

This is one of the common forms of pre-senile dementia. Onset is uncommon before the age of forty, and women predominate over men. In the first phase of the illness there is failing memory, muddled inefficiency over the tasks of life, and spatial disorientation. The patient may be apathetic, or perplexed and agitated. In the next stage the patient develops more rapid signs of intellectual deterioration and parietal lobe symptoms (see p. 160) and extrapyramidal symptoms may appear. Delusions and hallucinations may occur. In the final stage there is a profound apathetic dementia with the patient bed-ridden and doubly incontinent. The EEG is always abnormal.

Familial cases have been described with autosomal dominant inheritance but generally a multifactorial inheritance is suggested. The morbid risk of first-degree relatives of patients with Alzheimer's disease is increased four times.

Neuropathology – Cortical atrophy is generalized but most marked over the frontal and temporal lobes. *Loss of neurones in the neocortex, together with proliferation of astrocytes,* *senile plaques, and neurofibrillary tangles are striking,* and in greater number than in the normal aged brain. Clinical manifestations of dementia appear when the plaque count and neurofibrillary changes reach a certain threshold. In normal ageing the brain seems to have sufficient reserve capacity to withstand a limited amount of such changes and yet maintain normal function.

Neurochemistry – Although the neuropathological changes characterizing Alzheimer's disease have been known for most of this century, specific neurochemical changes have been identified only during the past decade. The most important of these is the **loss of cholinergic neurones** innervating the neocortex: the loss of these neurones is indicated by marked reductions in the concentration of the enzymes *choline-acetyltransferase* and *cholinesterase.* Much of the cholinergic innervation of the neocortex originates from the nucleus basalis of Meynert located at the base of the forebrain; neurones in this nucleus degenerate in Alzheimer's disease. The importance of cholinergic mechanisms has been demonstrated: cholinergic drugs, such as the cholinesterase inhibitor *physostigmine,* cause a transient improvement in memory functions in patients suffering from Alzheimer-type dementia, whereas anti-cholinergic drugs, such as the muscarinic receptor antagonist *scopolamine,* have the opposite effect. Since cortical postsynaptic muscarinic receptors remain relatively unaffected in Alzheimer's disease, attempts have been made to stimulate these receptors by *cholinomimetic agents* (choline, lecithin) administered to the patients: these efforts, however, have remained unsuccessful.

Apart from cholinergic neurones, noradrenergic and 5-hydroxytryptaminergic neurones innervating the neocortex can also degenerate, resulting in reductions in cortical noradrenaline and 5-hydroxytryptamine levels. Consistent decreases have been shown in the cortical levels of *somatostatin* indicating the degeneration of nerve cells containing this neuropeptide transmitter.

MULTIPLE-INFARCT DEMENTIA (ARTERIOSCLEROTIC DEMENTIA)

This results from repeated cerebrovascular accidents often from cerebral emboli. Other evidence of arteriosclerosis is found throughout the cardiovascular system and focal signs such as pseudobulbar palsy, increased reflexes, extensor plantar responses, and extrapyramidal features occur more often than in Alzheimer's disease. Marked cerebral softening occurs in this type of dementia and this differentiates it from Alzheimer's disease, where senile plaques predominate.

Onset is uncommon before the age of fifty, and the sex ratio is approximately equal. The most striking difference between this type of dementia and Alzheimer's disease is the step-wise progression, and the presence of other evidence of arteriosclerosis on physical examination. Patients may complain of somatic symptoms such as headache, dizziness, tinnitus, and syncope in addition to problems with memory. There may be transient attacks of hemiparesis, dysphasia, or visual dysfunctions which are at first followed by restitution, but which eventually lead to the dementia becoming more profound.

PICK'S DISEASE

This is less common than Alzheimer's disease, but a familial pattern is also well recognized. The frontal and temporal lobes are particularly atrophied. Personality changes and dysphasia therefore occur early in the disease. Neuronal loss occurs with gliosis but plaques and tangles do not and the EEG may be normal.

HUNTINGTON'S CHOREA

This disorder is characterized by a combination of pre-senile dementia, extrapyramidal features, and choreic movements. The transmission of this disease by a *single autosomal dominant gene* is well recognized, with half the offspring of an affected person being affected. It is now becoming possible to identify some of the carriers of the gene. Reduced levels of GABA in the basal ganglia and substantia nigra are thought to be responsible for the choreiform movements. The dementia often appears slowly and later in the disease than the neurological or psychotic features. The latter start with personality changes, such as becoming quarrelsome, slow, and apathetic, but schizophrenic symptoms and marked mood changes occur.

The frontal lobe shows greatest atrophy along with the caudate nuclei and marked dilatation of the ventricles.

CREUTZFELD—JACOB DISEASE

Cerebral atrophy is less marked in this form of dementia but a characteristic spongy appearance of the grey matter is seen microscopically along with neuronal loss and proliferation of astrocytes. This may occur in different parts of the brain accounting for the different clinical presentations. The *EEG is always abnormal* with increased slow-wave activity and bilateral spike-wave discharges which accompany the characteristic *myoclonic jerks*. It has been demonstrated that this disease can be transmitted from humans to primates experimentally, and some instances have occurred when 'natural' transmission has occurred. It is therefore believed that a slow virus or virus-like particle is responsible, and the illness has been related to Kuru. It is probable that the virus-like particle fails to invoke the usual inflammatory response in the brain and a similar aetiological factor is being sought in other forms of pre-senile dementia.

ALCOHOLIC DEMENTIA

There is increasing evidence that cerebral atrophy occurs in a proportion of those who have drunk heavily for many years. In the early years the chronic brain syndrome associated with alcoholism appears to be reversible.

Table 11   *Causes of chronic brain syndrome*

	systemic	*intra-cranial*
degenerative		see text, pp. 150–52 boxing encephalopathy
space-occupying lesions	secondaries	cerebral tumours* subdural haematomas* normal pressure hydrocephalus*
infections		neurosyphilis* (GPI or meningovascular) chronic encephalitis
anoxic	anaemia* congestive cardiac failure* chronic respiratory failure	carbon monoxide poisoning post-cardiac arrest
metabolic	uraemia* liver failure* remote effects of carcinoma	
endocrine	myxoedema* Addison's disease* hypoglycaemia* parathyroid disease*	
toxic	barbiturates,* bromides* manganese, carbon disulphide	alcoholic atrophy
vitamin deficiency	B_{12} and folic acid deficiency* thiamine deficiency* nicotinic acid deficiency*	

Note: * = potentially reversible cause for chronic brain syndrome.

Non-degenerative causes of dementia are shown as *Table 11*. Four *neurological diseases* are worth highlighting.

NORMAL PRESSURE HYDROCEPHALUS

A form of hydrocephalus in which there is an obstruction in the subarachnoid space to the free egress of CSF from the ventricles. Memory impairment, a stiff-legged shuffling gait, urinary incontinence, and slowness develop over weeks or months. The EEG is frequently abnormal; but the diagnosis is confirmed by CAT scan, which shows symmetrical ventricular enlargement but no enlargement of the subarachnoid space above the basal cisterns. Treatment is by insertion of a **shunt** with a low-pressure one-way valve, between the lateral ventricle and the superior vena cava. Results are variable, but sometimes impressive.

NEUROSYPHILIS

General paralysis of the insane (GPI) has become something of a rarity, but was at one time an important cause of a chronic brain syndrome accompanied by highly characteristic neurological signs (Argyll–Robertson pupils, trombone tremor of tongue, dysarthria, ataxia, and upper motor neurone signs). *Meningo-vascular syphilis* presents with headache and lethargy which proceeds to a dementia: there may be a basal meningitis with cranial nerve palsies and a wide variety of other neurological signs depending on the area involved.

PARKINSON'S SYNDROME

Arteriosclerosis may underlie both the dementia and movement disorders in Parkinson's syndrome. But dementia has also been reported in cases of idiopathic Parkinsonism, the aetiology of which is uncertain.

MULTIPLE SCLEROSIS

Minor cognitive impairment can be detected in the majority of patients with multiple sclerosis. Profound global dementia is uncommon but is rarely the presenting feature of the illness.

When investigating a case of chronic brain syndrome it is especially important to detect conditions which may be either arrested or partially reversed, and these have been asterisked in *Table 11*.

Differential diagnosis

DEMENTIA MUST BE DIFFERENTIATED FROM FUNCTIONAL ILLNESSES

1. **Depressive pseudodementia**. Old patients who are depressed may appear to be demented, in that they complain of defective memory, appear disoriented, have a poor knowledge of current events, and perform poorly on cognitive tests. A detailed history from an informant should differentiate the initial depressed mood leading to later disturbance of memory from the picture of dementia which starts with memory and behavioural impairments, but leads on to depression at a later stage. A past history of a depressive episode, depressive symptoms antedating other symptoms, and a more acute onset should put one on the right track.

2. **Hysterical pseudodementia**. A patient may be brought to a casualty department having been found wandering and unable to give his name and address (see **hysterical amnesia**, *p. 311). Alternatively a patient may be admitted with suspected dementia but close observation reveals inconsistencies between his poor performance on formal cognitive testing and his ability to find his way around the ward.

The **Ganser syndrome** consists of 'talking past the point' and giving approximate answers:

How many legs does a horse have?
Five.
What colours are the lights on a traffic light?
Red, yellow, and blue.

The patient's answers are markedly inaccurate, yet they indicate that the question has been understood. The absurd responses are given deliberately and with apparently serious intent. The playful, childish quality of some of the patient's answers is also seen in the 'buffoonery syndromes' associated with hebephrenic schizophrenia or chronic hypomania. The patient may also report hallucinatory experiences, have a fluctuating level of consciousness and demonstrate other hysterical phenomena (p. 220). Such states are most likely among those with low IQ and a history of previous head injury. Either hysterical mechanisms or conscious simulation (malingering; see p. 222) may be involved.

3. **Psychotic illness**. *Hypomania* may appear as a picture of dementia especially as formal cognitive testing is difficult or impossible. *Chronic schizophrenics* with prominent defect symptoms may also appear demented. The other characteristics of the illness should be clear from the history.

DEMENTIA MUST ALSO BE DISTINGUISHED FROM OTHER ORGANIC ILLNESS

1. **Korsakow's syndrome.** Here the disorder is confined to short-term memory and disorientation in time; whereas chronic brain syndrome is a global syndrome involving ability to think, lability of emotion, and changes of personality.

2. **Acute brain syndrome.** Here the onset is more acute, and there is clouding of consciousness. In chronic brain syndrome the patient is more in touch with his surroundings, and he attempts to cooperate despite cognitive difficulties. In acute brain syndrome the patient fluctuates, and can sometimes be shown to be cognitively intact in lucid intervals. Severe perceptual disturbances are more likely in acute brain syndrome.

3. **Focal brain syndromes**. Focal neurological signs are of great importance in localizing disease within the brain. In the degenerative pre-senile dementias neurological signs are usually symmetrical. If dysphasia is produced by focal disease patients have as much difficulty recalling objects from sight as from memory, whereas patients with diffuse chronic brain disease do much better if they can handle and see the object.

4. **Mental retardation**. A careful history will reveal that the patient's problems are not of recent origin, and psychometric tests will show a vocabulary in keeping with verbal and performance IQ, whereas in dementia there will be relative preservation of vocabulary.

Investigations of chronic brain syndrome

CONFIRMATION OF THE DIAGNOSIS

Psychometric testing (see p. 69) when patient is not physically ill, in pain, unduly depressed, or anxious.

INVESTIGATION OF POSSIBLE CAUSES

Interview an informant to obtain the following information:

1. Possible family history of dementia or Huntington's chorea.
2. Previous head injuries: even slight ones may be important.
3. Recent history of faints, fits, or episodes of collapse.
4. What drugs have been taken? Is there possible dietary neglect?
5. What is the patient's usage of alcohol?
6. Obtain description of the personality before illness. Ask about previous episodes of depression.
7. What is the duration of the patient's symptoms? (Short duration suggests tumour, covert infarction, or extra-cranial causes.)

PHYSICAL INVESTIGATIONS TO DISCOVER REMEDIABLE CAUSES

All patients should have the following:

1. Haemoglobin, full blood count, viscosity.
2. Wassermann reaction or equivalent.
3. Blood urea, electrolytes, calcium, and phosphate.
4. Liver function tests, cholesterol, and plasma proteins.
5. B_{12} and folate.
6. Thyroid function tests.
7. Urine should be examined microscopically, and cultured if necessary.
8. Chest and skull X-ray.
9. EEG.
10. CAT scan (if available).

THE FOLLOWING MAY BE CARRIED OUT IF INDICATED

1. Lumbar puncture (if no cause has been found from other tests).
2. Anti-nuclear antibodies.
3. ECG.

Treatment

This depends upon the aetiology. **Reversible causes** (see *Table 11*) must be **detected as early as possible** and vigorously treated.

Non-progressive disorders such as trauma may show improvement over the year following injury; and share with reversible causes a need for active rehabilitation. A decision on long-term care should be taken only when the patient has reached his optimal level of function.

Progressive causes of dementia (for example, Alzheimer's disease) will inevitably deteriorate, requiring progressive care facilities in the community and eventual residential care.

GENERAL MEASURES

Any physical illness that is present (this is common in the elderly) must be treated, and **hearing or visual deficits** corrected as far as possible. **Antidepressant treatment** is indicated if depression is severe. **Sedation** may be required for behavioural disturbance, but should be prescribed only if the patient is disruptive or is a danger to others. It may make matters worse.

Continuation of normal life at home should be aimed at if it is possible, since this provides sufficient stimulus and the familiar surroundings which help to preserve functions. Increased social support will become necessary and attendance at a day centre or day hospital can provide further systematic assessment and stimulating daily routine. The needs of relatives at home must be considered if they are to be able and willing to continue the care of an increasingly dependent person.

Course and prognosis

The course of dementia is variable. Creutzfeld–Jacob disease leads to the most rapid deterioration, with half the patients being dead within nine months. Alzheimer's disease usually leads to death within two to five years. With multi-infarct dementia the course is variable, with many patients dying within five years of the diagnosis. The latter dementia often has a step-wise deterioration determined by further cerebrovascular accidents.

FOCAL BRAIN SYNDROMES

Wernicke's encephalopathy and Korsakow's syndrome

Wernicke's encephalopathy is a subacute brain syndrome caused by a deficiency of thiamine. **Korsakow's syndrome** is a chronic brain syndrome with the same cause. The acute symptoms of the former syndrome may incompletely resolve leaving the clinical picture of the latter.

EPIDEMIOLOGY

The condition is found throughout adult life, most often in the forties and fifties, and is twice as common in men as in women.

CLINICAL FEATURES

Wernicke's encephalopathy is a subacute brain syndrome accompanied by ocular palsies (especially abducent palsies, conjugate deviation gaze palsies, and nystagmus) and ataxia of gait. There may be prodromal nausea and there will usually be a marked memory disorder.

It is not confined to alcoholics, and can occur with thiamine deficiency from any cause (that is dietary, carcinoma of the stomach, toxaemia of pregnancy, pernicious anaemia).

Korsakow's syndrome refers to the selective memory disturbance that is revealed once the generalized cognitive impairment of the acute state clears. Immediate recall (registration) is intact, but the *ability to form new memories* is grossly deficient (see p. 36). The patient is usually *disoriented in time*, but other modalities may also be affected. Long-term memories are relatively well preserved. The patient may provide plausible but incorrect answers to questions that he cannot answer: *confabulation*. There is also an apathy or air of blandness and lack of concern about the failure to answer the questions correctly. Other aspects of cognitive functioning are preserved and the patient does not show clouding of consciousness. Peripheral neuropathy occurs commonly with these disorders.

NEUROPATHOLOGY

Symmetrical lesions are found in the walls of the third ventricle, the periaqueductal region and the floor of the fourth ventricle; also the medial dorsal nuclei of the thalamus and the mamillary bodies. There is proliferation of blood vessels and glia, with petechial haemorrhages. Ocular signs are related to lesions in the third and sixth cranial nuclei, nystagmus to lesions in the vestibular nuclei, and ataxia to lesions in the vestibular nuclei and the vermis of the cerebellum.

Most cases are due to thiamine deficiency, but rarer causes of damage to this part of the brain are: bilateral temporal lobectomy, tumours of the third ventricle, anoxic brain damage, subarachnoid haemorrhage, tuberculous meningitis, and viral encephalitis.

DIFFERENTIAL DIAGNOSIS

Acute brain syndrome of other causes. The history of alcoholism is helpful but in Wernicke's encephalopathy the neurological signs confirm the diagnosis, while in

Korsakow's syndrome there will be absence of clouding. The neurological signs also help to distinguish the condition from delirium tremens, another acute brain syndrome resulting from alcoholism, which is four times more common than Wernicke's encephalopathy.

Chronic brain syndrome. The specific nature of the memory defect is the principal differentiating feature. Chronic alcohol ingestion may lead to a chronic brain syndrome because of cerebral atrophy (see p. 152).

INVESTIGATIONS

Psychometric testing will identify the specific memory impairment necessary to make the diagnosis. Take blood for pyruvate assay as soon as possible, and before giving intravenous parenterovite. Only if the expected history of heavy drinking is not obtained need the other causes be considered.

A lumbar puncture, EEG, and CAT scan would then be helpful. Investigations to identify other damage resulting from alcohol are appropriate.

TREATMENT

Wernicke's encephalopathy requires urgent treatment with large doses of thiamine, with the intention of treating the acute symptoms and modifying the memory impairment. The vitamin is given together with other vitamins of the B group intravenously initially ('parenterovite' contains 250 mg of thiamine in each ampoule) then intramuscularly. Other aspects of management are attention to infection, dehydration, and electrolyte balance. Bed rest is required initially. Sedation may be required and is similar to that used for delirium tremens.

COURSE AND PROGNOSIS

Sixth nerve palsies clear rapidly with prompt treatment, ataxia clears over a few months in many patients but the neuropathy resolves slowly if at all.

The subacute brain syndrome sometimes clears rapidly without lasting amnesia. Otherwise it clears over one to two months leaving the amnesia, which only shows any subsequent improvement in half of the patients. In this chronic state the retrograde amnesia is pronounced, there is apathy but confabulation is rare.

Temporal lobe lesions

Lesions of the *dominant temporal lobe* produce sensory dysphasia together with alexia and agraphia if the lesion extends posteriorly towards the parietal lobe. *Non-dominant temporal lobe lesions* may be relatively asymptomatic though visuospatial difficulties may occur. *Bilateral lesions of the medial parts of the temporal lobes* are those which cause severe memory deficits in the absence of other intellectual impairment.

Of special interest to the psychiatrist are temporal lobe lesions which present with personality change, unpredictable aggressive behaviour, and 'symptomatic schizophrenias' associated with chronic lesions. These have been recognized principally in relation to temporal lobe epilepsy (see p. 136).

Frontal lobe syndrome

Frontal lobe tumours may present to the psychiatrist because of the predominance of behavioural and mood changes over neurological signs. Lateral lesions have been associated with disturbances of volition and psychomotor activity whereas lesions in the medial and orbital areas affect the limbic system and reticular formation leading to disinhibition and mood changes.

The patient typically shows *lack of spontaneity* and initiative and a general diminution of motor activity, although when others provide the stimulus he may behave quite normally. The mood is one of rather inappropriate mild *euphoria* – sometimes described as a 'fatuous jocularity' – alternating with apathy, irritability, or even depression. *Overfamiliarity* occurs sometimes progressing to sexual disinhibition. The patient seems unaware of his unsocial behaviour and irresponsible attitude. Judgement and foresight are impaired. Cognitive functions are largely unimpaired although specific tests for frontal lobe function are available. Neurological signs include combinations of optic atrophy and papilloedema if the lesion involves the optic nerves, or contralateral spastic paresis, grasp reflex, increased tendon reflexes, and a positive Babinski response if the lesion extends posteriorly on to the motor cortex.

Parietal lobe lesions

There are changes in the cognitive and visuospatial spheres: *agnosia* is a disturbance of recognition without sensory disturbance or intellectual impairment. *Apraxia* is the inability to carry out motor activity when motor and sensory systems are intact. Lesions of either parietal lobe produce visuospatial difficulties.

Right (non-dominant) hemisphere lesions produce:

1. Neglect of contralateral sensory field and anosagnosia (failure to recognize disabilities on that side).
2. Disturbance of body image.
3. Dressing apraxia.
4. Visuospatial agnosia (constructional apraxia).
5. Inability to follow a route on map ('topographagnosia').

Left (dominant) hemisphere lesions produce:

1. Motor aphasia (anterior lesions).
2. Sensory aphasia (posterior lesions).

3. Difficulty in writing and drawing ('dysgraphia').

4. Difficulty in reading ('dyslexia').

5. Right–left disorientation.

HEAD INJURY

The severity of brain damage

A patient who has sustained a closed head injury will report a loss of memory from some time before the injury to the time of the injury itself – called the *retrograde amnesia, or RA* – and a loss of memory from the time of the injury to some time afterwards when consecutive memory resumes – called the *post-traumatic amnesia (PTA)*.

The RA is usually considerably shorter than the PTA, and does not in any case give a very reliable indication of brain damage. The two factors from the history which best correlate with the severity of organic damage are the *duration of unconsciousness* and the *duration of the post-traumatic amnesia*. Most of those who report a PTA of more than twenty-four hours will be fortunate if they recover without some degree of intellectual impairment.

The location of brain damage

The effects of location of brain injury on subsequent psychological dysfunction can be examined by studying soldiers who have suffered penetrating injuries to the brain. *Frontal lobe damage* causes severe effects on both mood and behaviour; with injuries to the orbital surface producing severe effects on the personality such as lack of perseverance, inability to maintain relationships, and disinhibition especially affecting sexual and aggressive impulses, while those on the convex lateral surface produce lack of drive, indifference, and incapacity for decisions.

Left hemisphere lesions are associated with global intellectual impairment as well as dysphasias and impaired memory; while injuries to the *right hemisphere* are followed by affective and behavioural disorders and by somatic complaints. Injury to the *parietal or temporal lobes* is associated with intellectual impairment and dysphasia.

Long-term psychological sequelae of closed head injury

Since there are many possible sequelae, we will organize our account by starting at the top of our hierarchy (see p. 49) and working downwards.

CHRONIC BRAIN SYNDROME

In very severe head injuries the chronic brain syndrome will be accompanied by dysphasias and quadriparesis, and the patient may be apathetic, slow, or even mute. Control of affect will be poor, and loss of libido is the rule. Such severe disabilities present formidable problems for rehabilitation, although assessment is usually straightforward.

The main problems of assessment are presented by minor degrees of global damage involving minimal degrees of intellectual impairment and claims for compensation.

POST-TRAUMATIC EPILEPSY

This develops in about 5 per cent of closed head injuries and over 30 per cent of injuries involving penetration of the dura mater. After closed head injury temporal lobe epilepsy (see p. 133) is the commonest form, and is the form most likely to be followed by psychiatric disability. Epilepsy developing in the year following injury is particularly likely to be associated with psychiatric disability.

PSYCHOTIC ILLNESS

A *post-traumatic psychosis* refers to a psychotic illness manifest as soon as consciousness is resumed after injury: these usually remit with treatment. There is an increased incidence of all types of psychotic illness after head injury, although the available evidence suggests that there is a constitutional predisposition in cases of schizophrenia and affective psychosis, so that the role of the head injury is to increase the likelihood of the disorder being manifested.

DEPRESSIVE ILLNESS

Symptoms of affective illness are very common after head injury, and all combinations of non-psychotic symptomatology occur. Indeed *suicide* accounts for 14 per cent of all deaths following head injury. A triad of persistent headaches, dizziness, and irritability is sometimes described as a *post-concussional syndrome*, although the longer it lasts the more it tends to merge with non-specific patterns of psychiatric disorder, and the less likely are such symptoms to be a pure expression of brain damage. Abnormal illness behaviours, such as hypochondriacal symptoms (see p. 219) and hysterical symptoms (see p. 221) commonly accompany such illnesses. Obsessional states (see p. 215) have also been shown to be more common after head injury.

One theoretically important study compared head-injured twins with their normal co-twins some ten years following the injury. Although the head-injured twin was found to be inferior to the normal co-twin on a variety of tests of intellectual function, such differences were subtle and unobtrusive in everyday life. The MZ twins were more concordant than the DZ twins for the 'post-concussional' symptoms described above; and those twins thought to have shown a 'change in personality' consisting of tension, fatiguability, and lessened ability to work were found to have co-twins with the same traits. Once more, it is clear that constitutional predisposition to such symptoms must play a major role, with the function of the head injury being to release the symptoms in the short term.

PERSONALITY DISORDER

The personality changes which go to make up the *frontal lobe syndrome* (see p. 160) have already been referred to, while another pattern consists of *explosive aggressive outbursts* on minor provocation. As you have seen from the twin study reported above, constitutional factors are likely to play a decisive role in the development of non-specific 'neurotic' symptoms.

FURTHER READING

Lishman, A. (1978) *Organic Psychiatry*. Oxford: Blackwell Scientific.

12 / SCHIZOPHRENIA AND ALLIED STATES

EPIDEMIOLOGY

There have been many studies of the prevalence of schizophrenia, some of which have provided widely differing figures. In the past, unstandardized diagnostic practices were largely responsible for this variation: modern studies have produced much more consistent figures.

Approximately 1 per cent of adults are diagnosed as schizophrenic at some time during their lives. The inception rate (new illnesses) is 15 to 20 per 100,000 in the UK, and the point prevalence is about 200 per 100,000. The large difference between these figures implies a mean duration of illness of approximately fifteen years; schizophrenia is often a chronic condition, but the course of the illness may vary greatly.

Recent studies have demonstrated that the incidence of schizophrenia is similar in countries all over the world but tends to run a less chronic course in the developing countries. The peak incidence occurs between twenty-five and thirty years of age and there is another smaller peak in the over sixty-five age group.

Although higher rates of schizophrenia are found in lower social classes and in central zones of large cities, these findings are the result of the illness rather than its cause. The social class distribution of fathers of patients with schizophrenia approximates to that of the general population and the downward social drift is accounted for by the many handicaps that accompany schizophrenia. These also result in people with chronic schizophrenia living alone in the cheap hotels and lodging houses that are found in the centres of large cities.

CLINICAL FEATURES

Schizophrenia is a term used to describe a syndrome of abnormalities in the history and mental state. This does not imply a particular cause or course of the symptoms which may be quite variable. The abnormalities occur in several spheres and are divided into *positive* and *negative* symptoms.

Positive symptoms

1. **Contact with reality** is reduced. The normal mental processes which allow clear differentiation between subjective experiences and the outside world break down. The patient may state that his thoughts are known to others or are not his own, that is caused by others (**disorders of thought possession**). His own movements, or his own feelings and impulses, may be experienced as being generated by, or under the control of, other people or forces (**passivity phenomena**). In **thought withdrawal** the patient feels that his thoughts are being actively removed from his head (*'My thoughts are removed by a phrenological vacuum extractor'*). These phenomena are sometimes described as **disintegrative delusions** (see p. 49).

2. **Hallucinations** are common, usually of the auditory type. Thus the person with schizophrenia may experience his own thoughts as coming from the outside world spoken aloud (**thought echo**). Another typical form is for the patient to hear himself referred to as 'he' or 'him' (**third-person auditory hallucinations**). (Other auditory hallucinations which are common in schizophrenia are voices which make obscene, threatening, or highly critical comments: *but these occur in other conditions as well.*)

3. **Thinking** may become disturbed so that the patient's speech shows unusual logic, idiosyncratic use of words, or made-up words, called **neologisms** (see p. 26). Associations between concepts become loosened so the usual flow of logical ideas is replaced by passages of speech which are difficult to follow ('knight's move' in thought, or 'derailment'). In **schizophrenic thought disorder** the patient's speech contains thoughts which do not directly follow from one another (p. 26).

4. **Delusions** of various types may occur. Delusions which cannot be derived from some other abnormality are called **primary delusions** (see p. 31). A form of primary delusional experience which is diagnostic of schizophrenia is called **delusional perception** (see p. 31). Such experiences usually have a vivid quality, and are well remembered by the patient.
   (As a result of abnormal experiences such as hallucinations the patient may develop **secondary delusions**, so that X-rays, computers, bugging devices, witchcraft, or hypnosis may be blamed for the occurrence of these phenomena. These should be thought of as the patient's attempts to make sense of his puzzling experiences, and they *are of no diagnostic significance in their own right*.)

5. The normal **control of emotions may be disturbed** with outbursts of laughter or anger without any appropriate stimulus (**incongruous affect**). This may occur spontaneously but may also reflect the patient's psychotic experiences – threatening

hallucinations, or the experience of being controlled by others – and may cause resentment or hostility in the patient.

Negative symptoms

1. **Poverty of speech**. The patient has little to say for himself and tends to give empty or laconic replies to questions. The patient's thinking has lost richness and complexity, and this is reflected in his speech.
2. **Slowness of thought and movement** also contribute to the picture of an unresponsive person and clear psychomotor retardation may occur.
3. **Emotional flatness** tends to accompany slowness and poverty of speech, and refers to the absence of normal modulation of mood, with lack of facial expressiveness and emotional responsiveness.
4. **Loss of volition** indicates that the patient seems unable to motivate himself to work satisfactorily or, in severe forms, even to be able to care for himself on a day-to-day basis. Movements and speech become slow. This lack of drive leads to under-activity and **social withdrawal** – symptoms which are greatly exacerbated if the patient lives in an understimulating enrivonment.

Many other psychotic phenomena may occur (see Chapter 3) but these are not characteristic of schizophrenia and may occur with any psychotic illness. In addition patients with schizophrenia may complain of depression, anxiety, irritability, and somatic symptoms of tension. However, in the presence of schizophrenic phenomena symptoms from lower down the diagnostic hierarchy (see p. 49) do not alter the diagnosis.

Type 1 schizophrenia

The **positive symptoms** are characteristic of Type 1 schizophrenia according to a recent classification. These symptoms are made worse by *over-arousal* and respond to medication with *neuroleptics*.

Type 2 schizophrenia

In Type 2 schizophrenia the symptoms are more chronic; **negative symptoms predominate** and the response to medication is less clear. It has been demonstrated that in some patients Type 2 schizophrenia is associated with enlarged cerebral ventricles on CAT scan and 'soft' neurological signs. The negative symptoms are exacerbated by living in an *understimulating environment* and contribute to the features of *institutionalization*.

Other clinical classifications of schizophrenia are more descriptive and reflect the different presentations of the syndrome.

Acute undifferentiated schizophrenia

This often follows a precipitating stress, florid positive symptoms are present, and the patient makes a good recovery.

Paranoid schizophrenia

In paranoid schizophrenia the patient shows marked persecutory or other delusions which may persist in moderated form even when the patient's general condition improves. In spite of this there is relatively little deterioration of personality and the patient may be able to live independently in the community.

Chronic schizophrenia

Chronic schizophrenia is characterized by a protracted course and the gradual development of pronounced negative symptoms. (see Glossary for other types of schizophrenia).

DIAGNOSTIC CRITERIA

There is no international consensus on the best way to diagnose schizophrenia. Most European definitions pay no regard either to the duration of the symptoms or to the presence of affective phenomena, and rely heavily on symptoms brought together by *Schneider*, and described as **first-rank symptoms**. Schneider said that *in the absence of epilepsy, intoxication, or other evidence of gross cerebral damage,* the presence of one or more of these symptoms indicates a likely diagnosis of schizophrenia. Most psychiatrists would now add *mania* to the list of conditions in which first-rank symptoms can occur.

The ten first-rank symptoms

Disorders of thought possession
1. Thought insertion or thought withdrawal.
2. Thought broadcasting.

Passivity phenomena
3. Emotions ('made feelings').
4. Impulses ('made impulses').

    5. Sensations ('made sensations').

    6. Acts . . . under some outside influence.

Auditory hallucinations in which the person hears

    7. His own thoughts echoed out aloud.

    8. Two or more people discussing or arguing about him in the third person.

    9. Voices that form a running commentary on his behaviour.
       (*Now he's drinking his tea.*)

A particular kind of delusional experience

    10. Delusional perception.

It can be seen that these are similar (but not identical) to the positive symptoms that have already been described. If schizophrenia is defined in this way, approximately one-third of patients will make a full recovery and have no further attacks. In the United States schizophrenia is currently defined in a more restrictive way than this, in order to delineate a condition which is more likely to run a chronic course. This is easily achieved by inserting a requirement that symptoms related to the illness should have been present continuously for at least six months, and that the illness should have affected social functioning or self-care.

Schizophrenia or mania?

Recent studies have demonstrated that approximately only 70 per cent of patients with schizophrenia demonstrate first-rank symptoms, and have confirmed that they also occur in mania. The differentiation between these two conditions rests on two sets of criteria.

> The first regards the **mental state** of the patient; the presence of pronounced elation of mood characterizes **mania**, together with the other features of that condition (see p. 191).
> The second regards the **course** of the illness. Repeated episodes of illness occur in both mania and schizophrenia but the latter is more likely to result in a gradual accumulation of negative symptoms.

DIFFERENTIAL DIAGNOSIS

Symptomatic schizophrenia

Sometimes psychoses resembling schizophrenia occur secondarily to known organic diseases or intoxications. Among the more important of these are:

    1. Amphetamine psychosis.

2. Temporal lobe epilepsy.

3. Huntington's chorea.

4. Neoplasms of the cerebral cortex.

The psychosis secondary to intoxication with amphetamine (or other sympathomimetic amines) can appear identical to paranoid schizophrenia. Since the patient does not always admit to taking drugs, a urine specimen should always be sent for amphetamines in any young person with an unexplained psychotic illness. (If the drug is withdrawn, these psychoses should remit completely within ten days.)

The psychoses secondary to temporal lobe epilepsy (see p. 133) usually follow some three to five years after the fits, while those secondary to Huntington's disease usually (but not always) follow the onset of the choreic movements.

Diagnosis of schizophrenia-like illnesses caused by cortical neoplasms depends on eliciting other neurological signs: it means that *every patient with an apparently schizophrenic illness must have a thorough neurological examination.*

Alcoholic hallucinosis (see p. 199)

Here the primary abnormality is an auditory hallucinosis, and any delusions are secondary.

Toxic psychosis due to hallucinogens (see p. 208)

A number of 'hallucinogenic' drugs – such as mescaline, lysergic acid, and psilocylin (the 'magic mushroom') can produce toxic psychoses which are superficially similar to schizophrenia. However, they are usually readily distinguishable because of the disturbances in time perception and in both colour and shape constancy.

Paranoid psychosis

This is an illness with persecutory delusions but without other evidence of schizophrenia. Such patients do not have an increased genetic loading for schizophrenia, but the illness often represents a development of a previous sensitive, suspicious, and rigid personality. The delusions may form a complex and logically elaborated system which leaves other areas of the personality intact. Morbid jealousy and erotomania are specific examples of this syndrome.

Cycloid psychoses

These should be regarded by non-psychiatrists as variants of manic-depressive illness (see p. 190). A number of such cyclic illnesses have been described, of which the best known is **schizo-affective disorder**. In this illness the excited pole has typically schizophrenic features, while the inhibited pole is depressed. Negative symptoms are usually absent and such illnesses tend to run a fluctuating course with complete remission between episodes.

NEUROCHEMISTRY

The most influential current biological theory of schizophrenia is the '**dopamine hypothesis**'. This hypothesis assumes a functional abnormality in the mesolimbic and mesocortical dopaminergic neuronal systems of the brain. This theory is based on the effects of drugs.

> Drugs leading to a *stimulation* of central dopamine receptors (L-DOPA, amphetamine) can cause paranoid 'schizophreniform' states.

> Whereas the most effective drugs in the treatment of schizophrenia, the neuroleptics, are potent *blockers of central dopamine receptors.*

Furthermore, there is a good correlation between the ability of neuroleptics to bind to central dopamine receptors and to exert anti-psychotic effects in schizophrenic patients. There is also evidence that some schizophrenic patients may have an *increased number of dopamine receptors in their brains*: on post-mortem examination an increased number of spiroperidol binding sites were demonstrated in some limbic areas – the nucleus accumbens and amygdala. (Spiroperidol is a butyrophenone neuroleptic which selectively labels dopamine receptors; see also **neuroleptics** – p. 82.)

AETIOLOGY

The aetiology of schizophrenia can be considered under several headings. The theories regarding aetiology are not mutually exclusive and evidence for each should be sought in examining the individual case.

Genetic causes

These have been repeatedly demonstrated. Whereas the lifetime risk for schizophrenia in the general population is approximately 1 per cent, that for a person who has a sibling or one parent suffering from the illness is about 12 per cent, and for the child of two parents with schizophrenia it is approximately 25 per cent. The concordance rate for dizygotic twins has been found to be roughly that of siblings whereas concordance rates for monozygotic (identical) twins is much higher: 50–60 per cent. This holds even for those twins who have been reared apart, which overcomes the criticism that the high concordance rates might reflect environmental rather than genetic effects. Adoption studies have confirmed the importance of genetic factors, as children of schizophrenic mothers adopted by families which are free of the disease show a similar chance of developing schizophrenia to those brought up by their own mothers.

No single genetic model can account for these findings, and certain subgroups of schizophrenia may have particularly strong genetic components in their aetiology.

Environmental factors

These are also necessary for the disorder to develop. Genetically identical twins can be discordant for schizophrenia and there is evidence that the affected twin has experienced *birth complications* which the unaffected twin has escaped. Such perinatal complications are associated with **enlarged ventricular size** on the CAT scan. Recent studies have shown an increase of ventricular size in one-third of patients with chronic disease who also show minor abnormalities of cognitive functioning. These findings were particularly prevalent among those with marked negative symptoms. It has been suggested that genetic factors and environmental factors interact. A sufficiently strong genetic loading may itself be sufficient for the disease to develop, but with lesser degrees of genetic loading environmental factors such as birth complications and severe childhood illnesses may be necessary in addition.

Neurological theories

These are stimulated by the fact that schizophrenic symptoms may be caused by organic brain disease. Of particular relevance is the fact that long-standing temporal lobe epilepsy may lead to the development of schizophrenic symptoms.

Psychological theories

Schizophrenic patients have been shown to be in an abnormal state of arousal which has been related to social withdrawal. This may be the necessary response if a schizophrenic is faced with an overwhelming amount of conflicting stimuli which he is unable to sort out. A reduction of arousal is brought about by drug therapy and this leads to improvement.

COURSE

Schizophrenia is generally considered to be an illness which has a characteristic chronic course and leads to the person's becoming progressively disabled. The exception to this lies in the recognition of acute schizophrenia, with positive symptoms (Type 1 clinical picture), from which the patient may make a complete recovery. Overall figures for the outcome of schizophrenia are as follows:

10% show rapid and permanent deterioration,
35% show mild and persistent symptoms which require continuing care either in a hostel or in the patient's home,
35% appear 'cured' for long periods of time but have relapses of their illness, and
20% are apparently 'cured' and stable.

Repeated episodes of psychosis together with hospitalization lead to a set of **secondary**

handicaps in addition to the negative symptoms of the illness itself. The patient's job will be disrupted by repeated absences through illness; the onset of psychotic symptoms at the place of work will further increase the chance that he may lose his job and find further employment difficult to obtain. Similarly personal friendships may be severed, and relatives may reject the patient if they have been involved in his delusions or affected by difficult behaviour during his illness. The patient may experience prejudice against him in his attempts to find independent housing or to arrange his finances. Increasing inability to work leads to a decline in skills which often leads to a slow movement down the social scale.

PREDISPOSING FACTORS

A well-recognized predisposing factor is a pre-morbid *schizoid personality*. Such people show a marked degree of shyness and reserve, they may be socially phobic, have few or no friends, and behave in an eccentric fashion. Other recognized predisposing factors include *birth trauma* (see p. 229). Impaired sensory input such as *deafness and blindness* predispose individuals (especially the elderly in whom such handicaps may be multiple) to develop persecutory states.

PRECIPITATING FACTORS

An acute episode of a schizophrenic illness may be precipitated in a predisposed individual by environmental stress. Stressful *life events* in the three weeks before the onset of psychotic symptoms are more frequent than would be expected by chance. This includes desirable (such as promotion) as well as undesirable events (such as redundancy), the common ingredient being some form of increased tension.

An increased chance of relapse of schizophrenia has been shown to occur if the patient lives in an environment where he receives much criticism. The relapse rate has been shown to be nearly four times increased if the patient returns from hospital to a family in which there is a high level of hostile or critical *'expressed emotion'* (EE). Tape recordings of conversation in such families reveal frequently expressed critical comments directed towards the patient. The chance of relapse in such a situation can be reduced by the use of phenothiazine medication and by ensuring that the patient spends less time in face-to-face contact with emotionally arousing relatives. It has been shown that family therapy can effectively reduce the expression of hostility in the family with a consequent reduction in the relapse rate.

INVESTIGATIONS

Investigations are aimed at confirming the diagnosis, and at elucidating aetiological and prognostic factors.

Physical

1. Drug screen for amphetamines.
2. Tests for organic illness if clinically indicated: e.g. EEG, lumbar puncture, CAT scan.

Psycho-social

1. History from relatives and other informants to confirm history of illness, assess presence of precipitating life events, and to supplement information about genetic factors.
2. Social worker or other team member to assess home environment concerning attitudes of the family, and their level of 'expressed emotion.'

TREATMENT

Although in the past many patients with schizophrenia were treated as long-term in-patients, the emphasis today is on brief hospital treatment for the acute episode followed by sustained treatment in the community. The aim of the latter is to prevent relapse and reduce the chances of negative symptoms and secondary handicaps developing.

Acute phase

MEDICATION

Treatment in the *acute phase* usually involves admission to the in-patient unit or day hospital for all the appropriate investigations to be performed and medication to be rapidly increased to therapeutic levels..

Oral neuroleptic medication is started in a dose that suppresses the psychotic phenomena and accompanying disturbances of behaviour and affect but without causing undue sedation (often chlorpromazine, in the range 300–900 mgs per day).

NURSING

Nursing at this time is aimed at keeping the patient in an environment which is reasonably free of stressful situations and conflict while maintaining as normal a daily routine as his clinical condition permits. If the patient holds ideas which render him a danger to himself or others it may be necessary to detain him in hospital compulsorily (see p. 305). Rehabilitation should start early. The patient is seen and assessed by the *occupational therapist* as soon as is practicable.

Long-term treatment

MEDICATION

Medication is usually changed to long-acting injections (flupenthixol or fluphenazine) which need to be given only every two to four weeks. The drug is dissolved in an oily solution from which it is gradually absorbed into tissue fluid. The drug passes straight into the blood stream without passing through the liver (where phenothiazines are metabolized); the absorption is such that a small quantity leads to a constant plasma level. This form of administration also increases compliance and allows the opportunity for the patient to be under regular supervision by the nurse who administers the injection.

Anti-Parkinsonian medication should be given only if extrapyramidal symptoms are present and it is not practicable to reduce the dose of the neuroleptic.

ACCOMMODATION

The patient should live in suitable accommodation, where relationships are smooth and the patient will be encouraged to lead a normal, active life. If this is to be his own home, a member of the team should help the other members of the family to understand the patient's illness and cooperate with his gradual return to a normal life style, which should include a good level of self-care, social activity, and occupation. If no such home environment exists and the illness is severe, the patient may be best placed in a hostel where his daily routine and independence may be preserved. It is useful to be able to offer care in a *day hospital* or in a *day centre* operated by local social services to help provide some useful structure to the patient's day, to reduce contact with emotionally arousing relatives, and to cover relapses which do not necessitate admission to the in-patient unit. *Voluntary organizations* such as the National Schizophrenia Fellowship may offer considerable support to the patient's family.

PROGNOSIS

Poor prognostic factors are:

Pre-morbid

1. Family history of schizophrenia.
2. Schizoid personality.
3. High EE home environment.
4. Poor previous work record.

Illness

1. Gradual onset without clear precipitating cause.
2. Absence of prominent affective or catatonic symptoms.
3. Pronounced negative symptoms.

A MODEL FOR SCHIZOPHRENIA

Many students or doctors other than psychiatrists view the diagnosis and treatment of schizophrenia as an exercise quite different from the rest of medicine. In fact the similarities with **diabetes** are numerous and the routine care of the schizophrenic patient in the community has many similarities with that of diabetics.

Both conditions are diagnosed by precise criteria (blood glucose level or the presence of first-rank symptoms) which have been chosen to correspond most closely with the other clinical characteristics of the condition. The aetiology of each condition includes genetic and environmental factors; an infection or large glucose load would correspond to stressful life events and are only important in predisposed individuals. In the case of diabetes, this predisposition may be clear early in life or may be evident only if the individual becomes obese. In the case of schizophrenia, individuals with a high genetic loading may develop it in adolescence in response to the very real life stresses of that developmental period, or the condition may develop late in life when the individual becomes deaf or blind, or develops cerebrovascular disease.

There are different types of the illness. 'Juvenile onset' diabetes with a poor prognosis would correspond to hebephrenic schizophrenia, while 'maturity-onset' is like paranoid schizophrenia with its later onset and preservation of personality. Each condition has a more modern classification into Types 1 and 2. The course of both illnesses is very variable; in the case of type 1 diabetes 50 per cent of patients die within twenty years but 10–15 per cent live forty years with few complications. As we have already seen, the course of schizophrenia is similarly variable.

The treatment of both conditions is similarly divided into acute and long term. Both conditions require very large doses of drugs in the acute phase but smaller maintenance doses.

The routine assessments in the maintenance phase of treatment are as follows:

1. Good control of the illness (glucose level and absence of psychotic symptoms).
2. Prevention of complications: maintenance on adequate doses of the drug, leading as normal a life as possible, avoiding severe stress (dietary restrictions/low expressed emotion environment).
3. Encourage a normal life: encourage interest and motivation for self-care and education about the illness and its treatment.

FURTHER READING

Wing, J. K. (1978) *Schizophrenia: Towards a New Synthesis*. London: Academic Press.

13 / AFFECTIVE DISORDERS

An affective disorder is a disorder of mood. **Anxiety, depression**, and **elation** are all associated with clinically important syndromes, although only the first two are common in general medical settings. In the interests of clarity we will describe anxiety states and depressive disorders separately, but it should be grasped from the outset that combinations of the two syndromes are very common both in general hospital and in general practice settings.

Affective illnesses occur in both psychotic and non-psychotic forms: we will first of all describe the common, non-psychotic form of illness (anxiety-related disorders and depressive illness), and then describe the severe, psychotic forms of illness, psychotic depression, and mania.

I. ANXIETY STATES AND RELATED DISORDERS

Epidemiology

Symptoms of anxiety and worry are among the commonest psychological symptoms encountered in the normal population: however, most worried people do not have enough other symptoms related to anxiety to justify a diagnosis of anxiety state. The prevalence of anxiety states has been estimated at between 2 and 4 per cent for men, and between 3 and 4.5 per cent for women in three recent surveys of the normal population. There have been no reliable estimates of inception rate. However, one study of inceptions of illnesses seen in general practice settings showed anxiety disorders to constitute about 10 per cent of all new illness onsets, and to account for about one-third of all those with a diagnosable psychiatric disorder. There are therefore grounds for supposing that the prevalence of anxiety states is considerably higher in medical settings than in the general population.

Most acute anxiety reactions are of relatively short duration, but in contrast phobic illnesses last longer and affect about 3 per cent of men and 6 per cent of women.

Neurochemistry

The syndrome of anxiety is characterized by increased arousal, increased sympathic activity (mydriasis, tachycardia, perspiration), and unpleasant subjective sensations of fear and apprehension. It is believed that both ascending **noradrenaline and 5-hydroxytryptamine containing neuronal pathways**, innervating the limbic lobe and neocortex, play important roles in mediating the symptoms of anxiety: while the noradrenaline containing neurones may be responsible for the increase in arousal, the 5-hydroxytryptamine containing neurones would mediate the suppression of some behaviours associated with the anxiety syndrome. Thus it has been shown that, in a behavioural model of anxiety (suppression of responding by aversive stimuli), 5-hydroxytryptaminergic drugs have an **anxiogenic** and anti-5-hydroxytryptamine drugs an **anxiolytic** effect.

It is thought that the monoamine-containing neurones are under the tonic **inhibitory influence of GABA-ergic neurones**: the enhancement of this inhibitory influence by GABA-mimetic drugs or by benzodiazepines produces an anxiolytic effect. Specific binding sites for the benzodiazepines ('**benzodiazepine receptors**') have been identified in the brain in close association with postsynaptic receptors for GABA ('GABA-benzodiazepine receptor complex'); especially high density of benzodiazepine receptors has been found in the neocortex and the limbic system. While the activation of benzodiazepine receptors by conventional benzodiazepines results in the enhancement of the inhibitory effects of GABA, this effect can be prevented by benzodiazepine antagonists, whereas newly synthesized '**inverse agonists**' of benzodiazepine receptors result in a decrease in GABA-mediated responses. Inverse agonists of benzodiazepine receptors have an anxiogenic effect both in animals and human subjects. (See also p. 85 in 'Drug treatments'.)

Symptoms

ANXIOUS RUMINATIONS

These often come about because the patient anxiously broods about the significance of the somatic symptoms (do the palpitations mean a heart attack, does the tiredness mean cancer?); or because he is afraid that others notice symptoms such as tremor. Such thoughts exacerbate the original anxiety, and in turn the somatic symptoms are magnified. Anxiety states are especially common in medical settings, for reasons that were explained in Chapter 10, p. 125. Patients who present with a single somatic symptom of anxiety such as tachycardia or tremor may present a diagnostic problem until it is appreciated that other psychological and somatic symptoms of anxiety are present.

In addition to anxious ruminations, the symptoms of **anxiety states** can conveniently be thought of in three groups:

autonomic symptoms of anxiety include	symptoms relating to motor tone include	symptoms of hypervigilance include
palpitations	shakiness	irritability
tachycardia	tremor	onset insomnia
cold, clammy hands	muscular aches	trouble staying asleep
sweating	lump in throat	easily startled
blepharospasm	distractibility	poor concentration
paraesthesiae	restlessness	feeling keyed up
dizziness	easily tired	
hot and cold spells	trouble swallowing	
frequency of micturition		
diarrhoea		
nausea		

PANIC ATTACKS

Sometimes patients experience episodes of severe, uncontrollable anxiety called **panic attacks**. These usually take the form of intense anxiety of sudden onset with both cognitive and somatic accompaniments. The patient thinks some misfortune will befall him: death by heart attack, madness, or just a nameless dread; typically accompanied by one or more symptoms such as sweating, tremor, palpitations, and paraesthesiae due to overbreathing. The attacks last from anything between a few minutes to some hours, and often present in the casualty department.

PHOBIC ILLNESSES

Patients with **phobic illnesses** become anxious only in particular situations and have no trouble providing that they avoid the object or situation that arouses their anxiety. However, their avoidance behaviour may become extreme.

Objects about which people develop specific phobias include spiders, snakes, dogs, rats, and moths; while **situations** include high places ('**acrophobia**'), enclosed spaces ('**claustrophobia**'), air-travel ('**air phobia**'), and social gatherings ('**social phobias**').

Agoraphobia commonly develops in women between the ages of eighteen and thirty-five and anxiety symptoms are experienced only in situations which share certain characteristics: being a long way from home, being in crowded places such as public transport, department stores, or cinema; shops where one must queue to pay before leaving, or any situation which is difficult to leave quickly. The anxiety may be reduced or be quite tolerable if a trusted person is with the patient: some women can manage even with a small child, others need an adult or cannot face the feared situation at all.

The patient may feel quite safe in her car, but is in real trouble if the car breaks down when she is on her own.

As time goes on the symptoms tend to progress and to generalize: panic attacks may occur even at the thought of going out, and eventually may occur without obvious provocation. By this time the patient is likely not to be going out at all, and is then said to be 'house-bound'.

Patients often develop depressive symptoms as well, but these will be described in the next section, and are not central to the agoraphobic symptom-complex.

Diagnosis

There is no natural dividing line between normal people and those with **anxiety states** that would enable us to lay down firm criteria for diagnosis. In this respect anxiety disorders resemble conditions like hypertension and anaemia in general medicine. There are various research criteria for the diagnosis, but they are arbitrary. In practical terms, any patient whose pronounced symptoms of anxiety are accompanied by three or more of the other symptoms given on p. 178 can usefully be thought of as satisfying the requirements for diagnosis, while with increasing numbers of symptoms there is increasing certainty that such a disorder is present.

Panic disorder should be diagnosed only if an individual describes recurrent panic attacks, and does not satisfy the criteria for either anxiety state or depression (see p. 186).

Phobias refer to a persistent, irrational fear with a compelling desire to avoid the objects or situations described above. The disorder should cause the patient significant distress, and the patient should regard her fear as excessive or unreasonable.

Agoraphobia should be diagnosed when there is marked fear in the situations described above and there is increased constriction of normal activities until fears or avoidance behaviour dominate the patient's life.

Differential diagnosis

OTHER PSYCHIATRIC ILLNESSES

Symptoms of anxiety commonly accompany more differentiated kinds of psychiatric disorders. Easily the commonest of these is **depression**; but such symptoms also occur in any **psychotic illness** (that is above anxiety state in the diagnostic hierarchy). Anxiety is also an integral part of an **obsessional state** (see p. 215). So, make sure that you have elicited all the patient's symptoms, and that those that you have elicited can be accounted for by morbid anxiety.

THYROTOXICOSIS (see p. 129)

Look for symptoms suggestive of hyperthyroidism. Atrial fibrillation, exophthalmos, or a thyroid bruit make thyroid function tests mandatory.

DRUG INTOXICATION (see p. 204)

Think of stimulants such as caffeine and methyl phenidate; also sympathomimetic agents such as bronchodilators.

DRUG WITHDRAWAL

Sometimes anxiety symptoms are caused by the patient's running out of sedatives – whether these be benzodiazepines, alcohol, or barbiturates. Diagnostic difficulties arise when the patient wishes to conceal his drug use, but wants help for the anxiety symptoms. (If drugs are obtained illicitly, and the patient thinks the doctor may prescribe a sedative as a treatment, he may be unwilling to give an honest history.)

PHAEOCHROMOCYTOMA

Thought of by every medical student, but in fact very rare indeed! The history of flushing attacks accompanied by diarrhoea alert one to the possibility.

Investigations

It is not necessary to carry out tests for thyrotoxicosis or phaeochromocytoma unless they are indicated by the results of the history and physical examination.

Aetiology

It is convenient to distinguish between long-term factors that predispose to symptoms of anxiety, and factors that release a particular episode.

PREDISPOSING FACTORS

Twin studies have shown that there is an undoubted genetic component in the propensity to anxiety state: however, it accounts for only a small proportion of the variance, and it seems probable that a polygenic mechanism is responsible.

The pre-morbid personalities of patients with anxiety states are heterogeneous, so that although they occur more easily in those with anxious temperaments, they can also occur in obsessional, dependent, and even in schizoid personalities. However, it seems likely that those individuals who score highly on questionnaires measuring neuroticism or 'trait anxiety' are more vulnerable to symptoms of anxiety than those with a more phlegmatic disposition.

Those with chronic social adversity are at greater risk, and this adversity may take the form of difficult interpersonal problems or unfavourable living conditions.

PRECIPITATING FACTORS

Anxiety states are usually in some understandable relationship to stressful life events.

In general medical settings anxiety symptoms are often related to worries about physical health, and it is therefore essential to allow patients to express their own fears about the nature of their illness before the doctor provides information from the medical viewpoint. Anxious ruminations are especially difficult to handle if the patient has no one in whom to confide, or is unable to find reassurance from people in his immediate social field.

However, in other cases the anxiety will not be related to physical health, but will be found to be a somatic expression of some interpersonal problem. It will often be the case that the patient has not connected the psychological problem with the physical symptom for which help is sought, so that taking a proper history not only helps us to understand the aetiology of the disorder, but also is an indispensable first step in treatment.

Treatment

GENERAL MEDICAL CARE

Taking a history, physical examination, and carrying out any essential physical investigations are all part of treatment, provided that they are done properly. The history must be taken in such a way that the patient has had an opportunity to ventilate problems and has received reassurance about any irrational fears: both these procedures are therapeutic. The physical examination should if possible be done in such a way that it reassures the patient: for example, if the doctor knows that the patient is afraid that he might have a gastric cancer, it is helpful if the doctor says that no mass can be felt, nor are there other signs that suggest cancer.

Finally, physical investigations can be therapeutic if they are carried out to produce final reassurance, but actively harmful if they signal to the patient that his doctors do not know what is wrong with him, but are prepared to go on and on because they can think of endless possibilities! Thus a patient who is told 'There isn't any evidence of cancer to account for this pain, but we'll put a tube in your tummy and look so that we can be quite certain' is likely to be reassured by the subsequent investigation showing no abnormalities; while a patient who, given no explanation for an endless series of physical investigations, will become more anxious as each normal finding is reported to him, because it looks as though the doctors are sure that there is something wrong, but do not know what it is.

ADVICE

All anxious people need advice, most don't actually want sedative drugs, and even fewer need such drugs. So, what advice should they be given?

First, an explanation that their various symptoms make up a common syndrome with which the doctor is familiar, and that the symptoms do not indicate serious disease. Next, advice on what to do during an anxiety attack: sit down if possible, try to relax and breathe no more deeply than usual, and the symptoms will pass off by themselves. Finally, advice on the advisability of going to relaxation classes, to meditation, or yoga, depending on the patient's interests. They may wish to read a book by Claire Weeks called *Self-help with your Nerves*.

In the course of taking the history the doctor will usually have heard about other related problems, and must use judgement to decide on whether the nature of these problems is such that help from others should be sought.

HELP FROM SOCIAL WORKERS

Patients with anxiety disorders often have social or interpersonal problems that can be helped greatly by a trained social worker. It should not be thought that only those with obviously soluble problems that can be 'talked out' should be referred: on the contrary, the social worker is often aware of resources that can be mobilized to help people with seemingly quite intractable problems, and should in any case be given the chance of making up her own mind about what might be done.

HELP FROM CLINICAL PSYCHOLOGISTS

People whose anxiety states do not remit with simple measures, or who are unable to learn relaxation from such local classes as are available, will sometimes succeed in learning relaxation in one-to-one treatment. If there is a pronounced element of anxious ruminations (see p. 178) then one should also consider the possibility of an 'anxiety management package'.

Patients with phobic illnesses should be treated with relaxation and graded in-vivo exposure (see p. 99).

DRUG TREATMENT

This should be avoided except in the management of short-term situations: for example, a patient who is anxious about some medical procedure despite reassurance, or someone who is very anxious about the outcome of a child's surgical operation and asks for help in staying calm. It will sometimes be necessary to offer benzodiazepines for a course of a few weeks at most, but the prescription should not be renewed, since these drugs produce dependence (see p. 87).

Course and prognosis

Most acute anxiety states remit, which is an excellent reason for avoiding dependence-producing drugs. Many of those put on to benzodiazepines and then thought to have developed 'chronic anxiety states' are experiencing anxiety symptoms when their drugs are withdrawn, but such symptoms often improve dramatically after a week to ten days. Some patients with chronic anxiety will be found to have social problems, but such problems should attract social interventions. In fact, most patients with persistent anxiety symptoms will gradually develop depressive symptoms as well: these will be dealt with in the next section.

II. DEPRESSION

Most patients in general medical settings with significant depressive symptoms will also have symptoms of anxiety as well, but the reverse is not true. There is therefore a sense in which depressive symptoms represent a more differentiated form of psychological illness than anxiety states, and for this reason we described anxiety states first. Some patients develop anxiety symptoms first, and if they persist they may go on to develop depressive symptoms as well. Others seem to develop both sets of symptoms simultaneously: it is not known why this happens.

There has been a long controversy about the best way to classify depressive illnesses, and the non-psychiatrist is well advised to ignore it. The common form of depression encountered in general medical settings is described here as **depressive illness**. There is also a more severe form of illness, which we have called **depressive psychosis**. These two forms of illness have been described elsewhere as 'reactive/endogenous' or as 'neurotic/psychotic', but neither set of terms is really satisfactory. It is now known that both sorts of depression are equally likely to be secondary to stressful life events, so the term 'endogenous' is actively misleading. The term 'neurotic' is best avoided, since it implies that people who become depressed are neurotic, and this is far from being the case. It is true that people who score highly on 'neuroticism' are more vulnerable to develop depressive illnesses when under stress, but with sufficient adversity depressive illnesses can develop in stable, phlegmatic people.

Epidemiology

Although depressive **symptoms** are somewhat less common than anxiety symptoms, they are nonetheless to be found in between 10 and 16 per cent of men, and between 20 and 24 per cent of women in community surveys. Once more, depressive **illnesses** – that is to say, people with more than a critical number of depressive symptoms – are very much less common, accounting for between 2.6 and 4 per cent of men, and about 7 to 8 per cent of women in surveys carried out in London, Canberra and the United States. The annual inception rate in the community is not known, although it seems likely that it is over half the point prevalence.

The prevalence of depressive illness is very much higher in consulting populations. Depressive illnesses are the commonest diagnosis in a study of inceptions of illness in general practice, accounting for 12 per cent of all new illnesses of any sort, and 45 per cent of all psychiatric diagnoses made in this setting. It is important to emphasize that most of these depressed patients were consulting their doctors either with somatic symptoms related to their depression, or with physical illnesses that they had in addition to their depression.

Neurochemistry

According to the **monoamine theory** of affective disorders depressive illness is due to a functional impairment in central noradrenaline- and/or 5-hydroxytryptamine- containing neurones.

This theory is based on the action of drugs: reserpine, a drug which *depletes* central neurones monoamine stores, causes depression, whereas drugs, which *increase* central monoamine levels either in presynaptic stores (monoamine oxidase inhibitors) or in the synaptic gap (tricyclic antidepressants) relieve the symptoms of depression. A more modern version of this theory concentrates on *changes in postsynaptic receptors* brought about by long-term medication with antidepressants: antidepressant treatments of different kinds (tricyclic and atypical antidepressants, monoamine oxidase inhibitors, and also electroconvulsive treatment) produce a reduced sensitivity (**'down-regulation of β-adrenoceptors'**).

There have been attempts to demonstrate changes in central noradrenergic and/or 5-hydroxytryptaminergic functions in depressed patients. Thus it has been shown that some depressed patients have a reduced metabolic turnover of central noradrenaline as evidenced by reduced urinary excretion of the noradrenaline metabolite 3-methoxy-4-hydroxyphenylglycol (MHPG), whereas other patients have reduced levels of 5-hydroxyindole-acetic acid (5-HIAA) in the cerebrospinal fluid, probably reflecting a reduced turnover of central 5-hydroxytryptamine. It has also been demonstrated that some patients have a reduced sensitivity of central adrenoceptors involved in neuroendocrine regulation: thus depression can be associated with

1. High resting cortisol levels and a reduced effectiveness of dexamethasone in suppressing cortisol secretion (*'dexamethasone suppression test'*), and/or

2. A reduced effectiveness of clonidine, an α_2-adrenoceptor stimulating drug, in enhancing growth hormone output.

There have been reports of *decreased concentration of 5-hydroxytryptamine* in the brains of suicide victims in whom a depressive illness could be inferred, and of a *reduced uptake of 5-hydroxytryptamine into blood platelets*, which are neurochemically analogous to 5-hydroxytryptaminergic nerve terminals, in depressed patients. (See also 'antidepressants' (pp. 88–91.)

Symptoms

These will be described under four headings: **emotional changes**, **cognitive changes**, **motivational changes**, and **neuro-vegetative symptoms**. Symptoms of anxiety, restlessness, and agitation may also be present.

EMOTIONAL CHANGES

In the early stages of a depressive illness the patient may notice that he no longer derives pleasure from life: this **anhedonia** may precede experience of sadness or unhappiness. Sense of humour is often lost, so that although he may see the point of a joke, he doesn't find it funny. Eventually the mood becomes one of **sadness** and misery, with the content of the patient's thought accompanying his mood. Thus the past supplies evidence of failures and wrong decisions, what is dismal about the present is dwelt on inordinately, and the future is seen as threatening or **hopeless**. This sadness is often accompanied by **crying spells**, although some patients report that they feel like crying but are unable to do so. The patient may feel that life isn't worth living, and begins to think of ways of ending his life. Feelings of affection for those close to him are often reduced, and the patient may lose his religious faith.

COGNITIVE CHANGES

These include feelings of **self-dislike** with an exaggerated assessment of current life problems. Changed self-concept and **self-blame** should be assessed by asking how the patient compares himself with other people, and whether he blames himself for being like he is. Depressed women may complain that they are ugly, or find their bodies repulsive. **Ideas of reference** may occur in which the patient feels that others look critically at her or make disparaging remarks about her. Religious patients may feel that they are **wicked or sinful**. There may be **difficulties about making decisions**, either because of **lack of confidence** or because of subjective **difficulty in thinking**. In severe forms of depression ideas of **guilt and worthlessness** appear. **Suicidal ideas** are particularly serious in the presence of such other symptoms. **Nihilistic ideas** take the form of saying that she has no money, no feelings, is already dead, or the world does not exist.

MOTIVATIONAL CHANGES

Low energy, fatigue, apathy, and inability to concentrate may occur secondarily to depressed mood, and are especially common in depressive states following infectious diseases such as glandular fever, infectious hepatitis, influenza, or brucellosis. Depressed patients tend to escape responsibility and to avoid demanding tasks. They may do this because their usual tasks seem boring or meaningless, or because they lack confidence to make the right decisions. Failure to complete tasks may reinforce ideas of self-blame or worthlessness. They are often said to be 'dependent' because they become willing to allow others to take over responsibility for giving them guidance.

NEURO-VEGETATIVE SYMPTOMS

These include disturbances of **appetite, weight, sleep rhythm, libido, energy level, and posture**. Depressed mood may influence the way the patient speaks, walks, and sits. In minor depressive illnesses increased appetite with weight gain is almost as common as anorexia and weight loss, but the latter symptoms predominate in severe depression. There is diminution of sexual interest and performance. Sleep is hard to come by, light, and unrefreshing. Emotional energy no longer flows outward to the world of people and events, and the patient bcomes lost in miserable self-absorption with his discomforts. In this way the patient may present the doctor with **headache**, **backache**, or some other **regional pain**, and the doctor may be so distracted by these symptoms that the depressive syndrome of which they form a part goes unrecognized. In severe depression the patient may report **early waking**, and **diurnal variation of mood** with his worst mood in the mornings.

Diagnosis (of depressive illness)

As with anxiety states, there is no point of discontinuity between normality and depression, so the dividing line between the two must be arbitrary. One widely used criterion requires depressed mood to be prominent and fairly persistent, and to have had at least four of the following eight symptoms on each day for the previous two weeks:

1. Poor or increased appetite/weight loss or gain.
2. Insomnia or hypersomnia.
3. Agitation or retardation.
4. Loss of interest or pleasure in usual activities.
5. Loss of energy or fatigue.
6. Feelings of worthlessness, guilt, or self-reproach.
7. Poor concentration/slowed thinking/indecisiveness.
8. Thoughts of death or suicide attempt.

Diagnosis (of psychotic depression)

(Also called *affective psychosis*, and *melancholia*. *'Endogenous depression'* is often used to refer to a similar kind of depression, but the term is misleading.)

This is a severe form of depressive illness with pervasive or unresponsive depressed mood; usually early morning waking and diurnal variation of mood; anorexia and marked weight loss; psychomotor retardation even to the point of depressive stupor, or marked psychomotor agitation. There may be **depressive delusions** in which the patient is convinced that he is wicked or worthless; the latter may take various forms: that he has no money, has a disease, or has already died. It **can** occur without a precipitant (thus the original name), and the patient often has a stable pre-morbid personality.

Differential diagnosis

SYMPTOMATIC DEPRESSION

Depression may be secondary to a systemic illness, or to the effects of a toxic substance like alcohol. Illnesses causing secondary depression may be either endocrine like myxoedema, thyrotoxicosis, Cushing's syndrome; infective like glandular fever, infectious hepatitis, brucellosis, or influenza; or neoplastic like carcinoma of the pancreas or bronchus.

ACUTE AND CHRONIC BRAIN SYNDROMES

The patient's depressive symptoms may be secondary to organic cerebral damage of various types (see pp. 144, 154, and 278).

BEREAVEMENT

Depressed mood, disturbed sleep, and crying occur in over 50 per cent of bereaved subjects, but there is no disturbance of self-esteem. However, about one-third have feelings of guilt concerning the dead person. Morbid grief reactions are described on p. 292.

SCHIZOPHRENIA (see p. 166)

Patients with schizophrenia may develop pronounced depressive symptoms. Persistent non-affective delusions or hallucinations, and even depressive hallucinations that are continuous rather than occasional suggest schizophrenia.

Aetiology

PREDISPOSING FACTORS

For **depressive illness**, most twin studies have not shown a genetic component, although the condition undoubtedly tends to run in families. It has been shown that first-degree family members who have not had episodes of depression tend to be not only more emotionally stable than those who have been affected, but also more stable than the general population. In contrast, those who develop depressive illnesses are more likely to be high on neuroticism, to have low self-esteem, and are rather more likely to be introverted and obsessional.

Although the evidence is not beyond doubt, many studies have shown that early bereavement – especially loss of mother by death or separation – makes people more vulnerable to later loss experiences.

For **psychotic depression**, there is persuasive evidence from both twin and adoption studies of a genetic element, but no specific mode of inheritance has been established.

Morbid risks in relatives of unipolar depressives vary with age of onset and severity of precipitating factors. There is some data to suggest a deficiency of cross-sex transmission.

Loss events, physical illness, and stressful social circumstances all favour the release of depressive phenomena:

Loss events may be bereavements, threatened future losses, as when a near relative develops a fatal illness, the loss of a relationship, or even a failure to be promoted. These are especially likely to precipitate depression in those with low self-esteem, in those without intimate confidants, and in those with some pre-existing conflict that is exacerbated by a stressful event. The loss may precede the episode of depression by as much as one year.

Physical illness commonly contributes to the genesis of depressive illnesses seen in general medical settings. The patient may have been mildly dysphoric before the onset of such illnesses, but experiences a marked exacerbation of depressive symptoms after the physical illness. Although the association between depression and infections like infectious hepatitis, influenza, and glandular fever has been recognized for many years, it should be appreciated that other infectious illnesses such as herpes zoster and urinary tract infections often seem to contribute to the development of depressive disorders. It has been shown that those with a lower self-esteem are at higher risk for developing depressive illnesses after episodes of infectious illness.

Stressful social circumstances – the third group of factors – are protean in their manifestations. Patients may have very little in the way of social support, or they may have lost what little that they had. Unsatisfactory living conditions, chronic illness in close relatives, and poor interpersonal relationships are recurrent themes in individual case histories.

Treatment

There is good evidence that antidepressant treatment shortens the course of depressive illness: the more severe the depression, the more likely are antidepressants to be helpful. Patients with lesser degrees of depression are more likely to remit spontaneously, and are likely to be helped as much by non-specific aspects of therapy as by antidepressant medication. However, in order to regain his normal adjustment the patient must be kept alive, so we will first deal with suicidal threats.

SUICIDAL THREATS (see p. 278)

One should establish the extent to which the patient has been preoccupied with ideas of suicide, and whether any concrete steps have been already carried out. Has the patient decided when, where, and how? A serious view should be taken of plans which involve a painful method such as hanging or swallowing disinfectant, or one which is likely to be successful, such as jumping from a high building. Have materials been especially obtained? If the patient intends to take an overdose, has he handled the bottle, or tipped the tablets out and looked at them? If it turns out that some of these events have occurred, then what has so far prevented the patient from carrying out his plans? If the patient is to be allowed to go home, one must consider the environment to which he will return. Has the patient anyone in whom he can confide? Will he be under surveillance from others? Has he a past history of self-injury or self-poisoning? Is he prepared to give an undertaking that he will not harm himself before his next appointment?

There is no evidence that asking about suicide increases the likelihood of an attempt: on the contrary, many patients report relief of feelings of anxiety and guilt after they have had such a discussion. It would be quite impracticable if all those who thought of suicide were to be referred to a psychiatrist, but it is reasonable to refer those where there is doubt, or where the risk to life is thought to be real. Patients with symptoms of psychotic depression should all be referred to specialist treatment: the risk of suicide is great, and so is their suffering.

SPECIFIC PHARMACOLOGICAL TREATMENT

Antidepressants are dealt with on pp. 88–91. However, it is worth noting that if the decision to prescribe an antidepressant is made, compliance will be very much greater if the doctor anticipates possible side-effects, predicts the likely duration of treatment, and explains that the drug will not produce dependence and that cessation of treatment will be an easy matter when the time comes. Will the patient give you an undertaking not to take an overdose of the antidepressant? It is irresponsible to give tricyclic antidepressants to patients who are likely to do this, since they are cardiotoxic in overdose. Consider asking a spouse or parent to look after the tablets, and remember that *tetracyclic antidepressants* are much less toxic, and only slightly less effective! If there is a real risk to life, the patient should be offered admission to hospital.

SPECIFIC PSYCHOLOGICAL TREATMENTS

It is usual to discover that depressive illnesses are in an understandable relationship to the patient's life situation and to the way in which he handles interpersonal relationships. Rather than endlessly dwelling on his symptoms, provide the patient with an opportunity to tell you about these problems. Most depressive illnesses will remit on a combination of antidepressants and kindness; if material arises which cannot be handled consider referral to a psychiatrist.

Cognitive therapy for depression (see p. 101) is given by some clinical psychologists, and is useful for patients whose depressive illnesses have not responded to antidepressants but in whom there is no risk to life, or are recurrent and accompanied by depressive ideas about the self. It has been claimed to reduce the relapse rate.

ELECTROCONVULSIVE TREATMENT

This is the treatment of choice for psychotic depression, as it produces improvement very rapidly. Severe depression is an appalling experience for the patient; any treatment which shortens it is a major benefit. It is described fully on pp. 94–7).

NON-SPECIFIC ASPECTS OF TREATMENT

In drug trials of antidepressants in primary care settings, many patients improve on placebo medication. It is naive to suppose that all these patients would have got better without treatment, although many would probably have done so. The *doctor's confidence that he can help his patient* – whether based on his own personal qualities or his faith in the content of his pills – *promotes hope*, and with it *an expectancy that improvement will occur*. By his offer of return visits, he effectively offers to monitor the patient's return to effective social functioning, and makes the patient feel that he has a powerful ally, so that the way becomes clearer for the resolution of both hopelessness and helplessness. The doctor's power to remove both social and occupational obligations may allow the patient to *rest without a sense of failure*; and if *sleep* can be restored there is often a major improvement in how the patient feels.

Course and prognosis

There is much variation in outcome of depressive illnesses seen in general medical settings, and although many will become symptom free within four to six weeks, about a third are likely to follow a protracted course. Illnesses following severe loss events in those with stable pre-morbid personalities are likely to have a good outcome, while those associated with chronically adverse social and interpersonal circumstances are likely to have a poorer outcome. **Depressive illnesses** associated with abnormal personalities, especially those described as manipulative, unstable, or highly dependent are likely to have a poor outcome, with hostile depressive outbursts accompanied by dramatic behaviour and impulsive suicidal attempts.

Depressive psychosis is highly responsive to treatment, but there is a high likelihood of recurrent episodes: when this happens the patient is thought of as a variant of manic-depressive illness where the episodes have so far been of the same type, and are sometimes called 'unipolar' illnesses.

III. MANIC-DEPRESSIVE PSYCHOSIS

In this illness the patient typically has episodes of depression – often psychotic in intensity – and at other times has episodes of psychotic excitement. In severe degree this illness is called mania, in milder degree hypomania. The sections which follow on symptoms, neurochemistry, diagnosis, and differential diagnosis will be confined to excited episodes since depressive psychosis has already been covered; the sections on epidemiology, treatment, and course and prognosis will be concerned with manic-depressive (or 'bipolar') illness.

Epidemiology (of bipolar illness)

The lifetime morbid risk for bipolar illness is approximately 1 per cent, with an annual inception rate of about 10 in 100,000 for men, and 15 in 100,000 for women. This means that in a standard catchment area of 250,000 there will be approximately 30 inceptions a year.

Neurochemistry (of mania)

A corollary to the 'monoamine theory of affective disorders' states that the biological abnormality in mania is the opposite to that found in depression: while in depression there is a lowered activity in central monoaminergic neuronal systems, an **increased monoaminergic activity** could be found in mania. This hypothesis of mania is based partly on the clinical observations that the symptoms of the depressive and manic syndromes are often polar opposites, and partly on the ability of drugs which can induce increased levels of noradrenaline and/or 5-hydroxytryptamine to produce manic reactions. These drugs, however, do not have consistent effects; they include *L- DOPA, amphetamine, monoamine oxidase inhibitors, and tricyclic antidepressants.* Dopamine has also been implicated in mania since the most effective anti-manic drugs are the neuroleptics which are potent dopamine receptor antagonists. Biochemical studies in manic patients have not produced consistent results: some studies show evidence of increased central noradrenaline turnover (increased urinary excretion of 3-methoxy-4-hydroxyphenylglycol (MHPG)); other studies, however, show normal values.

Symptoms (of mania)

The central features of mania are **elevation of mood, increased activity**, and **grandiose ideas**. The elevation of mood may take the form ranging from **euphoria** to **elation**, and in such patients there may be an infectious gaiety. Others are not so lucky. Some are **irritable** rather than euphoric and the irritability can easily turn to anger. As with depression there may be diurnal variation of mood, and there may be brief episodes of depressed mood between episodes of high spirits. The elevation of mood is part of a **disinhibition** which affects social, sexual, and financial behaviour.

Thus the patient may make tactless or rude remarks in social situations, may make inappropriate sexual advances to strangers and fail to take precautions against pregnancy, and expensive goods that are not needed may be ordered from shops.

Increased activity involves motor behaviour, speech, and appetite, with sleep being correspondingly reduced. In lesser degree the increased activity may be associated with getting more done, but as the patient restlessly moves from one activity to another they surround themselves with chaos. **Speech** is rapid and **thoughts are speeded**. Eventually the thoughts come faster than they can be uttered, and ideas become more loosely connected with **punning** and jumping from one topic to another using rhymes – or **'clang associations'**. Eventually speech may become completely unintelligible.

Appetite is increased and at first food is eaten greedily and with poor manners; eventually the patient becomes too over-active either to eat or to sleep.

These symptoms often cause patients to abandon good jobs and steady sexual partners: they may embark on hair-brained schemes and become progressively more **grandiose**. The patient may believe that he has some special mission, is extremely rich, or has some special message for others. Such **delusion-like ideas** are congruent with the patient's mood, so that if the predominant mood is one of irritability and suspiciousness they can be persecutory, if of elation they are expansive and grandiose. Schneiderian **'first-rank symptoms'** (see p. 167) can occur, including delusions of reference and passivity experiences. **Hallucinations** may also occur but once more are congruent with the prevailing mood; taking the form of voices giving advice or telling the patient of his special powers, and occasionally visions of an ecstatic or religious character. None of these symptoms tends to last long (hours rather than days): one is struck by a kaleidoscope of psychotic experiences which vary with the mood disorder. **Insight** is almost invariably impaired, with the patient seeing no need for treatment. However, others with whom he comes in contact rarely have doubts!

Diagnosis (of mania)

A period of elevated or irritable mood lasting at least a week with at least three of the following:

1. Increased activity or restlessness.
2. Pressure of words.
3. Subjective increased speed of thought.
4. Increased self-esteem, or grandiose ideas.
5. Decreased need for sleep.
6. Abnormal distractibility.
7. Disinhibited behaviour (see above).

Differential diagnosis (of mania)

SYMPTOMATIC MANIA

A manic illness does not always indicate a bipolar illness, since mania can be produced by drugs such as sympathomimetic amines, steroids, isoniazid, or L-DOPA; or it may be secondary to metabolic disorders such as renal failure or thyrotoxicosis; or it may follow cerebral insult such as encephalitis or a cerebral neoplasm.

SCHIZOPHRENIA (see p. 168)

The differentiation can be very difficult, especially as manic phenomena may occur during the course of a schizophrenic illness. If allegedly 'schizophrenic' phenomena have only occurred at times of elation and over-activity, the patient should be diagnosed as manic.

CYCLOID PSYCHOSES AND SCHIZO-AFFECTIVE PSYCHOSIS

These are psychotic illnesses which have episodes of various types of psychotic phenomena. They allow complete recovery between episodes of illness, and should be regarded by non-psychiatrists as variants of manic-depressive illness.

CYCLOTHYMIC PERSONALITY (see p. 61)

This is a normal personality variant where the individual recognizes variations in energy and outlook which appear like *formes frustes* of bipolar illness. The diagnostic criteria given above should assist in the differentiation.

Aetiology (of bipolar illness)

GENETIC FACTORS

Family and twin data indicate that bipolar affective illness is aetiologically distinct from most cases of unipolar depression. However, the genotype underlying bipolar illness may sometimes produce unipolar illness, and sometimes cyclothymic personality. While genetic factors are undoubtedly important, no specific mode of inheritance has been established. With manic-depressive probands (although not with probands with depressive illness), there is an increased incidence in sibs reared under unfavourable conditions. The genetic predisposition is very much greater in early onset cases.

PERSONALITY

People with cyclothymic or depressive traits in their personality are at greater risk of bipolar illness.

DRUGS

Some patients have their only episode of manic illness during treatment of a depressive episode with an antidepressant. Some people tolerate vast doses of amphetamines without developing psychotic illnesses, while others develop a manic illness on relatively small doses: in both cases, we are probably dealing with an interplay between genetic factors and environmental releasing factors.

STRESSFUL LIFE EVENTS

First episodes of mania often follow the same sort of stressful life events as precipitate episodes of depression. Once more, the stressful event is probably a releasing factor responsible for the timing of the episode.

Treatment (of mania)

NEUROLEPTICS

Haloperidol (p. 84) and chlorpromazine (p. 84) are drugs of choice for the symptoms of excitement and for suppressing any hallucinations.

LITHIUM CARBONATE (see pp. 92–4)

Lithium is used both to make attacks less frequent and to lessen the severity of attacks. It also has some value in the treatment of mania, although it is not a drug of first choice.

ELECTROCONVULSIVE TREATMENT (see pp. 94–7)

This is not usually necessary, but can be helpful in cases that do not respond to drug therapy.

ADMISSION TO HOSPITAL

This will often be necessary to contain episodes of mania which are very difficult to manage without specialized nursing care. It must not be forgotten that there is an increased risk of depression during mania: especially after the more excited symptoms have responded to treatment, while the patient is still active and disinhibited but during the brief episodes of depressed mood that have already been described.

Treatment (of recurrent illnesses)

Prophylactic lithium (see p. 93) is recommended for both bipolar (manic-depressive) illnesses and recurrent, unipolar psychotic depressions (see p. 190).

Carbamazepine (see p. 80) can be tried for 'rapid cycling' illnesses.

Course and prognosis

The natural history of bipolar illness is for the patient to have episodes of increasing frequency and duration over the course of his lifetime. However, lithium treatment has made a great impact on the course of the disorder and there is good evidence that it reduces both the intensity and the frequency of attacks. However, even without lithium there were always some people who recovered from a single attack of either mania or depressive psychosis and never had a recurrence: so lithium should only be offered after it is clear that a pattern of recurrence has been established.

FURTHER READING

Brown, G. and Harris, T. (1978) *The Social Origins of Depression*. London: Tavistock.
Paykel, E. (1984) *A Handbook of the Affective Disorders*. Edinburgh: Churchill Livingstone.
Williams, J. M. (1984) *The Psychological Treatment of Depression*. London: Croom Helm.

14 / MALADAPTIVE BEHAVIOURS

The apparently heterogeneous conditions described in this chapter have a number of features in common:

1. Each of the behaviours considered represents an *exaggeration of normal behaviour*: consumption of alcohol, the taking of drugs, dieting, and overeating are normal behaviours, and obsessional traits are common in normal people. They are **maladaptive** in the sense that they cause the individual to suffer, and usually place him at a biological disadvantage: there is a *morbidity* associated with all of the conditions described in this chapter, and many also have an increased *mortality*.

2. *Response to anxiety*. Each behaviour tends to become worse with increased anxiety, and there is a component of each which is associated with reduction of anxiety. The consumption of alcohol or drugs relieves anxiety, and washing the hands relieves the anxiety that results from the obsessional idea that they may be contaminated. In each case this reduction in anxiety is only short-lived, and in the longer term further anxiety is generated which leads to the repetition of the behaviour causing a vicious circle. Thus the alcoholic feels better after a few drinks but is left in a more anxious (withdrawn state) the next morning. This leads to further anxiety and further drinking.

3. A sense of subjective *compulsion* is experienced by the patient in most of these conditions. However hard he tries to resist, the person feels compelled to drink, starve, binge, or perform a certain act. The doctor must understand this so that he doesn't simply expect the patient readily to stop the behaviour.

ALCOHOL DEPENDENCE AND ALCOHOL-RELATED DISABILITIES

The concepts of dependence and alcohol-related disabilities are first defined.

Dependence

Alcohol becomes a drug of dependence when there is a compulsion to take it on a continuous or a periodic basis. The concept of dependence has three components.

1. Subjective awareness of a **compulsion to drink**.
2. **Increased tolerance**.
3. **Withdrawal symptoms**.

Awareness of a **compulsion to drink** is reported by the person, so that the first drink after a period of abstinence inevitably leads to a return to the previous level of consumption. The desire for a further drink is seen as irrational, the desire is resisted, yet the further drink is taken. If he tries to abstain, he may experience cravings for alcohol.

Increased tolerance develops so that large amounts of alcohol can be consumed without inebriation. The patient may have derived confidence from this, when in fact it indicates that dependence is beginning.

Withdrawal symptoms occur when there is an abrupt drop in the blood alcohol in someone who has maintained a high intake over a prolonged period of time. These typically occur in the morning, since this is the time when blood alcohol is at its lowest. They consist of shaking of the hands ('morning shakes'), nausea, sweating, and agitation. They are relieved by taking an alcoholic drink. More severe withdrawal symptoms include illusions, a sense of dread, and jumbled auditory hallucinations. *Generalized epileptic seizures* may occur, and after some forty-eight hours *delirium tremens* (see p. 146).

After a while, drinking begins to take priority over everything else: work, family life, social life, and even health. The *drinking repertoire* is restricted to a stereotyped pattern each day and drinking acquires salience over other activities. The concept of dependence leads to the discussion of whether someone is 'an alcoholic' or not. This is seldom a useful discussion. *It is better to ask whether a dependent individual has developed any related disabilities.*

Alcohol-related disabilities

These include physical, psychological, and social problems that result from persistent heavy drinking. Since alcohol-related disabilities may occur in the absence of dependence, this term includes many who come into contact with the medical services but would not be regarded as 'alcoholics'.

Epidemiology

Problem drinkers are greatly over-represented among medical in-patients. In general medical and orthopaedic wards 8 per cent of women and 29 per cent of men have been found to be problem drinkers. Higher figures will be found in casualty departments, because accidents often involve those with a high blood alcohol, and in gastro-intestinal clinics, since these deal with many of the physical complications of alcohol. Yet most alcohol abusers in the general hospital go undetected.

General population surveys of alcohol abusers are notoriously difficult but also demonstrate that many problem drinkers are not known to any form of helping agency. However, it is probable that the prevalence of alcohol dependence is between 0.9 and 1.4 per cent in England; while perhaps as many as 5 per cent of the adult population drink to excess. Figures for alcohol abuse are consistently higher among men than women. Highest rates are found in those twenty to thirty years old but patients hospitalized for alcohol-related illness tend to be in their forties. Lowest rates are found in the middle classes. Upper social classes often have a pattern of prolonged heavy drinking, while lower classes drink heavily at weekends.

Clinical features

PHYSICAL DISABILITIES

Cirrhosis of the liver is the best-recognized complication. Deaths from cirrhosis have risen in the UK recently because of the marked increase in alcohol consumption. For men the risk of cirrhosis increases as a result of drinking four pints of beer a day (or a quarter of a bottle of spirits or one bottle of wine), for women two pints of beer or equivalent is sufficient. Persistent heavy drinking is most likely to lead to cirrhosis, which will occur in 80 per cent of those who drink ten or more pints a day for fifteen years. **Hepatitis** is also common among heavy drinkers and may lead on to cirrhosis. **Hepatic encephalopathy** occurs in liver failure.

Half the cases of **chronic pancreatitis** occur in heavy drinkers, especially chronic calcifying pancreatitis. **Acute gastritis** is common among heavy drinkers, and peptic ulcers are three times more common than in non-drinkers. These illnesses together with **oesophageal varices** and **oesophagitis** mean that a problem drinker may present with abdominal pain, with a haematemesis or an iron-deficient anaemia. **Macrocytosis without anaemia** occurs as a result of folate deficiency. **Megaloblastic anaemia** may result from folate or vitamin B_{12} deficiency, or a direct toxic effect of alcohol. **Haemolytic anaemia** or **thrombocytopenia** may arise from cirrhosis.

The risk of **ischaemic heart disease** and **cerebrovascular accidents** is increased with alcohol abuse. **Cardiomyopathy** is more specifically linked to alcohol, which is associated with 50 per cent of cases of primary degeneration of the heart muscle.

Peripheral neuropathy occurs in 10 per cent of dependent drinkers and affects both sensory and motor systems especially in the lower limbs. It is due to thiamine deficiency but rarely responds to treatment. **Cerebellar degeneration**, **myopathy**, **Wernicke's encephalopathy** (see p. 158) occur. The alcoholic is at greater risk of **subdural haematoma** and **traumatic neuropathy**, as well as as injuries of all kinds due to accidents at home and at work, to road traffic accidents, and to episodes of violence.

Many of these physical disabilities are due to, or made worse by, dietary deficiencies and general poor health which predispose the alcohol-dependent patient to develop infection.

PSYCHOLOGICAL DISABILITIES

Depression is common among alcohol abusers. Three patterns may be discerned:

1. Alcohol has a *direct depressant effect* and the alcohol abuser may have a persistently depressed mood that responds to abstinence.
2. Alcohol abuse leads to *social problems*, such as unemployment, divorce, and debts, and these lead to the person becoming depressed.
3. Depression, occurring for some other reason, may be *relieved temporarily* by drinking. This is one way in which heavy drinking starts, with an eventual worsening of the depression.

The depression may lead to deliberate self-harm. Nearly half of the men who take overdoses are dependent upon alcohol. The risk of **suicide** is increased many times among the population of alcohol abusers admitted for treatment.

Anxiety is related to alcohol abuse in a similar way to depression. In addition, anxiety is marked during alcohol withdrawal.

Alcoholic hallucinosis is a rare condition separate from the acute effects of withdrawal. In the setting of clear consciousness auditory hallucinations occur which are generally in the second person and may be derogatory. They are often in the form of a conversation about the patient. The phenomenon usually occurs when prolonged heavy drinking ceases or is considerably reduced. It generally clears within a few days. If not, a state similar to schizophrenia develops. In this case it is likely that latent schizophrenia is released by the heavy alcohol intake.

Antisocial personality disorder (see p. 65) may lead to alcoholism, but a normal personality may be evident before persistent heavy drinking leads to mood changes, inability to hold a job, and disruption of personal relationships.

MEMORY IMPAIRMENT

1. This occurs during acute intoxication with alcohol. Although the person may function quite normally during an evening of heavy drinking the next day there will be a dense amnesia for those hours (**alcoholic amnesia**, or 'palimpsest').
2. A specific memory impairment occurs, **Korsakow's syndrome** (see p. 158).
3. **Alcoholic dementia**, which may resolve if the person stops drinking.

SOCIAL DISABILITIES

Marital problems occur because the alcohol abuser is late coming home, may be abusive or violent while drunk, incur debts, lose his job, and become impotent. The spouse may be disgusted by her drunk husband and embarrassed by his social behaviour. She may therefore become depressed and anxious herself, or even take an overdose, and the astute general practitioner may detect alcohol abuse in this indirect way. Effects on the children may predominate if it is the wife who is abusing alcohol.

Work problems develop if the person attends late, is drunk and argumentative at work, and fails to perform at his former standard. Alcoholics miss much time from work and lose their jobs more frequently than their sober colleagues.

Alcoholics often come into contact with the **police** because of antisocial behaviour while intoxicated, either being disorderly or committing a petty crime.

Vagrancy has many causes but alcohol abuse often combines with other factors to lead to this state. Such people may present very considerable problems to the health services because of their multiple physical illnesses, their poor living conditions, and their insistence on continued drinking.

The detection of alcohol-related disabilities

Doctors do not detect alcohol abuse in general medical practice because they fail to ask the appropriate questions.

WHEN TO SUSPECT A PROBLEM MAY BE PRESENT

1. When any of the physical problems mentioned on p. 198 present (do not be satisfied with diagnosing a peptic ulcer: ask yourself whether alcohol could be responsible).

2. When the patient seems evasive or unclear while describing his complaint (this might represent concealment of heavy drinking or indicate a memory impairment).

3. When the patient is in a high risk occupation. (Barman, publican, wine merchant, or brewer carries a high risk; well above average are company directors, commercial travellers, the armed forces, journalists, entertainers, and doctors).

4. When another family member has alcohol-related problems.

5. When investigations provide evidence of pathology which may be due to alcohol (for example, an unexpected elevation of the γ-GT).

THE CAGE

In any of these circumstances, you may find that the CAGE questions are useful. (See 'The Card'.)

C. Have you ever felt you ought to CUT down on your drinking?
A. Have people ANNOYED you by criticizing your drinking?
G. Have you ever felt bad or GUILTY about your drinking?
E. Have you ever had a drink first thing in the morning to steady your nerves or get rid of a hangover (EYE OPENER)?

If you get positive replies to any *two* of these questions, it is worth taking a proper 'drinking history'. (Probability of being a case if score is 2 or > 2 = 45%; probability of being a non-case if score is 0 or 1 = 97%.)

TAKING A DRINKING HISTORY

Start by asking the patient (and later an informant) to describe a **typical drinking day**. One starts with the morning and proceeds through the day establishing what is drunk and when.

1. Establish if the first drink of the day is taken to combat withdrawal symptoms.
2. Does the patient drink throughout the day without getting drunk, or in bouts – usually at lunchtime and the evening?
3. How much is drunk at each session?
4. Does a single drink always lead to many more, and the person generally become drunk? If so, has this led to blackouts or falls?
5. Establish whether drinking takes place alone, and whether the person drinks only in response to certain moods or situations.

In this way the doctor and patient together estimate how much is being spent on drink each week. This is compared to the patient's previous estimate of expenditure per week and is often an eye opener(!) for the patient.

Having established the current drinking pattern one then tries to ascertain the **development of heavy drinking** over the years. There are often key points in the patient's life, such as working in the armed forces or in the wine trade where a great increase in drinking occurred. The patient may recall his daily drinking pattern at times when he lost a particular job or when his marriage broke up. Contacts with the police may also be dated. In this way the doctor establishes the duration of heavy drinking, and which of the related disabilities have developed.

Aetiology

GENETIC FACTORS

The prevalence of alcoholism amongst parents and siblings of alcoholics is two and a half times that of the general population. This is not solely an environmental effect as sons of alcoholic fathers adopted away are just as likely to become alcoholics as those who remain in the original parental home.

PSYCHOLOGICAL

Prospective studies have shown that although neurotic traits in childhood do not relate to the later development of alcoholism, children who were impulsive, aggressive, and hyperactive are more likely to become alcoholic as adults.

However, alcohol is a potent anxiolytic and agoraphobics, social phobics, and other neurotic personalities are likely to use alcohol in this way. In some this will lead on to clear dependence upon alcohol. The relief of tension or distress by alcohol can be viewed as a reward in behavioural terms. If this happens repeatedly the consumption of alcohol becomes a self-perpetuating habit. Any difficulties that arise from heavy drinking, including withdrawal symptoms, increase anxiety which can once again be relieved by the ingestion of alcohol. Thus a vicious circle with increasing consumption is set up.

SOCIAL FACTORS

Several *occupations* have more alcoholics than would be expected, and these have been listed above. Predisposing effects of these occupations include availability of cheap or free alcohol, strong peer pressure to drink, lack of supervision at work, and estrangement from the stabilizing influences of home life.

Cultural factors are important as the taboos against drinking among Muslims and Mormons, and against drunkenness among Jews, lead to very low rates of alcoholism compared to cultures where drinking is equated with masculinity.

Availability of alcohol is being increasingly recognized as a factor. There is evidence for a direct relationship between per capita consumption in a population and the number of people with alcohol-related problems. The former is determined by the real price of alcoholic beverages and as this is reduced the mortality rate from cirrhosis increases.

Investigations

TO ESTABLISH THE DIAGNOSIS

Physical – test blood or urinary alcohol to detect alcohol in the patient's blood stream when he denies having drunk; or abnormal liver function in someone who denies drinking very much.

Social – interview an informant to establish the patient's true drinking pattern and extent of related disabilities when these are not clear from the patient. Assessment of family relationships, financial position, and job situation will reveal the true extent of social disabilities which are often more serious than the patient has led the doctor to believe.

A knowledge of these social factors may allow the doctor to understand the aetiology of the person's heavy drinking (this may be years previously) but also allow him to assess the factors which reinforce his current consumption.

TO ESTABLISH THE EXTENT OF ALCOHOL-RELATED DAMAGE

PHYSICAL

Test liver function, especially γ-glutamyl transpeptidase (γ-GT) which is raised in 75 per cent of dependent drinkers.
Blood film for macrocytosis in the absence of anaemia.
Thereafter test to detect the physical sequelae of heavy drinking listed above.

PSYCHOLOGICAL

Test for memory impairment (see p. 71).

Treatment

PHYSICAL

Drug treatment is required for withdrawal symptoms. *Diazepam* or *chlormethiazole* for one week is usually sufficient (typical daily doses of chlormethiazole would be 6 g for two days, 4 g for two days and 2 g for two days). Treatment for delirium tremens is described on p. 147.

Parenterovite injections are given if there is any possibility that the person might be thiamine deficient.

Serious depression or anxiety occasionally requires drug treatment, but usually depression improves as the person is detoxified.

Any accompanying physical illnesses must be treated.

Disulfiram ('Antabuse') or *citrated calcium carbimide* ('Abstem') can be given daily and will help the impulsive drinker who knows that he will become acutely ill if he drinks during the subsequent twenty-four hours. The patient must be motivated to take the tablet each day for this to be a useful adjunct to other treatment.

PSYCHOLOGICAL

Supportive psychotherapy is essential. This alone may be the appropriate treatment for mild alcohol abuse in general practice or the general medical clinic. Often the assessment procedures described above may enable the patient to realize that his drinking is causing physical or social damage. If this motivates him to reduce his drinking, he is asked to keep a *daily diary* of his consumption. A gradual reduction will avoid withdrawal symptoms and drug treatment will be unnecessary. The major complaint is likely to be of insomnia, but hypnotics can be avoided if the patient is warned of this beforehand and encouraged to do without.

The doctor should ask the *patient's spouse* to encourage and help the patient especially at times of wanting a drink.

SOCIAL

Involvement of the family to understand the nature of the problem, provide support for the patient, and to help him cope.

Activities other than going to the pub or mixing with drinking friends should be encouraged.

The doctor must use his judgement as to whether total abstinence or controlled social drinking should be the aim of treatment. If alcohol-related problems are severe, or the patient has relapsed after previous periods of abstinence, total abstinence should be the goal.

With more serious cases *admission to a psychiatric ward or alcohol treatment unit* is recommended so that the commencement of psychological treatments occurs together with the detoxification. *Group therapy* is useful to help the person to be honest about the nature of the problem and find ways of coping without alcohol.

Alcoholics Anonymous is very helpful for many patients. It advocates a strict abstinence policy, provides a social structure to replace drinking, support is available at all times and often from ex-alcoholics with whom the patient can identify.

DRUG DEPENDENCE

Most of what has been written about alcohol-related problems applies to drug-related problems, so only a few points will be highlighted in this section.

Opiates

These drugs in the UK come from three sources: legal prescriptions, theft from chemists, and smuggled oriental heroin.

The addict takes the drug by mouth ('dropping'), inhales the fumes of burning heroin ('chasing the dragon'), nasally inhales it ('snorting'), injects it intramuscularly ('fix'), subcutaneously ('skin pop'), or intravenously ('main-lining'). Initially the drug-taker experiences a 'rush, thrill, buzz, or flash' following intravenous heroin. This is described like a rather superior sexual orgasm and is the reason for taking heroin at first. Appetite and sexual desire are decreased, and constipation is common.

As tolerance develops larger doses are required, dysphoria and somatic side-effects are experienced and the person takes the drug increasingly to avoid withdrawal symptoms.

WITHDRAWAL SYMPTOMS

The latter start eight to ten hours after the last dose with **rhinorrhoea, lacrimation, yawning, sweating,** and **craving. Nausea, vomiting, diarrhoea, abdominal cramps,** and **muscle pains** develop.

Central nervous system *rebound excitability* is shown by **mydriasis, tachycardia, hypertension, flushing,** and **involuntary movements**.

These symptoms ('cold turkey') are much feared by addicts because they are so unpleasant but in fact recede after seventy-two hours and do not carry the same risk to life as delirium tremens.

MORTALITY AND MORBIDITY

Mortality among opiate addicts is almost *fifteen times* that of the non-drug-taking population. This is accounted for by the *morbidity* associated with opiate dependence, itself mainly related to:

1. *Dirty injection technique* leading to **sepsis, hepatitis, endocarditis, tuberculosis,** and **nephrotic syndrome**.
2. *Drug overdosage* may cause **respiratory failure**.
3. Feelings of *desperation and depression* often lead to **suicide**.

CLINICAL FEATURES

During withdrawal, the patient will have widely dilated pupils, tachycardia, and pilo-erection as well as the symptoms listed above. Look for thrombosed veins, and other complications of dirty injections.

TREATMENT

As with alcohol-related problems this is largely concerned with helping the individual to develop a new life style free of the drug. This may involve changing the social group in which the person mixes if this includes other drug abusers. Financial and family problems and involvement with the law will all require social help.

It is often the general practitioner, casualty officer, or general physician who is initially faced with an addict claiming to be in withdrawal. *It is illegal to prescribe narcotics to those who are dependent upon them unless you have been approved by the Home Office.* When deciding whether to prescribe **methadone** – this drug is used because it can be given orally, it prevents withdrawal symptoms, but does not produce the pleasurable 'buzz' of heroin – it is best to err on the side of caution; there are some heroin-takers ('chippers') who take the drug only occasionally and are not dependent.

In the GP surgery and casualty department it is generally better not to prescribe in the absence of clear withdrawal symptoms or without the patient's signing a *treatment contract*. This defines a withdrawal regime or reducing doses over a two to three week period and states conditions which the patient must fulfil (for example, abstinence from additional drug-taking checked by urine samples each visit) if the doctor is to continue prescribing. Without such precautions the doctor may find himself becoming obliged to continue prescribing.

For serious cases of dependence, admission to a *specialist treatment unit* is advisable so that withdrawal symptoms can be avoided but a rapid detoxification can take place and the social aspects of treatment can commence immediately.

A minority of patients have developed dependence on opiates as a result of prescriptions from a doctor ('iatrogenic drug dependence'). In the case of terminally ill patients this does not matter. For the remainder opiates have usually been prescribed for a painful condition so alternative methods of controlling the pain must be sought before the opiate can be withdrawn gradually.

Barbiturates

These drugs are now very little used (see p. 78), but there has been a rise in young multiple drug-abusers who still manage to obtain these drugs through medical channels.

Barbiturate abusers may develop *tolerance*, but the risk of **respiratory depression** increases with large doses and these may be fatal. Drug-dependent individuals are particularly likely to take an overdose of barbiturates. A *withdrawal syndrome* similar to that of alcohol is recognized, **epileptic fits** and **delirium** are common.

CLINICAL FEATURES

The younger barbiturate addict may have injected these highly irritant drugs in aqueous solution, and so produced phlebitis, indolent abscesses, and sloughing ulcers. He may be unkempt, dirty, and malnourished. He may appear drunk, with slurred speech and incoherence, or be sleepy. Nystagmus is usually present, and depression is a common complication.

TREATMENT

Replacement with a short-acting barbiturate (for example, pentobarbitone) is recommended for those dependent upon high doses, with 10 per cent reduction of dosage per day and possible concurrent cover with an anticonvulsant. Subsequently prolonged difficulty with sleep occurs and **nightmares** result from REM rebound.

Benzodiazepines

These widely prescribed drugs are increasingly recognized as causing dependence. They cease to be effective anxiolytics once the user is habituated to them, yet severe symptoms of anxiety will be experienced if withdrawal is attempted. The *withdrawal symptoms* also include **giddiness**, **trembling**, **faintness**, **insomnia**, and **hypersensitivity**.

These can be minimized by using a long-acting drug, such as diazepam, and withdrawing it very slowly. Irritability and insomnia are severe in the first two weeks after withdrawal, but have virtually disappeared three months later.

The following drugs do not cause physical dependence but are of importance to psychiatry because of the abnormal mental states that they produce. They are often used with barbiturates or opiates, and they may precipitate psychotic illness.

Amphetamines

These drugs are still occasionally prescribed for hyperkinetic children and adults with narcolepsy. (Amphetamine abusers sometimes claim to suffer from the latter condition.)

They are usually obtained on the black market and are taken to produce a state of increased awareness, energy, and concentration, together with reduced hunger and fatigue. Taken intravenously they may produce a short-lived 'flush' and are used in this way by opiate addicts. These effects are followed by depression, anxiety, irritability, and anergia. Barbiturates may also be taken to combat the insomnia produced.

CLINICAL FEATURES

The patient will be talkative and over-active if intoxicated, sleepy or depressed if withdrawn. He may be malnourished because of the anorexia, and lick his lips because of the dry mouth. The pupils are dilated, there may be sweating, tachycardia, high blood pressure, or arrhythmias, and there is usually a generalized hyperreflexia.

Amphetamines may produce a **symptomatic schizophrenia** (see p. 168) in otherwise normal people, with persecutory delusions, accompanied by visual, tactile, and auditory hallucinations in a state of clear consciousness. It will also exacerbate schizophrenic symptoms in those vulnerable to the disorder. In other patients a **symptomatic mania** (see p. 192) can be precipitated. The mental state usually returns to normal over five to seven days as the drug is excreted, but occasionally a persistent psychosis requires treatment with phenothiazines.

Cocaine

Cocaine is 'snorted' into the nostril and absorbed through the nasal mucosa. It is a central nervous stimulant with effects similar to amphetamine but said to be less sharp and more subtle. It may produce disorientation and depression.

It resembles amphetamine in its ability to produce a symptomatic psychosis. Because the drug is expensive and hard to acquire it is generally used by those who also abuse other drugs.

CLINICAL FEATURES

The intoxicated patient may be excited, with dilated pupils and tremulousness. He may report a feeling of insects crawling under his skin ('formication'). At later stages, dizziness, convulsions, and cardiac arrhythmias occur. Death may occur from cardiac arrest.

Hallucinogens

Mescalin, lysergic acid diethylamide (LSD or 'acid'), dimethyltryptamine ('angel dust'), and psilocybin ('the magic mushroom') are hallucinogens but at the time of writing LSD and psilocybin are most commonly used in this country.

CLINICAL FEATURES

Taken orally LSD causes perceptual changes within forty minutes. Sensation in all modalities is heightened and distorted, and may be translated from one modality to another so sounds may be seen and colour smelled: 'synaesthesia'. The body image may be terrifyingly distorted; the patient may regard himself as able to fly or to walk on water. Numerous deaths have occurred in this way. Extreme emotional changes may occur, which result in anxiety and terror of imminent insanity: these are described as a 'bad trip'. Such states are best managed by someone 'talking down' the patient, emphasizing that the alarming experiences are due to the drug.

The acute effects die down over twenty-four hours, but perceptual changes may last longer. A more prolonged **psychosis** may result as with amphetamines, although it may be that the drug has merely released the psychosis in a vulnerable personality.

Sometimes *flash-back experiences* occur some months later when, under stress or the effect of another drug, the person relives part of the perceptual distortion that occurred during an LSD trip.

Cannabis

Cannabis is widely abused by young people, notably students and members of some ethnic groups. 'Grass' refers to the dried plant, *Cannabis sativa*, while 'resin' is secreted by the female parts of the flowering plant. The effects largely depend on the circumstances in which the drug is taken, and it is generally used as a social drug. There is no withdrawal syndrome, nor is there evidence of tolerance.

Feelings of well-being, relaxation, and tranquillity are induced within minutes of inhalation but prevailing moods of anger or depression may be aggravated. Perceptual disturbances of time, sight, and sound may occur but the person generally retains insight throughout.

Acute psychotic episodes can occur with high doses, and these may last up to forty-eight hours.

Solvent sniffing

Euphoria may result from the sniffing of solvents which contain toluene and acetone, but continued inhalation leads to stupor and loss of consciousness as these toxic substances are powerful CNS depressants and may cause neuronal destruction. *Psychological dependence* occurs and this causes concern because it involves children, especially those from a deprived background. The mortality is considerable; about 50 per cent due to direct toxic effects of the solvent, the remainder mainly due to asphyxia from the plastic bag from which the solvent was inhaled, or from inhalation of gastric contents.

CLINICAL FEATURES

Look for glue on the hands, face, or clothes, and the *glue sniffer's rash* over the mouth and nasal area. The patient is usually a child or adolescent, and boys outnumber girls by thirteen to one. The glue may be smelled. There are rapid variations in the level of consciousness, disorientation, sometimes slurred speech, and an ataxic gait.

Non-opiate analgesics

Those who regularly take large doses of aspirin, phenacetin, and paracetamol may do so secretively, against medical advice, and with serious physical consequences.

Psychological dependence occurs, and women with chronic depressive illness or personality disturbance are particularly prone to use these drugs in this way. The principal physical related problem is *analgesic nephropathy*.

Multiple drug abuse seems to be the norm rather than the exception, especially if alcohol is included as a drug. Therefore a drug-dependent person who has taken an overdose may have done so with several drugs. An opiate-dependent person denied his normal dose will turn to other drugs.

ANOREXIA NERVOSA

This condition predominantly affects adolescent girls, and takes the form of **self-induced loss of weight**, so that body weight is at least 25 per cent below standard weight, accompanied by an intense wish to be thin. The patient has an intense **fear of fatness**, and this takes the form of an *over-valued idea* (see p. 30) that she is fat, although aware that others regard her as thin – this feature distinguishes anorexia nervosa from all other causes of either weight loss or anorexia. In women there will be **amenorrhoea**, and in men **loss of sexual interest**.

The patient may successfully conceal abnormal eating habits, and sometimes even be under intense medical investigation for somatic complaints such as diarrhoea, metabolic disorder, or amenorrhoea before the diagnosis is recognized.

Epidemiology

In Scotland the prevalence has been estimated at 10.8 per 100,000 for women in the fifteen to thirty-four age group. Over 90 per cent of patients with anorexia nervosa are female. Surveys in England have indicated that between 1 and 2 per cent of adolescent girls are affected, with highest rates for the age group between thirteen and twenty, and with a few cases starting either before puberty or during adult life.

Clinical features

Emaciation with a weight of 35–40 kilos is common. If the weight has dropped as low as 30–35 kilos the patient may present with fainting. She may wear heavy clothes to mask the thinness. This weight loss results from calorie restriction and selective exclusion of carbohydrate from the diet, but protein deficiency can develop in the chronic state, which may present as swelling of the ankles. *Abuse of diuretics* leads to dehydration and *purgative abuse* leads to diarrhoea and hypokalaemia in severe cases.

The patient's apparent unconcern about her condition may be balanced by her parents' being distraught; whereas she may cook for the rest of the family she starves herself. *Preoccupation with calorie counting, avoidance of all carbohydrate, vomiting after meals, vigorous exercising, and taking laxatives* are common behaviours. The patient may deceive those around her into thinking that she is eating adequately and often does so in the medical ward.

The anorexia may be interspersed with bulimic episodes when binge-eating is followed by vomiting and guilt. The underlying panic in relation to weight gain becomes obvious at such times. The patient may show signs of depression or obsessionality especially in relation to food preparation and consumption.

The body shows evidence of chronic starvation with:

1. Cold, blue extremities.
2. Fine, downy, hair – 'lanugo' – on back and face.
3. Slow pulse: 40–60 per minute.
4. Low blood pressure: 90/60.
5. Low body temperature.
6. Reduction of LH and FSH with amenorrhoea.

The amenorrhoea is usually secondary to the loss of weight, but occasionally precedes it.

Differential diagnosis

Dieting is to be distinguished from anorexia by the absence of amenorrhoea and over-valued ideas about being fat when the patient is actually very thin.

Weight loss may also result from psychological or physical illnesses; *hyperthyroidism* and *diabetes* are examples of the latter that occur at this age. Organic causes of diarrhoea, such as *idiopathic steatorrhea* or *inflammatory bowel disease*, may need to be considered.

Amenorrhoea may result from *ovarian or pituitary disease*, following use of the *contraceptive pill*, or from *psychological stress*.

Depressive and obsessional features may suggest these illnesses, and occasionally *psychotic illnesses* can present with avoidance of food, but in anorexia nervosa the central fear of weight gain and distorted body image generally indicate the true diagnosis.

Aetiology

Eating disorders tend to run in families so obesity and alcoholism among older relatives is common. Episodes of anorexia during the teenage years of female relatives may have occurred though not necessarily reached medical treatment.

The anorexic patient is often obese during her younger childhood years and may have been teased for being so. An early menarche and rapid growth may increase pubertal fatness. The subsequent dieting may start as a reasonable behaviour, but get out of control in relation to a precipitating event. More commonly there is a background of disturbed family relationships with a dependent and immature patient. There may be competition with other siblings for parental attention, or conflicts about leaving home with an avoidance of mature responsibilities. This avoidance often involves sexual behaviour.

Maintaining factors are sometimes very important in prolonging what might otherwise have been a brief episode of dieting. For example, there may be some crisis within the family, such as the parents' marriage breaking up, or psychiatric illness in one of the parents, or a family situation which the daughter seems to be able to control with her anorexia.

Investigations

Physical investigations may be necessary to exclude other conditions listed in the differential diagnosis. More important is the need to assess the extent of malnutrition and electrolyte disturbance due to vomiting. *Confirmation of the diagnosis comes from the patient directly expressing her fear of weight gain* to the doctor. The doctor must allow the patient to develop enough trust for this to occur, preferably at the first interview. The patient may also indicate to a sympathetic doctor that she has other fears about growing up even if she is not prepared to describe these in detail at an early stage.

Assessment of body image in a standardized way by a psychologist is possible but often unnecessary, as experience over a short time generally provides evidence that the patient is afraid of gaining weight and does not do so even when she has initially promised to do so.

Luteinizing hormone levels have been shown to be low, and to show an impaired response to LH-releasing factor. Even when weight is restored, cyclical LH activity may not resume – suggesting an abnormality of the hypothalamo-pituitary axis.

Social investigations – a member of the team attempts to identify any problems in the parental or other family relationships which might cause or exacerbate the anorexia of the patient. The possibility of family therapy or support for the parents is investigated.

Treatment

Treatment is aimed first at restoration of normal body weight, and then assistance with maturation and establishment of independence appropriate to the patient's age.

1. RESTORATION OF BODY WEIGHT

Out-patient treatment may be appropriate: sometimes separation of the patient from her parents leads to weight gain – so moving to another house or hostel may help to avoid hospital admission.

In-patient treatment may be required from the outset if the patient's weight is very low and secondary physical problems are severe. Rarely the emaciation is extreme and the patient refuses voluntary treatment, so admission under Section 3 of the Mental Health Act (see p. 306) has to be considered. Restoration of body weight in hospital can be achieved in various ways, but perhaps the simplest has regard to three points.

1. Bed rest.
2. Supervision during meals and for at least half an hour afterwards.
3. Controlled diet, avoiding excessive weight gain. Aim at increasing by 3–4 lbs per week.

Drug treatment is sometimes helpful. *Chlorpromazine* reduces anxiety and stimulates appetite, but occasionally leads to epileptic fits. *Antidepressants* are used if there is evidence of a concurrent depressive illness, which sometimes occurs in older patients. Correction of *hypokalaemia* may be urgent if vomiting has been a pronounced feature, and of severe dehydration if diuretics have been abused. Other dietary deficiencies may need attention.

Behaviour therapy may be used as an adjunct to restoration of body weight. A target weight is set, and the weight to be gained is divided into steps with a clearly stated reward for each intermediate target weight. The gaining of rewards must be very strictly related to weight gains. The patient is initially confined to bed and denied visitors, earning privileges such as getting dressed, going out, and having time at home only once she puts on weight. One must guard against patients' gaining weight quickly so that they can be discharged and then lose it again.

Psychotherapy. A relationship of trust with the patient from the first interview is essential. It is likely that the patient will attend the first interview eager to discover whether the doctor will side with the parents' wish for increased weight or the patient's desire to stay thin. In fact the doctor makes it clear from the outset that weight gain is essential for a full recovery, but that he or she understands the patient's fears of weight gain.

2. MATURATION AND ESTABLISHMENT OF INDEPENDENCE

Treatment in the longer term is principally by **psychotherapy** with the patient and/or her family. Once trust has been established the aim of psychotherapy is to encourage the patient to discuss those powerful inner feelings which she has been unable to express previously and which have led to the anorexia.

Course and prognosis

The disorder usually lasts for at least two years. Weight gain in the short term is usually satisfactory in most cases. This is maintained in approximately 60 per cent and normal menstruation is restored in a similar proportion. Eating habits can be regarded as returning to normal in only 40–50 per cent and some patients present later with obesity. Psychiatric illness occurs in approximately one-third; this is usually a depressive illness, but obsessional illness, anxiety, or phobias may also occur.

Approximately 15 per cent of cases become chronic, that is continuing over five years or more, and the chance of recovery in these cases is poor. The condition carries a **mortality** rate of up to 10 per cent; death occurs through emaciation or suicide.

Factors that indicate a *good prognosis* are an onset very soon after puberty, a brief illness with brisk response to treatment, and satisfactory family relationships. A poor prognosis is indicated by the presence of vomiting, purgative abuse, and bulimic episodes with extreme weight loss and development of a chronic illness.

BULIMIA

This is a form of eating disorder where the abnormality is of uncontrolled and excessive eating ('**binge-eating**'). During the eating binges – which tend to last less than two hours – there is a feeling of loss of control of the eating behaviour, and the binge is followed either by *self-induced vomiting*, by the use of *laxatives*, or by *rigorous dieting* to counteract the effects of the binge. The patient typically eats high-calorie foods on their own, and reports a relief from tension during the binge.

Binge-eating occurs in both anorexia nervosa and obesity, and can also be a mild intermittent behaviour that cannot be regarded as pathological. Occasionally it occurs with sufficient frequency to be regarded as an eating disorder.

Diagnostic criteria

1. Recurrent episodes of binge-eating.
2. A feeling of lack of control during binges.
3. Self-induced vomiting, purgation, or severe dieting afterwards.
4. At least two binges per week for at least three months.

The patients presenting with bulimia tend to be older than those with anorexia nervosa, but often report a previous episode of anorexia that may have gone undetected. Virtually all are women, and the psychopathology overlaps with that described in anorexia nervosa. However, body weight is often normal, menstrual disorders occur in only about a half of the cases, and most readily agree that they have an eating disorder even though the bingeing may always have been done in secret. They may complain about their preoccupation with food and weight changes. Mood disturbances are common. Again, the eating disorder tends to mask other psychological problems and a binge may be a repeated way of relieving distress.

Complications

These can occur due to vomiting and purgation which result in potassium deficiency with weakness, cardiac arrhythmias, and renal damage; teeth may become pitted by gastric acid.

Treatment

This differs from that in anorexia because the patient's weight is normal. A *behavioural assessment* is employed to examine the circumstances in which bingeing occurs. This is usually when the person is under stress, which triggers negative thoughts about herself. Alternative strategies to over-eating are then put into practice at such moments. *Psychotherapy* is aimed first at getting the patient to express verbally her underlying conflicts and problems, and secondly at finding ways of coming to terms with these.

OBESITY

Obesity refers to an **abnormally high proportion of body fat**, and can best be estimated by comparing body weight with height. (The *body mass index* is weight in kilograms divided by the square of height in metres; it should be between 19 and 25. An obese person has a body mass index greater than 25). About one-third of adults in Britain and the USA are obese by this definition.

Aetiology

The aetiology is partly constitutional, partly social – a combination of over-eating and under-exercise. In some obese people an additional contribution comes from *abnormal eating patterns* such as eating to deal with stress, comfort eating, night-eating, continuous snacking, and binge-eating. Those who were **overweight in childhood** are a special group, with a greater tendency for abnormal eating patterns, and a greater likelihood of self-loathing and disparagement of their own body image.

Community studies have demonstrated that there is no direct link between obesity and neurotic illness. However, obese patients seen in medical clinics who find it impossible to lose weight may be an unrepresentative sample. The excess in weight may enable the patient to deny problems in the personal and sexual spheres. If weight loss is successfully achieved these problems may become prominent and disrupt personal relationships whose precarious stability seems to have depended on the patient being obese. It is not uncommon for such patients to have a history of anorexia when younger, which may not have reached medical attention, when similar sexual or interpersonal problems were evident.

Treatment

All obese patients should be given *advice on diet and exercise*, and many benefit from self-help groups although relapse is frequent.

One should consider patients with abnormal eating patterns, low self-esteem, and a negative attitude towards their body image for a cognitive-behavioural approach. *Such an offer of treatment will be made only to a small minority*, since most moderately obese patients do not over-eat, are not unduly sensitive to food cues, and their eating style is no different from that of other people.

Appetite suppressant drugs have no place in the treatment of obesity: they produce dependence and such effect that they may have on body weight is likely to be short-lasting.

Good results have been reported by surgical procedures in the treatment of severe obesity (body mass index > 40). Both *gastric resection and jejuno-ileal bypass* are followed by weight reduction as a result of decreased food intake, and there may be psychological benefits including increased self-confidence, elevation of mood, and decrease in negative self-image. The former operation is technically difficult, but associated with fewer post-operative complications.

OBSESSIONAL STATES

An obsessional illness is a state in which the outstanding symptom is a sense of subjective compulsion, which the patient feels must be resisted, to carry out some action, dwell on an idea, recall an experience, or to ruminate upon some abstract topic. The obsessional urge or idea is seen to be senseless but recognized as arising from within oneself, rather than being imposed from outside. Attempts to dispel the inner thought, or to resist the compulsion to carry out some act, usually lead to anxiety. (See definitions of both *obsessions* and *compulsions* in the Glossary.)

Obsessional phenomena include:

1. **Thoughts** of an unpleasant or obscene nature.
2. **Images** in the form of disgusting but vividly imagined scenes.
3. **Impulses** to perform acts of a violent or embarrassing nature.
4. **Rituals** such as hand-washing or elaborate ways of dressing or cleaning oneself.
5. **Ruminations** (see p. 29) about the pros and cons of everyday actions.

6. **Doubts** concerning whether or not actions involving safety (locking doors, turning off gas-taps and switches) have been completed.

Diagnostic criteria

An obsessional illness refers to symptoms as described above, in the absence of symptoms higher in the hierarchy (such as organic states, schizophrenia, or depression), when they cause significant distress and interfere with the individual's social or occupational functioning. Related phenomena include *slowness* and *depersonalization* (see p. 316).

Approximately two-thirds of patients who develop obsessional illness show *obsessional personality traits* (see p. 63). Indeed, those with such traits often experience some obsessional symptoms, but if they are able to function socially and occupationally they are not said to be *ill*. Such patients often experience a great increase in such symptoms if they develop a depressive illness, but in that case they are described as depressive illnessess – since depression is higher in the hierarchy, and the obsessional symptoms will remit with treatment of the depression.

Epidemiology

Estimates vary between 0.1 and 2 per 1,000 per year. Obsessional illnesses do occur without depressive symptoms, but they are comparatively rare. Obsessional illness accounts for only 2 per cent of the illness seen by psychiatrists.

Differential diagnosis

Obsessional symptoms may occur secondary to depression, schizophrenia, or organic brain disease – in which case treatment is usually directed at the precipitating condition.

Treatment

Behaviour therapy is the treatment of choice and consists of **response prevention** (see p. 101) for compulsive rituals and **thought-stopping** for obsessional thoughts. In the latter treatment the patient is helped to substitute neutral or pleasant thoughts for the distressing thought.

Tricyclic antidepressants, especially clomipramine, may be helpful even in the absence of marked depression. Anxiolytic drugs provide only temporary relief from the worst anxiety. Supportive, rather than interpretive, psychotherapy is helpful at times when the symptoms are worst.

FURTHER READING

Beech, H. R. and Vaughan, M. (1978) *Behavioural Treatment of Obsessional States.* Chichester: John Wiley.

Edwards, G. (1982) *The Treatment of Drinking Problems.* Grant McIntyre.

Hore, B. D. (1976) *Alcohol Dependence.* Butterworths.

Kessel, N. and Walton, H. (1986) *Alcoholism.* Harmondsworth: Penguin.

15 / ABNORMAL ILLNESS BEHAVIOUR

NORMAL ILLNESS BEHAVIOUR

Illness behaviour has been defined as *the ways in which given symptoms may be differentially perceived, evaluated, and acted (or not acted) upon.* This is an extremely broad definition which includes all aspects of thinking, emotion, and behaviour related to the symptoms of disease, whether or not these are associated with objective evidence of physical or mental illness. The more important aspects of illness behaviour are listed in *Table 12.*

The term 'illness behaviour' does not imply that the behaviours are necessarily pathological. It includes behaviours that are regarded as being entirely appropriate to any disorder that the subject may have and also those that are regarded as inappropriate because they seem to be either excessive or insufficient, or take an unusual form.

For individuals, illness behaviour includes both *traits* (for example, the lifelong tendency to have either a low or a high threshold for consulting doctors) and *state* (the behaviour at a particular time). There is evidence that such traits are acquired during childhood, by learning the patterns of illness behaviour that are characteristic of the culture or family, and these may have considerable value as defence mechanisms in later life. The majority of consultations, particularly in general practice, are determined to a considerable extent by current social and psychological factors. Thus many of the behaviours related to illness are not directly determined by disease processes but by the psychological and social state of the patient.

ABNORMAL ILLNESS BEHAVIOUR

The term **'abnormal illness behaviour'** is used to refer to illness behaviours which are

Table 12 *Aspects of illness behaviour*

1. symptom perception:	quality and intensity
2. evaluation of significance of symptoms (morbid risk)	
3. verbal communication:	complaint behaviour
4. non-verbal communication:	posture, gait, use of aids
5. consultation behaviour:	the numbers of medical and non-medical people consulted and the number of consultations
6. self-treatment:	number and frequency of medications
7. treatment compliance	
8. maintenance of customary activities and roles	
9. mood states:	including denial of negative affects

Source: Benjamin, S. (1984) The Effect of Illness Behaviour on the Apparent Relationship Between Physical and Mental Disorders. Reprinted with permission from *Journal of Psychosomatic Research* 28: 387–95. (Pergamon Press.)

regarded as inappropriate. This includes hypochondriasis, hysteria, factitious illness, and malingering; and also the denial of disease as, for example, in the case of a person who suffers a myocardial infarct but refuses to consult a doctor or to accept the need for treatment.

In the case of somatization, we have seen that there are a number of reasons why patients choose to focus on somatic rather than psychological components of illness. However, within the group of somatizers there are patients who will not accept either that they have psychological problems, or that they do not have physical disease that will account for their symptoms: in such cases, it seems reasonable to conclude that their illness behaviour is inappropriate, and to include them as examples of 'abnormal illness behaviour'.

HYPOCHONDRIASIS

Hypochondriasis is characterized by preoccupation with disease (either physical or mental). The term is used in several ways. Hypochondriacal **personality traits** include a lifelong tendency to be over-concerned with health, food fads, and physical fitness, as well as fear of illness. Hypochondriacal **symptoms** can take the form of ruminations, over-valued ideas, or delusions. (The term 'hypochondriacal' indicates only the content.) They have little diagnostic specificity. **Hypochondriacal delusions** can occur in almost any psychotic syndrome, including schizophrenia and dementia. When they occur in depressive illness they are usually secondary to the disorder of mood and related to ideas of pessimism and impending death. They may then include, for example, the patient's belief that he is dying of cancer, or in extreme cases the belief that he is already dead: such **nihilistic delusions** are a feature of **Cotard's syndrome**. However, 'hypochondriasis' is also used in a more specific way to refer to a syndrome, sometimes also called *'primary hypochondriasis'*, and this can be thought of as an example of abnormal illness behaviour.

Primary hypochondriasis

In this condition the characteristic feature is the presence of over-valued ideas about illness. The patient has rather vague but pervasive and persistent beliefs that he is suffering from an unidentified (usually physical) disease, despite the fact that he is likely to have been intensively investigated by many physicians and surgeons over a period of months or years with negative results. Depressive symptoms are either absent or inconsistent and subjective: for example, the patient may complain of poor appetite and sleep but the weight is steady and the spouse confirms that the patient is sleeping well. Perhaps because patients with this disorder regard themselves as physically ill, they are reluctant to see psychiatrists, and it appears to be an uncommon disorder in psychiatric practice but is more common in other medical settings.

Hypochondriasis can be thought of as 'chronic somatization'. Indeed, rather similar presentations are called **Briquet's syndrome** in the USA (also called 'somatization disorder' in the DSM III). By definition, this is a chronic disorder – continuing for at least several years – starting before the age of thirty, characterized by multiple physical complaints in the absence of relevant abnormal physical findings. At least fourteen of thirty-seven specified symptoms must be present. Although hysterical symptoms, as described below, are usually present, there are also prominent hypochondriacal features. Patients with this disorder are usually characterized by the weight of their medical records and their visits to many different departments of the hospital.

Dysmorphophobia

This is a more circumscribed condition which involves the belief that the body is deformed in some way; particularly the nose, but sometimes other parts of the body such as face, hair, breasts, or genitalia. The form of the belief is either an over-valued idea (see p. 30), which occurs most commonly in a setting of severe personality disorder; or a **delusion** (see p. 30), usually in the setting of schizophrenia. Patients with such beliefs commonly and repeatedly consult plastic surgeons but are unlikely to be helped by surgery.

HYSTERIA

This term too has been used in different ways and it is particularly important to clarify its meanings. 'Hysterical' is sometimes used by lay people to describe dramatic or histrionic behaviour: however, these latter terms are more appropriate. 'Hysterical' personality is an old-fashioned term for **histrionic personality** (see p. 64). The term 'hysteria' has also been used to refer to '**Briquet's syndrome**' (see p. 220), but these are a very different group. *These usages have nothing to commend them, and the word should be reserved for the following.*

Hysterical symptoms

Hysterical symptoms, which are *unconscious simulations of the signs of disease*, involve a disruption of normal functions, particularly those of the central nervous system, which are usually under voluntary control. Amongst the commonest are astasia–abasia (inability to stand and walk), fits, tremor, anaesthesia, paralysis, amnesia, and dysphonia. An important difference between hypochondriacal and hysterical symptoms is that patients with the former present with verbal complaints but the latter have primarily a non-verbal presentation.

Conversion (see p. 59) is the defence mechanism regarded as responsible for the production of simulated 'physical' symptoms, which are therefore called **conversion symptoms** (e.g. anaesthesias or pareses); **dissociation** (see p. 59) is the defence mechanism thought to result in the simulation of 'mental' symptoms (e.g. amnesia) and these are termed **dissociative symptoms**.

There are **two criteria** by which hysterical symptoms can be identified:

First, they mimic the phenomena of neurological and psychiatric disorders but *reflect the patient's concept of how such disorders present.* Thus a hysterical paralysis will not show the range of features of a typical upper or lower motor neurone lesion and an anaesthesia will fail to show the distribution of either a central or peripheral sensory loss: commonly a hysterical anaesthesia is of 'glove' or 'stocking' distribution on perhaps a single limb, rather than conforming to the distribution of a dermatome, a peripheral nerve, or the symmetrical distribution of a peripheral neuropathy.

Second, the function that appears to be lost *can often be demonstrated to be intact* in conditions which the patient does not associate with the symptom. For example, a leg which is 'paralysed' when the patient attempts to walk may show normal tone and reflexes in the relevant muscle groups and may be raised against gravity from the examination couch. Similarly a patient with hysterical dysphonia may phonate normally if coughing or laughing. It is often possible to remove hysterical symptoms by hypnotic suggestion and this may be helpful diagnostically but it is important to ensure that the underlying disorder is treated.

The patient is not conscious of either his simulation of symptoms or the reason for it. In this respect hysterical symptoms differ from **malingering** (see p. 222).

Hysterical symptoms, like hypochondriacal symptoms, have little diagnostic specificity. They can occur in almost any diagnostic setting and diagnosis depends on the identification of associated symptoms and signs. They occur particularly in the *affective disorders, personality disorders, and schizophrenia*. They also have an important association with *organic brain disease*, which results in the selective loss of inhibitory functions and the release of an underlying hysterical predisposition.

Transient hysterical symptoms are probably common in childhood but first onset becomes less common with increasing age. When appearing for the first time over the age of about forty they are particularly suggestive of a *neurological disorder*, such as disseminated sclerosis, and this requires investigation. *It is a common error to suppose that hysterical symptoms are incompatible with organic disease.*

Hysteria

Hysteria is a syndrome characterized by the presence of hysterical symptoms in the absence of any other demonstrable physical or psychiatric disorder. It should be possible to demonstrate that the symptoms have some adaptive value for the patient. For example, anxiety is relieved when the development of a symptom removes the patient from conflict.

> *A student who feared he might fail his exams developed a paralysis of his arm which prevented him from completing his course and sitting the exams.*

The primary cause of his symptom was anxiety about failure, and the symptom effectively relieved this. This relief of anxiety is therefore referred to as the **primary gain** of his illness. Because of their value, hysterical symptoms often result in a surprising lack of distress and the patient may pay little more than lip service to the wish to overcome his disability. French physicians have referred to this bland lack of concern as '**la belle indifférence**'. Subsequent use of the symptom to manipulate others, for example to be inappropriately cared for and financially supported, is called **secondary gain**: this is of course by no means confined to hysteria, and indeed may be a consequence of any physical or mental disorder.

Like other disorders, hysteria is diagnosed only if one can exclude conditions higher in the diagnostic hierarchy that might account for the hysterical symptoms. It should not therefore be made in the presence of organic disease of the brain, or depressive illness. It is a more convincing diagnosis if *gain* can be demonstrated.

Mass hysteria

Mass hysteria involves the epidemic spread of hysterical symptoms usually amongst adolescents and young adults who are in close proximity. There are generally several accounts of outbreaks, for example in schools or at 'pop' concerts, reported in the national press each year, sometimes masquerading as some new or mysterious disease. One interesting facet is the widespread vulnerability of the general population to the development of hysterical symptoms by suggestion, given 'favourable' conditions; they are by no means limited to a few 'weak' or abnormal personalities.

MALINGERING

Malingering closely resembles hysterical symptoms except that in the former the subject is both conscious that he is simulating the symptoms of disease and also of the purpose (the nature of the gain), for example this may be to get time off work or to avoid responsibility for some criminal action. In practice it can be extremely difficult to differentiate between them. Often they overlap, as in the case of a patient with a hysterical symptom who gradually acquires insight and then consciously maintains his symptom in order to 'save face'.

FACTITIOUS ILLNESS

Some patients produce the physical signs of disease, in order to deceive doctors, by self-injury or other subterfuge ('factitious' means artificial). They may present with many different signs, including rashes – **'dermatitis artefacta'**; infections, for example of the urinary tract or septic arthritis, due to the introduction of infected material; 'pyrexia of unknown origin' which results, for example, from putting the thermometer in a cup of tea; or lapses of consciousness due to the injection of insulin. Usually the patients are well aware of the deception but may have little or no insight into the motives for their behaviour. In this respect they differ from malingerers. Their motives in general are to maintain themselves in the role of invalidism, from which they derive comfort and care: they either fail to receive these normal human requirements from the more usual sources, or they are dependent personalities with excessive needs. Formal psychiatric assessment rarely leads to any diagnosis other than personality disorder.

Munchausen syndrome

Baron Munchausen was a fictional character who was famed for his fanciful stories. This form of factitious illness, sometimes referred to as 'hospital addiction', tends to present to surgical units, usually as an emergency, for example with signs of an 'acute abdomen' or with haematemesis, complete with blood-stained vomitus. The patient may give a polished history, which can include a false name and past medical history, and this often has the desired result of major surgery. Characteristically the patient bears the scars of many previous episodes. If the suspicions of staff are raised and the patient's history is checked by contacting other hospitals he is often found to have mysteriously left the ward and is never seen again. Such patients tend to roam the country, from one hospital to the next, using different names at each admission. They rarely wait to be seen by psychiatrists but if assessed appear to have grossly disturbed personalities.

Meadow's syndrome

Meadow's syndrome has also been described as 'Munchausen syndrome by proxy'. It consists of factitious illness in children caused by a parent, almost always the mother. Apart from demonstrating the abnormal needs of the mother it often results in serious physical and psychological abuse of the child. It has been described only recently but is thought to be relatively common and sometimes results in the child's death, for example due to hypoxia, caused by the mother, in order to induce fits. The range of presentations is as broad as those resulting from factitious illness in adults. It is important to be aware of this if you work in a paediatric unit.

THE MANAGEMENT OF 'ABNORMAL ILLNESS BEHAVIOUR'

1. Remember that anyone may have a physical disease, however obviously they show features of abnormal illness behaviour or an abnormal mental state. Frequently both physical and mental disorders occur in the same patient, so always look for evidence of both. All patients must be physically examined and, if necessary, investigated.

2. Carry out only those physical investigations which are essential and are indicated by the clinical history and examination. Remember that few physical diagnoses are made as a result of further investigations more than six months after the initial presentation. Repeated and inappropriate investigations add an iatrogenic component by reinforcing the patient's morbid ideas and behaviours, and also result in delay in initiating the appropriate psychiatric management.

3. At this stage it is essential to have a full psychiatric assessment and the purpose should be explained to the patient and his cooperation sought. (If the patient refuses, this is not an indication for repeating all the physical investigations!) The first step is to identify any associated mental illness, particularly an affective disorder, which should then be treated in the usual ways (see Chapters 7 and 10).

4. Patients with 'hysteria' or 'primary hypochondriasis' are difficult to treat because they don't regard themselves as mentally ill: often they show little motivation to change and pursue further inappropriate physical management. It is necessary for all doctors involved to work closely together and to take a consistent approach towards psychiatric management.

5. The cause of these disorders is primarily psychological and therefore the management should be psychological. However, the specific causes of a patient's illness will rarely be evident from the initial history: the effect of somatization is that the patient is unaware of underlying problems and relates all his difficulties to physical disease. Other factors will usually come to light only after taking detailed histories from the patient and others.

6. Insight-oriented psychotherapy can help the patient to face underlying problems and find more constructive ways to adjust to them. Behavioural psychotherapy can help the patient to give up inappropriate disability, by using a structured rehabilitation programme, and to change inappropriate attitudes and perceptions of himself through cognitive therapy.

7. Often inappropriate attitudes and behaviours are reinforced by family members who are over-solicitous. They must therefore be included in the treatment plan to modify the effect they have on the patient. Sometimes they have a particular need

to care for an invalid and are unable to tolerate the patient's recovery. Inappropriate medical 'treatment' can have a similar effect.

8. These disorders are generally resistant to treatment, perhaps because they are rarely seen by psychiatrists in the early stages and due to poor compliance by patients and/or their families. Those that fail to improve within the first year or two often run a chronic course subsequently.

FURTHER READING

Merskey, H. (1979) *The Analysis of Hysteria*. Baillière: London.
Trimble, H. R. (1981) *Post-traumatic Neurosis*. John Wiley: London.

PART 3
DISORDERS PECULIAR TO STAGES OF THE HUMAN LIFE CYCLE

16 / DISORDERS OF EARLY LIFE: MENTAL RETARDATION

The structure and functional efficiency of the brain can be affected from the moment of its earliest development, or it can become impaired by a variety of processes occurring in prenatal or early postnatal life. Mental retardation refers to the intellectual impairment to which the disorganization of cerebral function gives rise, and which is evident from early childhood. Obviously it is unlikely that intellectual functions alone are affected and other manifestations of brain disorder will be evident. High rates of social incompetence, problematic behaviour, and mental disorder have caused psychiatrists to be involved in the care of the mentally retarded.

There are numerous possibilities for damage and disorganization of the developing brain between conception and early postnatal life. Abnormalities might derive from either or both the parents' own genes – either dominant or recessive disorders; in the chromosomes of the foetus; in exposure of the foetus to intoxicants, drugs, alcohol; or to infections from viruses, bacteria, or protozoa; from mechanical injury by accident or by violence; from abnormalities of neuronal migration or of neural tube closure; from abnormal placentation or placental insufficiency; from multiple pregnancy; from prematurity and low birth weight with their attendant dangers; from traumatic birth with cerebral injury. Some of the aetiology will be multiple and additive. Mentally retarded persons will be encountered in all aspects of medical practice. Remember that they are also impaired in communication of their health care needs for both their physical and mental health and that they require special consideration, and usually the help of someone who knows them well to give a history.

EPIDEMIOLOGY

The distribution of measured intelligence has been so contrived as to distribute approximately normally around an IQ of 100 with a standard deviation of 15. On this basis about 2 per cent of the population would score 70 or less. Among this group of people are included many with obvious impairments of cerebral function, and these impairments are generally more obvious with decreasing IQ. Various ways of describing the severity of handicap have been used since 'moron', 'imbecile', and 'idiot' were abandoned. Currently **mental retardation**, *mild*, *moderate*, *severe*, and *profound*, is used. Nearly 80 per cent are in the mild group, and they mainly live unremarked in the community, though they will often have received special education. Progressively severe groups look more obviously impaired, are less likely to work and to live independently, and are more needy of special accommodation, support, and mental health care.

In actual practice, mental retardation is used as a category for human beings depending upon their capacity to meet the expectations of others in their social context rather than purely on the basis of measured intelligence so that social factors – such as poverty, over-crowding, poor nutrition – influence who is categorized. For administrative purposes only half of the total possible prevalence actually requires services. The most severely handicapped people, and those with epilepsy, also tend to die young.

Some obvious forms of disorder which are strongly predictive of mental impairment, such as *Down's syndrome*, or certain motor or speech difficulties, reveal the individual irrespective of his actual success or failure in social functioning, and are thus *stigmatizing*. Among the problems of mentally handicapped people are the prejudicial assumptions that are made about their potential level of functioning because of these stigmata.

MODES OF PRESENTATION

All doctors should be responsible for monitoring the mental competence of their patients and for ensuring that proper provision is available to those who seem intellectually impaired. The usual modes of presentation vary with chronological and developmental age as outlined above. Thus in the newborn period specific diagnosis of certain disease states is made both on the basis of routine chemical testing: PKU, thyroid deficiency (cretinism), or characteristic appearance; Down's (trisomy 21), Edward's syndrome (trisomy 18), confirmed by chromosome analysis. Apart from their abnormal appearance, it would be hard to say that these babies were 'retarded'. Some severe disorders are not apparent at birth – such as Hurler's syndrome – and some forms of cerebral palsy. The majority in the 'mild' group show no evidence of causative disease (see *Table 13*).

Table 13 *Some causes of mental retardation*

type of disorder	epidemiology	description
genetic disorders		
metabolic disorders		
(enzyme defects which create auto-intoxication or disorganization of tissues)		
• carbohydrates (galactosaemia)		
• fats		lipoidoses – gangliosidoses; Niemann-Pick; Gaucher's disease
• proteins (phenylketonuria)	1:10,000	fair hair, blue eyes, flapping hands (treatable)
multi-system abnormalities		
(autosomal dominants with variable manifestations)		
• tuberose sclerosis	1:10,000	infantile spasms; depigmented patches *adenoma sebaceum*, lesions of heart, brain, and kidney
• neurofibromatosis		*cafe-au-lait* patches in skin tumours beneath skin and in brain
chromosome disorders		
autosomes		
• trisomy 21 (Down's)	1: 600	small round head; large tongue; epicanthus, almond-shaped eyes; hypotonia; heart disease; gut atresias
• trisomy 18 (Edward's)	1: 8,000	
• part deletion of 5		*cri-du-chat* syndrome
sex chromosomes:		
• fragile X		frontal bossing, supra-orbital fullness, long thin face, large ears, small mandible, high-arched palate, macro-orchidism
• Klinefelter's syndrome XXY	1: 1,000	
• XYY syndrome	1: 1,000	
• multiple X	1: 1,000	
• Turner's syndrome XO	1:10,000	
infections		
rubella		cataracts; deafness; small eyes; congenital heart disease; 'autism'
cytomegalovirus		
toxoplasmosis		retinopathy; hydrocephalus, calcified lesions in brain
syphilis		depressed nasal bridge notched teeth
intoxications		
foetal alcohol syndrome		flat nasal bridge; 'poorly'; long philtrum, low birth weight
drugs (e.g. phenytoin)		hypertelorism; short nose

cont.

type of disorder	epidemiology	description
migrational, structural hydrocephalus spina bifida heterotopias (e.g. megalencephaly)		usually associated; handicaps from hydrocephalus may have epilepsy may be seen on CAT scan
malformations e.g. microcephaly		
mechanical anoxic placental – insufficiency – twins injury at parturition postnatal		'cerebral palsy' – spastic, ataxic dystonic, athetoid, hemiplegic

A further opportunity for diagnosis arises when a baby or toddler fails to reach its **developmental milestones** such as smiling, sitting, walking, talking, at an appropriate time:

6 weeks	social smiling
6–8 months	sits up
11–17 months	walks
about 1 year	talks words
about 2 years	small sentences

Subsequent enquiry may reveal a known disease – but it is not always possible to identify the cause of mental handicap. This could be because the family has expressed a unique recessive disease, or the child may have a hitherto unknown condition, or have suffered from the severe ill effects of some infectious illness which has been unnoticed. Certain of these children come to attention during routine clinic checks, or on school entry, or on proving in school to be quite incapable of making expected progress. Or else a predicament might arise which precipitates a mentally handicapped person into medical attention for the first time, perhaps because of a change in their mental health, their social circumstances, or their physical health. Extreme care should be taken by doctors, at such times of crisis, not to presume that a radical solution, such as hospitalization, is required when all that might be required is alternative accommodation.

MANAGEMENT

Parents

Making an appropriate diagnosis and telling the parents properly are the vital medical obligations.

Parents must be told as soon as mental retardation is recognized. They must be told together with careful exposition and a chance to question the doctor. The doctor should be skilled at telling. The parents' reaction is predictable and similar to bereavement: grief, shock, denial, anger, depression, and coming to terms. **Denial** (see p. 58) is the most persistent feature and may be the only form of accommodation for some people, but it means that the diagnosis of the handicap is, for them, always in doubt and the question of management and schooling will be opened repeatedly in a child's life. Multi-disciplinary teams for the assessment and management of mental retardation should exist in each District and all retarded children should be reviewed regularly by the team at the Development Assessment Centre. Parents might be encouraged to join *mutual support groups*, should be made knowledgeable about all the available *support services*, and should be encouraged to participate in improving their child's development to the best possible level for their child. Parents may require substantial support over many years and should repeatedly be given the chance to consider alternative management strategies, whether from home to community home or vice versa. Real independence means a move away from the parental home at some time.

Mentally retarded persons

There is an increased risk for:

1. Epilepsy – up to one-third of the population.
2. Physical handicap.
3. Oesophageal reflux.
4. Skeletal abnormalities.
5. Faecal and urinary incontinence.

These physical problems require skilled management, which is now often in the hands of the GP who visits the community home where they are resident.

There are also four sorts of behavioural abnormalities.

1. All forms of psychiatric disorder.
2. Hyperkinetic syndrome.
3. Self-injurious behaviour.
4. Socially inappropriate behaviour.

Schizophrenia and **depression** also occur in the retarded, but their classic symptoms may be modified by the retarded patient's capacity to express them. Significant change in the behaviour requires the attention of the consultant psychiatrist in mental retardation. These disorders are treated with the same drugs as would be used for non-retarded people, but they must be carefully monitored because of the patient's difficulty in explaining side-effects.

The **hyperkinetic syndrome** is a restless, joyless, endless pursuit of stimuli from which no satisfaction appears to be gained, and very little learned. Water play may be enjoyed, but children are otherwise highly distractible. Their mood is dysphoric and if baulked their reactions tend to be irritable and aggressive. It is aggravated by sedative drugs especially barbiturates and benzodiazepines.

It must be differentiated from the 'over-active child syndrome', or *attention deficit disorder*.

Self-injurious behaviour ranges from self-slapping to severe self-destructive biting or head-banging, which can form a pattern of continual self-stimulation, combined with rocking, finger-waving and flapping, and 'hand regard' (the child tends to inspect his hands). This is a common problem, and causes much distress to parents and care-givers. Solutions to the problem are not easy, but behaviour therapy and sedatives are usually tried. The *Lesch–Nyhan syndrome* is notably associated with self-mutilation.

Treatment

Problematic behaviour may be reduced by providing decent homes and normal surroundings. Socially unacceptable behaviour and self-injurious behaviour may need to be 'trained' with *behavioural techniques* specially modified for the handicapped. *Drugs* may be required for retarded people, just as for normal people, but care must be taken to observe *side-effects* to which retarded people may be specially susceptible, and which may be manifested by alterations in behaviour.

Epilepsy is common and requires sensitive treatment to avoid over-sedation or producing excitement. Certain forms of epilepsy – drop attacks, persistent infantile spasms, myoclonus, or status epilepticus – may be very demanding of care, and hospital provision may be required from time to time.

Placement

For a variety of reasons, some parents do not have their mentally handicapped children at home. Current policy is community placement in home-like settings. Certain special forms of education – for those who are both deaf and blind, or for autistic children may be arranged in boarding schools through the Education Authority on a special statement of need for special education to which all children with educational problems are entitled.

Mentally handicapped people should be encouraged in their personal growth towards independent living, though this may require some supervision. Some hard-to-manage mentally handicapped persons may require some supervision and rather special care to replace the older facility, which was largely a relatively benign abandonment in a long-stay hospital.

Services are provided by nurses, psychologists, care staff, and teachers with help from general practitioners, consultant specialists in handicap, paediatricians, and physiotherapists.

FURTHER READING

Kirman, B. and Bicknell, J. (1975) *Mental Handicap*. Edinburgh: Churchill Livingstone.

17 / CHILDHOOD AND ADOLESCENCE

THE VICISSITUDES OF CHILD-REARING

The ordinary mother, hoping for a child, has a notion of what the child will be like and what her relationship to the child will be, of how she will be because of the child, and how the child's father will *help* her. These fantasies generally accord with reality or they are smoothly modified with the arrival of the child, for instance with respect to the sex of her child. But for a variety of reasons there may be painful differences between what was hoped for and what occurs.

These differences are at their most obvious with the birth of a physically abnormal child or a mentally handicapped child, but at all stages of development and with each successive period of childhood, problems may arise from within the emergent child, or within the relationship between parent and child, or from the intrusions of a hostile or depriving environment. These are the sorts of problems that arise in child and adolescent psychiatry.

Consider first the mother's mental state and her circumstances at the time of the child's birth. Maternal depression is common, especially in women who are poorly supported by their spouse and those with several small children. Early separations because of sickness in mother or child create further difficulties in establishing a good relationship.

Vulnerable mothers are helped by having a person to support them through their labour and by spending ample time with their baby. The relationship is two-sided, and attributes of the baby, his *temperament*, will interact with those of his parents. Temperament can be 'difficult' (an irregular biological rhythm, withdrawn, unhappy, intensely reacting baby), or 'easy' (the reverse features), or just 'slow to warm up' with the parent. Mostly parents adapt or cope with their problems but *crying* and *sleeplessness* may become so intrusive as to disrupt family life. *Feeding* may be affected by maternal anxiety which is further enhanced by failure leading to *failure to thrive*. These issues may disrupt the process of *attachment* between mother and child by which they would form a close and secure relationship. They require prompt attention through understanding the parent's situation, explanation, and retraining the child to more normal habits while supporting the parent's capacity to 'parent' rather than taking over their role.

TODDLERS

Crawling, creeping, bottom-shuffling, and walking provide the opportunity to explore the environment and its objects. But this inquisitiveness may be too intense for mother's comfort leading to problems of control. 'Disobedient' and 'over-active' are parents' descriptions of how they experience their child. Feeding difficulties may reach severe dimensions with *faddiness* threatening to restrict diet severely. When confronted the child may exhibit *temper trantrums* which can be frightening to parents because of their intensity and the total loss of control that then ensues. Certain children with difficult temperaments and developmental delay may experience unusually severe frustration, and careful evaluation of their developmental status is advisable. Poverty of behaviour, or *non-emergence of expected behaviour*, is also a source of complaint. Obvious delay in the achievement of milestones suggests global mental handicap, but specific failures of development are also seen.

Early infantile autism

Sequentially, from earliest childhood, a *lack of responsiveness, cuddliness, and communicativeness via gaze response, babbling, and speech*, taking its onset before thirty months, suggests **infantile autism**, which is characterized by *failure of communication, socialization, and symbolic play*.

Pervasive developmental disorders

Other disorders such as **Asperger's syndrome** and **disintegrative psychoses** may not be evident before thirty months: the latter is likely to be the psychiatric aspect of severe, and sometimes relentlessly progressive, brain disease. Neurological impairment is more clearly the basis of acquired aphasia in childhood but more subtle deficits are seen in the **receptive or expressive dysphasias**. Schooling problems develop later and affect *reading, spelling, and arithmetic*, often quite specifically. In early childhood these children may show *delay in acquiring speech*.

SCHOOL AGE

Although bowel and bladder control are acquired by 90 per cent of children by school age, referrals for treatment tend to be delayed until forced by circumstance. **Nocturnal enuresis**, with or without daytime wetting, is not necessarily a psychiatric disorder but rates of behavioural problems are increased especially in girls and in association with daytime wetting. Enuresis has been called **primary** where there has never been established dryness or **secondary** where there is a lapse, but there seems little to distinguish these types by aetiology or association of outcome. Child psychiatrists tend to be referred the more obdurate cases and the more difficult and disturbed patients.

Most children have achieved bowel control by two and a half years. **Faecal soiling** (encopresis) continuing through school age is not normal and is socially unacceptable. Fewer than 1 per cent soil by adolescence. Sometimes a physical factor such as a painful fissure may originate the disturbance which persists as an aspect of child–parent distress. But the more coercive and rigid patterns of potty training provide the occasional opportunity for stubborn battles over opening the bowels leading to retention and overflow and a source of child power. Bear in mind the possibility of missed Hirschsprung's disease – variable lengths of lower gut segment without ganglia which remain atonic and preclude proper defaecation.

School refusers and truants

The characteristics of school refusers and truants underline the differences between the two largest groups of disorders in child psychiatry: the emotional disorders and the conduct disorders.

The families of **school refusers** are smaller, more neurotic, and generally achieved high standards at school. School refusers are usually more concerned about not leaving home than not going to school. Health care concerns, complaints of illness, are often used to secure staying at home. Younger children normally 'refuse' school quite suddenly and dramatically out of the blue, prompted by some incident. Older adolescents school refuse more gradually, clocking up time off over longer periods of time. School refusers mainly stay at home. Rates of depression are high in school refusers and the alternative term **school phobia** describes the frantic emotional state of tears and panic which appears when such children are forced to attend.

The **truants** come from larger indisciplined homes with parental absence and poor achievement. Truants are neither at home nor at school and are at risk of other conduct disorder.

Emotional disorders

Some of the emotional disorders of childhood severely impair the lives of the children and their families.

DEPRESSION

Depression can occur in children of all ages though it increases sharply in frequency towards puberty. Sadness, apathy, anorexia, anxiety, and slowing up of thought and action occur. Children feel hopeless about the future and lose their self-esteem; they grieve and mourn things, persons, and prestige which they may have lost. **Suicide** is very rare before puberty but does happen. **Self-poisoning**, however, is more usually an impulsive act which draws attention to an unsatisfactory situation rather than to depressed mood. Rarely do **specific phobias** become a problem though fears of the dark, certain animals, and death are universal during development and may obtrude in sleep disorders or in anxiety states and depression. Anxiety varies in its expression in development; it may be *experienced somatically*, usually as a state of tension in muscles leading to complaints of *pains in head, abdomen, or limbs*, or be more evident behaviourally in the disruption of previously acquired skills, impairing concentration and social behaviour.

CONVERSION HYSTERIA

Conversion hysteria is a term which is likely to be superseded because of its archaic implications. It suggests a variety of degrees of illness behaviour in the absence of apparent disease. Some symptoms, such as recurrent abdominal pain, may be somatic manifestations of tension, others such as *limb paralysis, unusual gaits, and aphonia*, may arise through inadvertent over-concern with a minor symptom. The resultant concern and cosseting might meet a psychological need in the child or his family, and the resulting medical involvement might be hard to withdraw from gracefully. Real disease may be overlooked if its presentation is unusual and it arises in a fraught predicament.

CONDUCT DISORDER

Conduct disorder describes a variety of problematic behaviours to which most children are given, to an extent, but may be extreme in degree and persistent in manifestation. The conduct disorders may occur in groups – *socialized* – or as lonesome pursuits – *unsocialized*. The children may also experience various degrees of emotional disorder. Aggressiveness, stealing, lying, cheating, and fire-setting are among the principal issues involved. The children appear rude, surly, or cheeky at interview; often protesting indifference to their fate and unconcern about their offences. Occasionally they might seem over-polite, charming, or eager to please. Such children have usually been brought up in depriving environments and with poor models of social behaviour at home, at school, or in their neighbourhood.

Long-term prognosis is generally poor with delinquency, high rates of adult psychiatric disorder, and criminal behaviour. The children with conduct disorders are also often regarded as over-active children who show marked attention deficit in school or even in the clinic. There is a marked overlap between what some people call conduct disorder and others regard as over-activity. One issue is to what extent is the problem intrinsic or reactive to aspects of its environment, another concerns drug treatment since certain over-active children respond to methylphenidate, amphetamine, or even to amitriptyline, which are not useful in conduct disorders.

TICS

Tics in children are commonplace and may be shown by 20 per cent of children transiently at some stage. More persistent *tics, usually eye blinks, or head jerks* may be precipitated by acute stress or a vulnerable background. Severe tics associated with grunts, obscene vocalization, or gestures onsetting between two and fifteen years, around ten years, form the **Gilles de la Tourette's syndrome**, a much rarer (1 in 2,000) event. The disorder may be socially incapacitating.

Child abuse, deprivation and neglect

Managing a child is difficult and, at times, frustrating. If the rewards are low and the stress high, adults caring for the child may not be able to cope. In such situations they may be very coercive to the child, limiting his freedom, physically assaulting him, tormenting, abusing, maltreating, or misfeeding him. Abuse may be a sudden excess of violence, or in some parents with severe personality deviations it is very prolonged, systematic, and sadistic.

Physical abuse is more likely to occur to young children of pre-school age, especially those with such depressed, young, immature, or unseasoned parents. Separations and sickness in the child may add to the risk. Poverty, disharmony, single status, and a background of violence in the parents' up-bringing increase the risk of abuse. *All doctors must recognize the possibilities of deliberate harm being done to children*, including the presentations of factitious illnesses for which bogus evidence is provided and which lead to painful and serious investigations, and to potentially dangerous treatment (see p. 000).

Sexual abuse is more likely to occur to older girls. The perpetrator is usually an older male, often a stepfather or living-in male friend of the mother's.

Emotional and physical abuse and neglect are often associated with poor physical growth. This, once called '**deprivation dwarfism**', is largely due to the family policies controlling the amount of food actually made available to the child. The children grow on adequate diets in hospital or in care. All doctors must be suspicious about possible child abuse, and be prepared to allow police, social worker, and NSPCC investigation of the case if they suspect abuse of any sort. *It is crucial to note the evidence and to take direct action to secure a **place of safety** if the child is in danger.*

ADOLESCENCE

Sexual changes of puberty, the growth spurt, and chronology, go to make up 'adolescence'. But adolescence has its developmental components; the realization of **personal identity** (self-hood) and the subsequent **separation from parents**, the need for **attachment** to others, the need to become **financially self-supporting**, and the wish for **heterosexual relationships**. The pangs created by meeting these needs colour the sorts of issues that adolescents raise and may contribute to the sharp increase in referrals which comes with adolescence.

Adolescent psychiatry refers to a series of problems, seen both in child psychiatry and in adult psychiatry, with puberty being a fulcrum for change in the modes of presentation. At interview the adolescent must be given the opportunity to present himself and he may benefit from the supportive history from a parent – although he may resent it.

Particularly frequent disorders of adolescence include *anorexia nervosa, self-poisoning and attempted suicide, drug-taking and experimentation, depression, and schizophrenia.* Special in-patient treatment facilities are available. They have a variety of treatment orientations and usually include aspects of group living which promote the general goals of adolescence described above.

Anorexia nervosa

Pre-pubertal anorexia nervosa (see p. 209) does occur. It usually shades in from extreme food faddiness, and oppositional behaviour about eating. Parents are usually heavily drawn in to the behaviours and rituals surrounding the child's self-deprivation of food. Anorexia nervosa becomes more frequent with puberty and seems to serve as a device for denying growing up into a potentially sexual being.

HISTORY-TAKING AND INTERVIEWING

In child and adolescent psychiatry the situation is usually that persons in care and control of the child – often the mother – want the doctor to understand how the child is unsatisfactory. The story will be told as if it is a medical story and you, because of your training, are most likely to hear it as a medical story. But it is not necessarily a medical story in the usual sense. A complaint is being filed. The sources of the complaint may indeed stem from some intrinsic fault within the child, the child may have a disease or an illness, or the child, because of previously faulty management or unsatisfactory experiences, may now be expressing his distress in one of the ways which, at his state of development, is open to him. But equally, the complaint being made might say more about how the child is being perceived or being managed by the complainant. In any event, your witness cannot be detached, since she feels that she is responsible, in one way or another, for the situation that she wishes to describe. This makes the interview extremely taxing and, since the interview is also potentially a therapeutic intervention, it needs to be managed with extreme care. A first interview is likely to take at least an hour.

Since the complaint is often being made somewhat reluctantly and prompted by others, it is necessary to spend time *engaging* the complainant.

To do this, she must be heard first in telling what she wishes to say and listened to with warmth and empathy. What precisely is the problem behaviour or in what way is the child failing her expectations? When did the problem first arise and why has it come to the fore now, and how does she come to be here? All too often referrals to child psychiatrists are somewhat furtive because the referring agent did not clearly indicate that a referral to a psychiatrist was being made, nor what the purpose of the referral was.

Who is experiencing the problem most acutely? Where and in what situation does it manifest itself? Who else suffers? What has been said about it: by teachers to the parents, by neighbours, or by other children? Try to clarify precisely what the parent means by apparently technical terms such as 'temper tantrums', 'depression', 'sleeplessness', 'naughtiness', 'failure to talk', or even 'bed-wetting'. (Only after painful, prolonged probing did a mother explain that a child, referred for 'bed-wetting', would stand on his bedside locker and hose the bed down with his pee.)

Among the complaints will emerge the sorts of solutions which have been attempted. It is important to note what has been tried, how sensibly, and for how long these attempts were made.

In what context does the complaint occur? Is it continuous or sporadic, is it worsening or static or improving? Has the referral itself already affected the behaviour? Is the problem limited to the home or does it extend to school and the neighbourhood? Can some people (one of the parents, for example) cope much better with it or even scarcely perceive it?

It is next necessary to *understand the situation of the child*. This is best done historically, or developmentally, by building up a picture of the whole family. First the *current situation*: who is living with the child and where do they live? Who are the child's natural mother and father? Where are they now?

Draw a picture of the family using a *family tree* like the one a geneticist might use (see p. 70).

Ask what pregnancies the mother has had, where the children were born, where they are now, and how each one is faring. Name the children and obtain their birthdays. Briefly outline their development before turning to the details of the referred child. How does this child fit into the family? Are both parents and both sets of grandparents alive? Where are they? Have any significant family members died? When and how did they die? Many families will have been reconstituted as a result of illegitimacy, death, divorce, or broken common-law relationships. A substitute parent may have brought his own children into the home.

As this history emerges, it will do so with *feelings* and with expressed emotions. These must be acknowledged, empathized with, and noted. The emergent history may create tensions or division or disagreements between the informants. You will see how they actually function in dealing with the problem of handling the interview. This may be revealing.

The *emotional cost* of the child will become apparent, what trouble it was to conceive, to bear, to raise, to nurse through illness. The child may have threatened the family in a variety of ways – by being less than entirely welcome, by threatening the health of the mother, by 'causing' her depression, by failing to give the expected sort of reward, by revealing the parents' inability to provide the parenting they had hoped to give – or by being severely ill and 'threatening to die'.

In the course of raising their children, parents re-experience some of their own childhood traumas and so their relationships as children themselves may be touched on at this time. Their own place in their own sibships may reveal that they were obliged to parent their siblings or that they never dealt with a baby until they had one themselves.

Out of all this, the particular *predicament* of the child will begin to emerge, his own particular unique life situation. Where he stands today, in the context of his own family.

THE EXAMINATION OF THE CHILD

The examination which follows is based on one developed at the Park Hospital, Oxford. It may be possible with older children to follow something like the same procedure as used to examine an adult's mental state but, particularly in young children, formal examination of the mental state is impossible. Every opportunity should be taken to observe the child's behaviour and this should be recorded systematically and objectively. Avoid global clinical impressions. Do not forget to obtain the *child's view of the situation*, including his likes, dislikes, and hopes for the future. Establishing a useful conversation with the child requires you to show warmth, interest, and respect for the child. Approach emotive topics gradually and carefully and use language that is appropriate (including use of play material for younger children).

When you require the child's cooperation ask for it directly. Do not ask *'Would you like to . . . ?'*, because if the child would not like to, you are sunk.

THE MENTAL STATE

General behaviour

> Dress and appearance.
> (*Is the child appropriately and cleanly clad?*)
> Parent–child interaction and separation.
> (*Do the parents seem able and willing to manage the child; was there a tantrum on separation?*)
> Emotional responsiveness and relationship with the doctor.
> (*Describe your own feelings about the quality of your interaction with the child.*)
> Habitual mannerisms
> (*Does the child have tics, or recurrent speech, or stereotypic mannerisms?*)
> Description of the course of interview.
> (*What went on: drawing, play, tears, temper?*)

Anxiety and mood

> Signs of tension and sadness:
> (*include facial expression, apprehension, tearfulness*)
> Whether preoccupied by fears, worries, depressing thoughts.

Whether restless, disinhibited, assertive, aggressive.
Whether apathetic, withdrawn, or shy.

Talk (form)

Spontaneity, flow.
(Is speech painfully difficult to elicit or does it flow ceaselessly; or is the flow and exchange of talk normal?)
Defects of prosody, articulation, or sentence structure.
Coherence.
(Can you follow what is being said, or does it lose its point?)

Talk (content)

Attention or persistence.
(Whether easily distracted; whether interrupted by hallucinatory experience.)
Degree and duration of interest in topics, activities, or objects.
(Does the child flit ceaselessly from one topic to another?)
Spontaneous interruptions of attention.
(Is speech suddenly arrested, the point lost?)

Activity level

Gross activity.
(In particular, whether 'over-active' or 'hyperkinetic'.)

Intellectual function

Rough assessment of reading level, spelling, arithmetic, writing, general knowledge.
Write name and address, draw a man, copy triangle, diamond, cross, and circle.
*Ideally, **testing by a clinical or educational psychologist** should be arranged including assessment of basic intellectual ability, educational attainments, and specific learning problems.*
*A **school report** about progress and general behaviour should always be obtained or, for younger children, an account from nursery school or play-group.*

TREATMENT

Discussion, clarification, diagnosis, reassurance

Most problems of child behaviour do not come to doctors and even fewer are referred to specialists. In the ordinary practice of medicine the chance to ventilate parental concern, seek guidance and clarification in problems of upbringing, or even face up to the ordeal of specialist referral will at times, of themselves, provide a basis for orienting to a problem or provide reassurance.

Psychotherapies

Various strategies for exploring the situation which has arisen, for providing support and for achieving some understanding and resolving problems in relationships and reducing stress. Allowing a child to talk, explain his feelings, confess, relieve guilt may be helpful. Young children need a comfortable place to play, to enact their distress to the therapist. For adolescents groups of various sorts are used. **Family therapy** entails working with the whole 'living group' to illustrate and clarify the sorts of interpersonal reactions and tensions which exist and to work out better ways of functioning as a family.

Behaviour therapies

Variously used to alter behaviour by eliminating unwanted and encouraging wanted behaviours – whether in encopresis, in conduct disorders, or in anorexia nervosa.

ENCOPRESIS

In encopresis after a physical examination to exclude organic factors such as Hirschsprung's disease or anal fissure, a baseline must be established of the exact frequency and the nature of the soiling. Attention should be paid to ensuring bulk in the diet. Agreeing to eat bran may indicate a willingness to change the habit. Stool softeners and laxatives can be helpful. Rewards are given for appropriately going to the toilet – stars or praise – and for defaecation. Soiling itself is cleaned up and otherwise ignored. Careful monitoring by 'the therapist' provides necessary rewards to the parents and to the child. The chart should be used as a basis for discussion and for clarification of the treatment.

ENURESIS

In enuresis a similar policy of charting and rewarding can be used providing it is closely monitored. Failing this the 'bell and pad' mechanism can be tried (see p. 102) if adequate explanation is given to adequately motivated people. Given these, success rates are high (80 per cent) but they cannot be presumed. The principle is that if the child wets the bed urine forms a connection between two metal plates otherwise separated by a cotton pad. A bell rings. The child is then aroused and may void urine in the lavatory. The reason this works is unclear. It is however *vital* to ensure that the family rehearse the procedure properly. Sporadic, and occasionally long-lasting, relief can be given by using amitriptyline or imipramine in doses of 25–50 mg at night. The effects are usually dramatic but ephemeral.

Drug treatment

Drugs are used sparingly and thoughtfully in child psychiatry, respecting our ignorance of their effects upon the immature brain, upon the developing child, and with regard to the problems relating to some of their side-effects.

ANTIDEPRESSANTS

Amitriptyline	depression
Imipramine	phobic states
	enuresis
Chlormipramine	obsessional states

MAJOR TRANQUILLIZERS

Chlorpromazine	schizophrenia
Haloperidol	Tourette's syndrome
	calming disturbed behaviour
	anorexia nervosa

STIMULANTS

Methylphenidate	{ hyperkinetic syndrome
Amphetamine	{ over-active child syndrome

LAXATIVES, STOOL SOFTENERS

Senna preparations	encopresis
Stool softening gels	retention of faeces

Placements

DAY HOSPITAL ATTENDANCE

This is useful to allow detailed observation, provide for longer duration treatments, allow certain systematic therapies to be given (play therapy, for example), and to provide relief to strained relationships.

IN-PATIENT ADMISSION

Admission to paediatric ward or to a specialist child psychiatry unit extends these possibilities.

RECEPTION INTO CARE

This may be needed for children whose problem behaviour brings them into severe conflict at home or in trouble with the authorities.

FURTHER READING

Rutter, M. (1975) *Helping Troubled Children*. Harmondsworth: Penguin.
Rutter, M. (1972) *Maternal Deprivation Reassessed*. Harmondsworth: Penguin.

18 / SEXUAL AND REPRODUCTIVE DISORDERS

This chapter will be concerned with human sexual development throughout the life cycle. We shall therefore start with gender identity disorders, since these take their onset in the pre-school child, and pass on to consider homosexuality since it appears that events in childhood and adolescence are of some aetiological importance.

The second part of the chapter considers the common sexual problems of adult life, with emphasis on their aetiology and assessment. The section on paraphilias is short, since these seldom request medical treatment.

The third part of the chapter considers disorders related to reproduction, once more arranged in sequence from menstrual disorders, through pregnancy to the puerperium, and ending with disorders relating to the menopause.

DISORDERS OF EARLY DEVELOPMENT

Gender identity disorders

A person's *gender identity* refers to his or her awareness of being male or female, and *gender role* refers to the public expression of such an identity in clothing and behaviour. The aetiology of gender identity disorders is not fully understood. Most of those with such disorders are anatomically, hormonally, and genetically indistinguishable from other members of their biological gender. It has been suggested that prenatal endocrine influences on the developing brain may be important, and it can be shown that if androgens are given to a pregnant rhesus monkey her female infant will behave as a male. However, hormonal abnormalities have not been demonstrated in humans. Patterns of early rearing are likely to be important: the 'assigned sex for rearing' refers to being called 'John', dressed as a boy, and given a toy aeroplane; or called 'Jane', dressed as a girl, and given a cuddly doll. However, once more, the parents of transsexual patients usually deny that they brought the child up in an unusual way. The available evidence suggests that the gender-related behaviours acquired in the pre-school child are critically important in determining later satisfaction with gender role: any deviant patterns learned before going to school tend to be reinforced rather than disturbed by experience at the infant's school. Minor degrees of *gender dysphoria* are relatively common at school, with effeminate boys stigmatized as 'pansies', and masculine girls ambivalently regarded as 'tomboys'. It seems clear that a developing child needs a satisfactory role-model with whom he or she can identify if an appropriate gender identity is to be developed.

Transsexualism

This rare disorder is characterized by the person's persistent sense of discomfort and inappropriateness about their anatomic sex together with a wish to be rid of their genitals and to live as a member of the opposite sex. These feelings take their origin in childhood. The patient wishes to be a member of the other sex and dresses in clothes of the desired sex without sexual arousal, but with a feeling of relief. The patients greatly dislike their genitalia, and request surgical removal of them. The idea of 'really' being a member of the other sex is an example of an *over-valued idea*. Men outnumber women by about three to one: the prevalence in England is 1 in 34,000 men and 1 in 108,000 women.

MEDICAL RELEVANCE

Such patients present to doctors requesting hormone treatment or sex-change operations. They should be referred to a specialist clinic. Sometimes previously normal patients can acquire all the features of the syndrome during a psychotic illness, most usually a schizophrenia. There is a strong association with depressive illness, and suicidal ideas and self-mutilation are common.

Homosexuality

It is a mistake to suppose that people are either homosexual or heterosexual, since many people are capable of either form of sexual activity. Figures from the USA suggest that approximately one-third of men have a homosexual experience leading to orgasm at some time in their lives, most usually during adolescence, to be compared with about 6 per cent of women. Only about 3 per cent of men and 2 per cent of women have an exclusively homosexual experience.

Homosexual behaviour becomes much more common in conditions where the other sex is not available, such as prison; and it is common in those few societies where it is not stigmatized.

AETIOLOGY

Genetic factors are of some importance, since the MZ concordance for homosexuality is higher than the DZ concordance. *Endocrine influences* during pregnancy may determine gender behaviour in childhood, as mentioned above. The importance of *parental role-models* has also been stressed: homosexual patients coming for treatment typically report disturbed relationships with the same-sex parent. A boy who has been unable to identify with a weak or absent father, and whose nascent sexuality has been influenced by an over-protective mother, may be expected to have difficulties in acquiring sexual feelings about women. At about puberty a developing child must bring three things together: his or her gender identity, the developing capacity for sexual responsiveness, and the ability to develop close interpersonal relationships. Thus effeminate boys are likely to develop a homosexual orientation at puberty, and those who are unconfident about their masculinity may be unattractive to the opposite sex, so that early attempts at striking up relationships are painful. The same boys may be more than usually attractive to males seeking 'unmasculine partners', so that the adolescent enters the rather less competitive homosexual world.

Similar arguments apply to the acquisition of female homosexual behaviour, although here additional factors might be fear or disgust at the sexual behaviour of men ('heterophobia'), deliberate avoidance of men as part of a feminist stance, and poor performance in heterosexual situations.

MEDICAL RELEVANCE

The most important aspect of male homosexuality that involves doctors is the high prevalence of sexually transmitted diseases. Up to 16 per cent of patients with sexually transmitted diseases attending clinics in London have been found to be homosexual, but much lower rates are found elsewhere in the UK. Anal, oral, and genital lesions occur.

Until recent scares about AIDS, the enormous number of partners made recurrent infections likely. (Female homosexuals do not present the same problem of frequent short-lived relationships as homosexual men and their forms of sexual behaviour do not put them at such high risk; they therefore do not present with more sexually transmitted diseases).

Although anxiety and depression have been reported frequently among homosexual men, there appears to be a truly increased prevalence only for those without a stable relationship. This inability to form lasting relationships may be indicative of interpersonal problems which go well beyond the patient's sexual orientation.

SEXUAL DISORDERS OF ADULT LIFE

The commonest forms of sexual disorders are those in which normal sexual activity is desired but not being achieved. **Primary sexual problems** are those which have been present since the onset of sexual activity, **secondary sexual problems** develop after a period of adequate sexual function.

Epidemiology

Few reliable statistics are available. One area with an established sexual problems' clinic serving a defined area reports an annual consultation rate of 64 per 100,000 at risk; but data from surveys suggest that the prevalence of sexual problems is very much higher than this.

Sexual intercourse

Intercourse can be divided into three phases: *desire, arousal, and orgasm*, all under different innervation. Sexual interest is mainly under limbic control, arousal mainly under the control of parasympathetic (cholinergic and peptidergic) systems, while orgasm is mainly under sympathetic (adrenergic) control. The various sexual problems which arise can most easily be classified under these three headings.

Both men and women can experience disorders of sexual desire. Problems with arousal lead in the man to erectile difficulties and in the woman to lack of lubrication and general sexual unresponsiveness. Difficulties in the orgasmic phase cause premature or retarded ejaculation in the man and orgasmic dysfunction in the woman.

Male sexual problems

LACK OF INTEREST

This can occur as a primary complaint, often accompanied by general anxiety about sexual intercourse both between one individual and another and also at different times of life. Although psychological factors such as inhibitions from the past or relationship problems in the present are often important, organic factors may also be present. An increase in prolactin secretion which may be due to a cerebral tumour will cause loss of libido in both men and women. The ratio of testosterone to oestrogen in both sexes affects desire; higher testosterone levels stimulate it.

ERECTILE FAILURE

This may be primary or secondary.

Primary erectile difficulties arise because of inhibitions about sex or difficulties experienced in early sexual encounters. There may rarely be a basic organic defect.

Secondary erectile problems may arise after occasional failures due to alcohol, fatigue, and so on, and this may lead to anxiety about the ability to perform, causing further failure and thus creating a vicious circle.

Organic factors may also be important and it has been estimated that up to 85 per cent of men with erectile difficulties have some physical problems, although even where these are present anxiety about performance is likely to make things worse. *Diabetes* and *multiple sclerosis* sometimes present with erectile failure, and problems are likely to increase with age. There are definite physiological ageing changes affecting the strength of the erection and the ease with which it is obtained; further impairment may result from *atherosclerotic narrowing* of penile arteries. Where there has been serious illness, for example a coronary, the patient may also be *anxious* about the adverse effects of the exertion needed in intercourse.

PREMATURE EJACULATION

This is common, affecting up to 6 per cent of all men at some time in their sexual lives. It often arises after initial sexual experiences in situations where intercourse has to be hurried, for example the back of a car or in the parental home, and is then perpetuated by the anxiety that it will recur. Occasionally it can occur after a period of normal control, perhaps after a traumatic experience of some kind.

RETARDED EJACULATION

This is very much less common. It often occurs after medication, especially with tricyclic antidepressants, but it may also occur in inhibited men who can usually masturbate normally to ejaculation.

RETROGRADE EJACULATION

This is ejaculation of semen upwards into the bladder instead of externally, and commonly follows prostatectomy, both transurethral and intra-abdominal.

PAINFUL EJACULATION

This is a rare complaint possibly due to infection and painful muscle spasm.

Female sexual problems

LACK OF DRIVE

In women this is often due to inhibitions passed on from parents and society in general, or from unfortunate past experiences such as rape or incest. It may also be caused by increased prolactin levels in the blood, and by a diminished testosterone/oestrogen ratio as in men. Many women experience different levels of desire at different phases of the menstrual cycle, and many lose interest in sex after childbirth for a time, probably due to a combination of factors. These may include changing hormonal patterns, dyspareunia after episiotomy, changes in the general marital relationship, and fear of further pregnancy.

LACK OF AROUSAL
(GENERAL SEXUAL UNRESPONSIVENESS)

Arousal in the woman, as in the man, causes vasodilatation of the blood supply to the genital area. In the man this results in the cavernous sinuses of the penis filling with blood, and in the woman produces a cuff of dilated blood vessels encircling the lower part of the vagina. Some of the fluid from these vessels goes as a transudate into the vagina producing the lubrication. A woman may not particularly desire sex but if adequately stimulated by a sensitive partner may be able to respond, lubricate, and reach orgasm. Inability to respond may be due to inhibitions from learned attitudes or past experiences, or to adverse conditions in the present, including difficulties in the marital relationship. Any kind of anxiety connected with the situation, for example intercourse in the parental home or anxiety about the baby, may affect her ability to relax and respond. Inadequate stimulation from an inexperienced lover is often a cause of early difficulties. Lack of arousal will in all these situations cause dyspareunia (see below) because of lack of lubrication, and this can easily produce a vicious circle leading to avoidance of all sexual encounters. This commonly occurs after childbirth.

Arousal in the woman may also be affected as in the man, by drugs and neurological and vascular disease, and in post-menopausal women lubrication may be diminished because of lowered oestrogen levels.

DYSPAREUNIA

Pain on intercourse from any cause will inhibit arousal and may be caused by *vaginal infections, pelvic inflammatory disease, endometriosis, episiotomy, and by operations affecting the cervix*, which may prevent the elevation of the uterus out of the pelvis which occurs in normal intercourse, leading to buffeting of the cervix by the penis.

ORGASMIC DYSFUNCTION

About 10 per cent of women never experience orgasm from any form of stimulation. About one-third of the rest reach orgasm in most acts of intercourse and most of the rest will respond to clitoral stimulation only. A small group respond to breast stimulation or even fantasy alone.

A few women lack the normal bulbo-cavernosus reflex (stimulation of the glans clitoris causing reflex spasm of the perineal muscles) and may be physiologically unable to reach orgasm. Many of the 10 per cent, however, may never have been adequately stimulated by their partners and have been too inhibited to masturbate themselves. Some women fear the momentary loss of control experienced during orgasm and are unable to 'relax and let it happen'.

VAGINISMUS

This is a spasm of the part of the pelvic masculature surrounding the lower part of the vagina, making penetration difficult or impossible. It may be primary or secondary. Primary vaginismus may rarely be due to a small or even absent vagina or a very strong hymen, but is almost always psychological due to phobic anxiety to penetration. These women may respond normally to arousal and be orgasmic with clitoral stimulation but cannot let anything, even their own finger or a vaginal tampon, into the vagina. Secondary vaginismus may arise after painful vaginal lesions of all kinds.

Aetiological factors in sexual dysfunctions

PREDISPOSING

Psychological – inhibited upbringing in relation to sexual matters, inadequate sexual education, and traumatic early sexual experience such as incest or sexual assault.

Physical – these are rare causes of primary sexual problems, but anatomical problems, such as hypospadias or Peyronie's disease, or hormonal problems may present in this way.

Physically disabled people may have sexual problems which can usually be overcome with a sympathetic partner.

Precipitating – The first attempts at sexual intercourse form the precipitating factor in primary problems.

Childbirth, infidelity, or other relationship problems commonly precipitate secondary problems. The onset of physical or depressive illness also do so, as can a sexual problem developing in the partner.

Physical illness may precipitate sexual problems directly – as with diabetes – or as secondary complications. Following myocardial infarction, impotence and ejaculatory difficulties are common; loss of interest may result from depression or from the unfounded fear that sexual activity will cause further infarction.

Other physical conditions that may cause sexual dysfunction are renal dialysis, abdominal surgery leading to ostomies, mastectomy, neurological conditions that cause spinal cord damage, or peripheral neuropathy.

Hysterectomy usually leads to an improvement in sexual functioning because of relief of menorrhagia, but if this symptom has been used as a convenient excuse not to have intercourse a more overt problem may present after the operation. Vaginal shrinkage following the operation may cause pain and ensuing sexual dysfunction.

Both psychological and physical factors may occur together. About half of diabetic males develop impotence, especially the older men. But in many men erections occur early in the morning and with masturbation so the mechanism cannot be entirely physical.

Maintaining factors – These are often important. Anxiety occurring with sexual arousal leads to vaginismus and impotence which often cause pain and shame. This can threaten the relationship so one or both partners may be afraid to attempt further sexual activity. If they do try they are anxious in anticipation which exacerbates the difficulty, further failure ensues, and the problem is perpetuated. Poor communication between partners about sex, inadequate information about it, and conflicts in the general relationship all maintain sexual problems.

Assessment of sexual dysfunction

Although sexual dysfunction may require specialist treatment every doctor should be able to recognize and briefly assess such problems.

1. The sexual problem may be *presented directly* by the patient or the partner. Often it *presents indirectly* to the gynaecology, family planning, or infertility clinics. Depression, anxiety, or general problems in the relationship may also be presented when the patient is ashamed or embarrassed to describe the sexual problem directly.

2. The *exact nature of the problem and its duration*. Is it the patient who experiences the difficulty or is it the partner? Is it primary or secondary? Which phase of sexual activity is affected? Can masturbation or sex with another partner occur satisfactorily? (If it can, organic causes need not be considered!) During such questioning the doctor will become aware of the patient's attitude to and knowledge about sex. A history indicative of *psychiatric or physical illness* in either partner must be sought as this could be responsible for a change in the sexual relationship. Similarly a drug history is required.

3. The patient must be *physically examined* to investigate the possibility of physical causes for the problem. It is especially important to examine the secondary sexual characteristics, the cardiovascular system, and to do a neurological examination of the lower limbs. Impotence may be the first sign of diabetes, so examine the urine and be prepared to examine the Valsalva response (see *Table 14*).

4. *The partner must be seen* so that a history of the problem and the partner's attitude to it may be assessed. When the two partners are seen together the doctor observes their ability to discuss sex, whether one partner blames the other, and their attitude towards treatment. It is essential to see each partner alone on at least one occasion so that the doctor can explore the possibility that one partner has had an extramarital affair. The upbringing and previous sexual experience of each partner is also evaluated individually. The couple's *general relationship with one another* should be assessed as well as their sexual relationship.

5. The expectations of, and preparedness to engage in, treatment must be assessed before it is commenced.

Treatment of sexual disorders

GENERAL MEASURES

Clarification of the problem and a full discussion of the sexual relationship will help the

Table 14 *The history and examination of the patient with secondary sexual problems*

history

sexually functional with another partner or by masturbation?		suggests psychogenic causes
is patient depressed?	*(men)* *(either sex)*	erectile problems loss of libido
is patient anxious?	*(men)* *(women)*	erectile problems delayed orgasm
recent illness or surgery?	myocardial infarct, ileostomy, colostomy, mastectomy	avoidance of sexual activity
problems with current sexual relationship?		lack of interest or enjoyment erectile problems
what drugs is patient taking • oral contraceptives, • corticosteroids • parasympatholytics	propanthiline, phenothiazines, tricyclic antidepressants	decreased arousal impaired erection
• sympatholytics	methyldopa, guanethidine, trazodone, thioridazine	impaired ejaculation

men

does history suggest autonomic neuropathy?	postural hypotension, bladder dysfunction	erectile problems
is there pain in buttocks on effort?	(refer to surgeon)	Leriche syndrome

women

does history suggest vaginal infection?		dyspareunia

on examination

general	look for hypertension, cardiovascular disease, diabetes	
loss of secondary sexual characteristics		hypogonadism, hypopituitism
autonomic neuropathy Valsalva response	no rate change	diabetes
neurological signs in legs (include cremasteric reflexes, perianal sensory loss)		spinal causes, cauda equina lesion

couple to discuss their difficulty more freely and this alone may lead to resolution of the problem. Improvement of the general relationship may be required before any improvement in the sexual relationship could be expected. However, this is not a medical problem.

Education and advice – A great deal can be done to help these patients by sex education, relieving anxiety, and by helping to overcome inhibitions by giving them permission to enjoy their sexuality. Increasing communication between the couple is also important. All trained professionals can give simple counselling on these lines and this may be all that is needed for the couple to sort out their own problems. Where more help is required specialist treatment needs to be directed towards increasing the positive stimuli to make the reverberating circuit fire off to orgasm where this is possible.

If there are fears of pregnancy, then *contraceptive advice* is needed. Sometimes fear of infertility interferes with normal sexual function and such fears must be dealt with before more specific treatment is attempted.

Reassurance that physical illness will not be exacerbated by sexual intercourse may allow the couple to resume their previous satisfactory relationship. Specific advice may be appropriate, for example taking a beta-blocker before intercourse for the angina patient. Any underlying *psychiatric or physical illness* must be treated. Although antidepressants can cause impotence, their appropriate use to treat depressive illness may lead to greatly improved sexual functioning.

Physical treatment – Administration of testosterone has been shown to be useful where there is definite impairment of gonadal function. It has also been shown to increase libido even where testosterone levels are normal but will not then improve function. Penile prosthetic surgery has been used in cases of neuropathy.

SPECIFIC PSYCHOLOGICAL TREATMENT

Specialist treatment is usually the province of sexual dysfunction clinics but may be performed by any suitably trained professional. After individual and joint assessment, the couple are seen together for a number of sessions with the understanding that between each session they will be required to do certain exercises together.

The treatment is based on a behavioural model. It is assumed that sexual arousal leads to anxiety and the new response of relaxation must be learned instead. Since the anxiety is usually greatest with penetration, the treatment programme begins with *an absolute ban on attempts at full intercourse* for the first few weeks. This means that instead of experiencing frustrating failed attempts the couple can enjoy mutual pleasurable stimulation. Initially this is solely non-genital stimulation, later genital stimulation is introduced provided that increasing sexual arousal can be achieved while both partners remain relaxed. This must be practised over several weeks and discussed fully both with the therapist and with each other before steps toward full intercourse are taken. Specific techniques are used for premature ejaculation, vaginismus, and orgasmic failure (see Further Reading, p. 269).

As well as the behavioural techniques, counselling and education are usually required. Commonly resentment or embarrassment has developed between the partners and this must be faced and dealt with during sessions. If the problem has been labelled as that of one partner alone, both must recognize their role in the development and treatment of it. Suitable literature is available to guide the couple through sex therapy and to increase their understanding of normal sexual functioning.

Psychotherapy may be appropriate, either in the form of marital therapy if the couple's general relationship requires help, or individual psychotherapy if one partner is found to have problems of their own which will be helped with this form of treatment (see p. 106).

OUTCOME

Treatment of patients attending sexual dysfunctioning clinics leads to a satisfactory outcome in approximately two-thirds of cases. The outcome is best with vaginismus and premature ejaculation (often primary problems). The outcome of treatment depends on the quality of the couple's general relationship and motivation for treatment.

Paraphilias

In these disorders sexual arousal is repeatedly obtained from non-human objects, or with humans but involving suffering or humiliation or non-consenting partners.

FETISHISM

In fetishism a piece of clothing or part of the body, such as hair or feet, is used as a means of obtaining sexual arousal and orgasm. It is essentially a male perversion and there are many grades, from using the fetish (often an item of female clothing) as an adjunct to normal sexual intercourse to using it as a sole means of gaining arousal.

PAEDOPHILIA

Paedophilia is the act or fantasy of engaging in sexual activity with young children as a repeatedly preferred method of achieving sexual arousal. Paedophilic acts usually take the form of immature sex play, with coitus or violence occurring only rarely. Paedophilia often involves a child previously known to the man and may be incest.

Aetiology – In adolescents paedophilia may be an exaggerated form of immature sexual activity. Among older men marital and social difficulties or social isolation are common, and alcohol may be involved in releasing the behaviour.

Medical involvement may be required to assess the man or aid the child and her family. The former may be a request from a court.

SADOMASOCHISM

Sadomasochism is sexual gratification involving fantasy or acts of cruelty either to the person (masochism) or to another (sadism). The phenomenon may remain entirely confined to fantasy or may accompany coitus either as a general humiliation or as a highly specific ritual. Sadism is generally performed by men on women, other men, or animals.

TRANSVESTISM

Transvestism occurs in both sexes and involves the persistent wearing of clothes of the opposite sex. This is initially for sexual excitement and the person becomes intensely frustrated if cross-dressing is prevented. There are different forms, with some men wearing female clothing in secret, others doing so overtly. If the purpose remains one of sexual arousal this is a kind of fetish; if the behaviour becomes continuous it may lead to a state resembling transsexualism. Both heterosexual and homosexual men and women cross-dress. It should probably be thought of as a minor form of gender dysphoria allied to deviant sexual practices.

Anxiety, depression, or marital problems may present to the doctor often with the spouse, rather than the patient, coming to the doctor. These are treated in the usual way, but if the cross-dresser is resistant to change, the future of the marital relationship may be in doubt. Clarifying this issue with both partners will then need to be a first step in treatment.

EXHIBITIONISM

Exhibitionism is the repetitive act of exposing the genitals to an unsuspecting stranger for the purpose of achieving sexual arousal. The desire to shock the innocent party is strong. The man may masturbate but experience intense guilt later.

Depression is an important cause in the elderly, and the behaviour is occasionally accompanied by schizophrenia, organic brain damage, or mental handicap. Exhibitionism may be a short-lived episode in an otherwise normal person but persistent offenders tend to come from troubled family backgrounds, are immature, and under-achieve as adults.

The medical task is to detect treatable psychiatric illness if it is present, to try and prevent stigmatization of the occasional offender, and refer for *behaviour therapy* those who are well motivated to stop the behaviour. The anti-androgen, *cyproterone acetate*, is occasionally used for short periods in conjunction with other treatments.

In relation to court reports the doctor must remember that the majority of convicted exposers do not repeat the crime; it is the repeated offender who seems to be neither easily treatable nor deterred.

VOYEURISM

Voyeurism is sexual gratification through looking at people (usually strangers) who are naked, undressing, or engaging in sexual activity. The observer does not attempt to engage the person whom he has watched in sexual activity but masturbates afterwards.

REPRODUCTIVE DISORDERS

Premenstrual tension

EPIDEMIOLOGY

Estimates of prevalence range from one-third to three-quarters of all women of reproductive age, depending on the severity and duration of the symptoms included within the definition. The frequency is such that it is probably inappropriate to regard this condition as pathological, but the extreme distress experienced by some women results in medical consultation.

CLINICAL FEATURES

The commonest physical complaints include breast tenderness and feelings of abdominal distension, and mental symptoms include depressed mood, anxiety, and irritability. These occur for up to ten days prior to a menstrual period and end one to two days afterwards.

DIAGNOSTIC CRITERIA

The physical symptoms are characteristic. The affective symptoms are limited to a maximum of eleven to twelve days of each cycle. The 'biological' symptoms of depression do not occur. The condition should be differentiated from the affective disorders, in which symptoms may be exacerbated premenstrually but are more persistent throughout the cycle.

AETIOLOGY

Despite the evident link between the timing of premenstrual symptoms and the menstrual cycle, various aetiological theories concerning imbalance of ovarian or pituitary hormones have not been substantiated.

TREATMENT

Progesterone, bromocriptine, anxiolytics, vitamin B_6, antidepressants, and diuretics have all been advocated but there is no evidence that any of these has more than a placebo effect: sympathetic explanation is probably equally valuable.

Disorders of pregnancy

EPIDEMIOLOGY

During the first trimester approximately 10 per cent of women experience a new episode of minor affective disorder. During the second trimester this rate falls and is probably similar to the frequency in the general population. There is evidence of an increase of minor affective disorders in the third trimester, which is associated with particular risk factors, such as being unmarried and lower socio-economic status.

CLINICAL FEATURES

Any mental illness can have its onset during pregnancy, or may occur as a continuation of a pre-existing disorder. There does not appear to be any increased risk for illnesses characterized by psychotic symptoms and the vast majority are typical of the minor affective disorders with a mixture of depressive and anxiety symptoms. However, thought content is likely to be focused on the pregnancy and its implications for the future, including the related social and psychological consequences.

AETIOLOGY

Minor affective disorders which have their onset during pregnancy are associated particularly with a previous history of mental illness, with marital conflict, and ambivalence about continuation with the pregnancy.

Onset during the first trimester is associated particularly with a previous history of termination of pregnancy, worries concerning the normality of the foetus, and fears of retribution. Onset in the second and third trimesters has been found to be associated particularly with recent bereavement.

INVESTIGATIONS

These will usually be limited to a search for evidence of particular aetiological factors which may play a part and the assessment should include interviews with the husband and possibly other informants. Particular attention should be paid to past history and pre-morbid personality, previous termination of pregnancy, the marital relationship, and available sources of support.

TREATMENT

Supportive psychotherapy and counselling may be valuable to women for whom there is evidence of particular psychological difficulties, especially those who have failed to adjust to previous termination. *Joint marital therapy* may be indicated where there is evidence of particular difficulties in the marriage which may be highlighted by the pregnancy. Women who have material social difficulties and inadequate social support will need help, which should be available from local social services departments. It is particularly important to follow up patients into the puerperium, to assess the development of bonding between mother and child, and ensure a satisfactory level of child care.

COURSE AND PROGNOSIS

The outcome of minor affective disorders which have their onset during pregnancy remains uncertain. Studies based on married women of higher socio-economic status suggest that most recover during the first three months of the puerperium; those based on less socially stable populations with lower socio-economic status indicate a more chronic course, with continuation during the puerperium and possibly for longer. It has been suggested that there are particular risks for subsequent child care and bonding between mother and child which may have long-term implications for child development.

Termination of pregnancy

In England and Wales approximately 100,000 women have terminations of pregnancy each year. Before the Abortion Act (1967) psychiatrists were frequently involved in assessing women prior to termination which was often carried out on grounds of suicidal risk due to depressive illness. Since the introduction of this Act recommendations for termination are usually made by the general practitioner and gynaecologist. Psychiatrists are involved mainly when there is a past history of serious mental illness or a particular need to assess the patient's likely response to termination.

Adverse psychological responses to abortion are rare. Although depression and anxiety are common during unwanted pregnancies these usually resolve within a few weeks after termination. However there is some increase in the risk of postnatal depression in women with a history of termination, when past feelings of guilt may be re-evoked. By contrast, studies of women refused abortion show they are more likely to suffer depression later on, have an increased risk of suicide, have difficulty in adjusting to their unwanted children, and have children who are at greater risk of delinquency and difficulties at school.

Disorders of the puerperium

There is a well-recognized *increase in the prevalence of mental illness following childbirth*. In recent years research has led to the classification of these disorders into three main groups which are considered separately below, but there is still much uncertainty about whether these conditions are related to each other.

'MATERNITY BLUES'

Epidemiology

Between 50 and 80 per cent of all women develop the 'maternity blues' during the first week following delivery and this has been a consistent finding in different countries, cultures, and ethnic groups. It is, therefore, doubtful whether this condition should be considered pathological, but it undoubtedly causes significant distress and requires medical recognition. No consistent relationship has been found to social class, parity, hospital as compared with home delivery, or obstetric complications.

Clinical features

Symptoms tend to develop in a predictable sequence starting on the *first post-partum day* with feelings of exhaustion, anorexia, and complaints of poor concentration. Mild perplexity and disorientation may occur. Weeping occurs in approximately 50 per cent of all women on the first day. However, about 80 per cent of all women also experience elation on the first day and this appears to be a normal response to childbirth, and in a minority (8 per cent) this persists or increases in the subsequent three days and is accompanied by garrulousness, over-activity, and excitability.

Symptoms which have their peak onset on the *third to fifth days* include depressed mood, restlessness, and irritability. Labile mood with swings from depression to elation on the same day is characteristic of this condition.

Weeping tends to be precipitated by minor events and in a substantial minority of cases depressive thought content includes low self-esteem, feelings of guilt, and pessimism concerning the future. Irritability and anger tend to be directed particularly towards the husband or to hospital staff and may lead to self-discharge from hospital.

Diagnostic criteria

'Maternity blues' invariably have their onset within the first week of parturition and last no longer than two weeks. The mood changes are characteristically brief and fluctuate rapidly, usually persisting for only a few hours at a time and at most for one to two days. For the majority there is sudden onset and sudden recovery lasting between one and three days.

Differential diagnosis

The disorder must be differentiated from **post-natal depression**, which starts later, is more prolonged, and includes more persistent affective changes; and from **puerperal psychosis** which has its onset at around the same time as 'maternity blues' and may have similar prodromal symptoms but then progresses with the development of psychotic features. **Acute toxic states** are suggested by evidence of clouding of consciousness or disorientation but are now uncommon where good obstetric care is available. Approximately 40 per cent of mothers experience either **lack of affection** or negative feelings towards their baby in the first few weeks or months of the puerperium but this is not necessarily related to 'maternity blues'. (It is associated with amniotomy and painful labour.) Mothers are usually extremely distressed by their lack of feelings, and may experience feelings of guilt. They may derive considerable benefit from reassurance that this is a common experience which rarely persists and is not indicative of either mental illness or inadequacy as a mother.

Aetiology

A biological contribution to the aetiology is strongly suggested by the relatively specific timing of onset and duration, the labile mood, and the lack of any relationship to psycho-social or cultural factors. While there is a strong suspicion that the profound hormonal changes occurring at this time are implicated, most studies so far have failed to show any association between the presence or severity of 'maternity blues' and hormonal status. In the first post-partum week there is a precipitate decrease in the circulating concentrations of oestrogens and progesterone. There are several sites in the CNS, including monoamine neurones and receptors, which are sensitive to these hormones. While no clear relationships have been established between various steroid concentrations and the 'blues', it is of interest that steroid-sensitive platelet alpha-noradrenergic receptors are reduced in cases of the blues. Such a receptor change in the CNS could be a basis for the affective changes. Increased **prolactin** and also increased **platelet monoamine oxidase** activity have been found to be associated with anxiety and depression during the first post-partum week. **Increased plasma cortisol** and **reduced tryptophan** in the last week or two of pregnancy have been found to be associated with more severe cases. At present the implications of these findings are uncertain.

There is a tendency for episodes, and particularly more severe episodes, to be associated with a past history of depressive illness, including postnatal depression, or affective symptoms in the third trimester of pregnancy.

Treatment

It is important to recognize the nature of the condition so that the patient and her family can be reassured about the likely course and outcome. Considerable tact and understanding are required by medical and nursing staff in their approach to the patient. Monitoring of the mental state should continue to ensure that complete recovery takes place, and that no other mental disorder is developing.

Course and prognosis

By definition recovery invariably takes place within two weeks without specific treatment; if this does not occur the diagnosis should be reviewed.

POST-NATAL DEPRESSION

Epidemiology

Between 10 and 20 per cent of women develop a depressive illness during the first three months following childbirth and the incidence is, therefore, increased compared with the general population.

Clinical features

Generally symptoms develop after the patient has been discharged from hospital two weeks or more after parturition. The patient feels despondent, is tearful, and distressed by feelings of inadequacy and inability to cope, particularly with the baby. There may be feelings of guilt, usually limited to self-reproach about not caring for the baby. The mood is often labile and depression tends to be worse in the evening. Commonly there is marked irritability, anorexia, fatigue, and feelings of exhaustion. Sleep disturbance is usually limited to initial insomnia. Almost always the patient exhibits excessive concern regarding the health of the baby and often shows hypochondriacal preoccupation with her own somatic symptoms.

Diagnostic criteria

The disorder is characterized by mixed symptoms of depression and anxiety which have their onset in the puerperium and persist for a minimum of two weeks.

Differential diagnosis

It must be differentiated both from the '**maternity blues**' and from **puerperal psychosis**, and also from other disorders characterized by neurotic symptoms which have their onset before or during the puerperium.

Aetiology

There is no evidence that biological factors play any major part in the cause of post-natal depression, despite some claims to the contrary. There is an increased frequency in primiparae over the age of thirty. There is also an association with a history of a disturbed relationship between the mother and her own parents during her childhood. As with non-puerperal depressed women, there is evidence that adverse life events interact with social and personality vulnerability factors to induce depressive illness in the postnatal period.

Some studies have suggested that there is a relationship between anxiety during pregnancy and post-natal depression. For some women childbirth presents a maturational crisis, imposing a new psychological and physical burden, and increased demands from others for dependency.

Investigations

No specific investigations are required, apart from establishing the time of onset of the disorder in relation to the puerperium and a careful assessment of the psychological and social significance to the patient of childbirth.

Treatment

Tricyclic antidepressants are occasionally required, based on the usual indications. Claims for the effectiveness of specific treatment with **progesterone** on its own or in combination with monoamine oxidase inhibitors have been made but are at present unsubstantiated. For the most part treatment should focus on counselling and **supportive therapy** of the patient and her family by the general practitioner and health visitor, who should be particularly aware of difficulties that may occur in the process of bonding.

Course and prognosis

The majority of patients recover within six to twelve months, but one follow-up study suggests that nearly one-half of patients, most of whom were untreated, were unimproved one year after childbirth. Chronic non-psychotic illnesses starting after childbirth are not uncommon, tend to include poor libido and hypochondriasis, and may remain unidentified for many years.

PUERPERAL PSYCHOSIS

Epidemiology

Between one and two women per thousand deliveries develop a new episode of illness characterized by psychotic symptoms. The majority of these have their onset within the first two weeks of parturition. There is an increased risk particularly for primiparous women (double that for multiparous women) and possibly after caesarean section. No definite relationship has been found with other obstetric factors, with social class, or marital status.

Clinical features

Symptoms generally have their onset between three and ten days after childbirth although a small proportion start in the subsequent two weeks. Usually they develop rapidly over the course of a few days. Any of the syndromes of the functional psychoses may occur but there is a particular tendency to find mixed states, with both **affective and schizophreniform** symptoms, and marked fluctuations in the type and severity of symptoms during the course of the disorder. **Depressive symptoms** predominate in over half these episodes and **manic symptoms** in about a third. Often these are mixed with **'first-rank' symptoms of schizophrenia**. **Perplexity** occurs in the majority and a substantial minority are **disoriented** at some stage.

Diagnostic criteria

Any mental illness which includes psychotic symptoms and has its onset within four weeks after parturition is included in this category. It should be differentiated from episodes of illness having a previous onset but continuing into the puerperium and from acute toxic states (delirium).

Aetiology

There is an increased risk of psychotic illness generally (although not of puerperal illness) in the first-degree relatives of women with puerperal psychosis. Thus there appears to be some general genetic predisposition. There is an increased risk of psychoses at times other than the puerperium after an episode of puerperal psychosis and this also supports the probability of a constitutional predisposition. It is generally believed that these disorders are caused by the rapid and extreme changes in the hormonal state following parturition but confirmation has proved elusive. Recently comparisons of psychotic puerperal women with non-psychotic puerperal women have shown the former to have higher levels of **thyroxin** and **prolactin** (and possibly oestrogen) and lower levels of **luteinizing hormone** and **progesterone**. Even if these findings are confirmed it remains uncertain whether they are a cause or effect.

Investigations

Careful monitoring of the physical and mental state is required to rule out the possibility of an acute toxic state. Details of the patient's social circumstances and the available sources of support will be important in planning her treatment.

Treatment

It is usually necessary to admit the patient to a psychiatric unit and wherever possible this should be with her baby to a specialized mother and baby unit. Patients with a predominantly depressive syndrome in the puerperium tend to respond less well to antidepressant drugs than those with depressive illnesses at other times. **Electroconvulsive treatment** is particularly effective and therefore tends to be used earlier than in other depressive illnesses. Those with predominantly manic or depressive illnesses are usually started on a **major tranquillizer** (chlorpromazine or haloperidol are suitable) and if there is no definite improvement within four weeks then ECT is started. Despite claims for the value of treatment with oestrogen and/or progesterone there is little evidence to support their efficacy. Expert nursing, including attention to nutrition and fluid balance, is important and should also include the mother's supervised **access to the baby**. As her mental state improves she should take increasing responsibility for the baby's care. Her ability to do this will require careful assessment which will determine the amount and nature of supervision needed once they are discharged from hospital.

Course and prognosis

With treatment virtually all patients improve or recover within three months. Of those patients who have further pregnancies about **30 per cent have a recurrence** of puerperal psychoses. If the patient has a *bipolar illness* the risk in subsequent pregnancy is as high as 50 per cent. However the risk of recurrence is by no means limited to the puerperium and about 40 per cent of all women who suffer a puerperal psychosis will have another episode of psychotic illness at some time.

INFANTICIDE

Depression in the puerperium carries a small but definite risk that the mother will kill her child. If this occurs within twelve months of the birth and there is evidence that 'the balance of her mind was disturbed' at the time, this act is described as infanticide and dealt with in British law as manslaughter rather than murder. Approximately half the women who kill their children in the puerperium also commit suicide.

The therapeutic use of drugs during pregnancy and the puerperium

1. Drugs taken by women of child-bearing age may have a teratogenic effect if they become pregnant.
2. Drugs taken at the end of pregnancy may result in withdrawal symptoms in the baby following delivery.
3. Drugs taken during lactation may result in toxicity in the breast-fed child.

In view of these possible effects it is desirable to avoid the use of any medication for the treatment of mental illness during pregnancy, and – if the mother wishes to breast-feed her child – during the puerperium. However, if there is a strong clinical indication for medication, this must be balanced against the risks.

TRICYCLIC ANTIDEPRESSANTS

There is probably no evidence of a teratogenic effect when tricyclic antidepressants are taken in therapeutic doses. Withdrawal effects occur in neonates and if possible it is preferable to stop these drugs a few days before delivery is expected. Tricyclics are excreted in the milk only in very small quantities and, therefore, **breast-feeding is not contra-indicated** when the mother is being treated with these drugs.

BENZODIAZEPINES

There have been reports of congenital malformations, particularly cleft-lip and palate, in children born to women taking these drugs during pregnancy. Although the risk is probably small, the potential value of taking these drugs is unlikely to warrant their continuation during pregnancy and they should be avoided. Diazepam has been used for the treatment of pre-eclamptic toxaemia. This may result in toxicity in the neonate causing the *'floppy infant' syndrome*, as well as withdrawal symptoms due to prior physical addiction and both require specialized neonatal care. These drugs are excreted in milk and their **use should be resisted during lactation**.

PHENOTHIAZINES AND BUTYROPHENONES

There is little evidence that these drugs have a teratogenic effect and it appears that toxic effects in the neonate are rare. When taken by the lactating mother these drugs are absorbed by the baby in very small quantities and there is no evidence that this has a detrimental effect. Although best avoided during pregnancy and the puerperium, these drugs **may be used if there is a strong clinical indication**.

LITHIUM

It is well established that **lithium has a teratogenic effect**. It should, therefore, be stopped prior to a planned pregnancy and contraception should be practised at other times. If essential it may be taken during the third trimester, but special precautions must be taken to control the serum level of the drug, which must be stopped before delivery. Lithium **passes into breast milk** and this can result in toxicity, but there is little evidence of any long-term effect.

Sterilization and hysterectomy

Recent prospective studies indicate that these procedures rarely contribute to the aetiology of mental illness. Sexual enjoyment is often enhanced by sterilization and regrets are uncommon. In a small proportion of cases there are prolonged difficulties in adjustment, including symptoms of anxiety and depression, and these are virtually limited to women in whom there is a past history of similar symptoms. Sometimes these procedures are embarked on as an unrealistic way of trying to deal with other problems, particularly in the marriage or in sexual adjustment. Therefore, a past history of mental illness or current interpersonal or social difficulties indicates a particular need for cautious assessment before surgery.

The menopause

There is no evidence that serious mental illness of any kind is commoner in women around the time of the menopause than at other times.

The term 'involutional melancholia' was used in the past to describe severe depressive illness which was thought to be specifically linked to the menopause. The term is now obsolete, because this form of the disorder is related to the effects of age on depressive illness, rather than to the menopause.

EPIDEMIOLOGY AND CLINICAL FEATURES OF MENOPAUSAL SYMPTOMS

Symptoms commonly complained of by menopausal and post-menopausal women fall into two main groups. Complaints of *hot flushes and excessive sweating* are commonest one or two years after the cessation of periods, when they are experienced by up to 90 per cent of all women and then gradually dwindle in frequency over the next few years. These are caused by vaso-motor changes, are closely related to reduced ovarian activity, and respond to treatment with oestrogen.

In the year following the end of menstruation approximately one-third of women complain of symptoms including *irritability, anxiety, fatigue, and headaches* and this is approximately 10 per cent greater than the frequency in pre-menopausal and post-menopausal women. These symptoms do not differ in quality from affective symptoms occurring in women at other times, or in men.

AETIOLOGY

There is no evidence that the affective symptoms are related to reduced oestrogen production: they are primarily psychological in origin. To some extent they appear to be determined by the *meaning of the experience* of the menopause. The end of potentially reproductive life is mourned by many women and regarded as a sign of ageing. However, it is welcomed by others, particularly in those cultures where contraception is not practised.

It is also a time when many other changes commonly occur in a woman's life, including the loss of children who leave home and the death of parents. These changes require considerable adjustment and it is not surprising if symptoms of minor affective disorder are commoner at this stage of life, particularly in those individuals who generally have difficulty in making appropriate adjustments to change.

Careful assessment of the nature and duration of symptoms will help to determine the possible value of medication. Each patient will require an individual appraisal of her current social circumstances and her psychological response to recent events.

TREATMENT

Symptoms of minor affective disorder occurring at the menopause do not respond to oestrogen any better than to placebos. Both tricyclic antidepressants and benzodiazepines have been found to relieve some symptoms better than placebos, but their use should be restricted to the usual indications for these drugs. Most patients will benefit from supportive psychotherapy.

FURTHER READING

Bancroft, J. H. J. (1983) *Human Sexuality and its Problems*. Edinburgh: Churchill Livingstone.

Belliveau, F. and Richter, P. (1975) *Understanding Human Sexual Inadequacy*. London: Hodder.

Hawton, K. (1982) Sexual Problems in the General Hospital. In F. Creed and J. Pfeffer (eds) *Medicine and Psychiatry*. London: Pitman.

Brockington, I. F. and Kumar, R. (1982) *Motherhood and Mental Illness*. London: Academic Press.

Christie-Brown, J. R. W. and Christie-Brown, M. E. (1976) Psychiatric Disorders associated with the Menopause. In R. J. Beard (ed.) *The Menopause*. Lancaster: MTP.

Gath, D. and Cooper, P. (1982) Psychiatric Aspects of Hysterectomy and Female Sterilisation. In K. Granville-Grossman (ed.) *Recent Advances in Psychiatry*, vol. 4. Edinburgh: Churchill Livingstone.

19 / DISORDERS OF OLD AGE

There has been a progressive increase in life expectancy this century throughout the western world. This has meant that more and more people survive into old age and the proportion of the population of the United Kingdom aged over sixty-five years has risen from 5 to 15 per cent. Similar changes in the age structure of populations throughout the rest of the world are occurring at an even more dramatic rate so that an understanding of the special characteristics of illnesses and the way that they present in old age is very important. Women survive into late life more often than men and in the years beyond the age of seventy-five men are outnumbered by two to one. In the last fifteen years of this century the number of people who are over seventy-five will increase by 25 per cent, and by 40 per cent in the age group who are over eighty-five.

Illnesses of all sorts and disabilities that arise from them are more common among the elderly than in other age groups. Old people are thus more likely to consult both general practitioners and hospital clinics. It is important to appreciate that most of these old people are not suffering from psychiatric disorders. Nor should the word 'senile' be used to indicate great age: most old people are not demented. It is unfortunate that although the noun 'senium' refers to the last part of the normal life cycle, the adjective 'senile' means demented in normal colloquial English!

However, it is also important to appreciate that changes in normal psychological functions are a necessary accompaniment of ageing. Old people are not involved in as wide a range of activities as young people, and this can be explained only partly by externally imposed factors such as retirement with a consequently reduced income, upper age-limits for some activities, or failing health. Drive and ambition are usually reduced, and there is a tendency to become less involved with new ventures.

Impulses and emotions are usually better controlled so that intemperate outbursts are uncommon. Specific skills and information acquired over a lifetime of experience are usually well preserved, but the acquisition of new skills or the response to new situations is not so good as it used to be. These normal changes of ageing bring with them a need for more time to cope with new tasks or situations, and there are limits to the amount of change that the individual can tolerate.

It should be remembered that the retired population tend to live alone. Those who stay on in the family home may find it difficult to maintain, and it may also lack modern amenities; while those who move into 'sheltered accommodation' often find it cramped and don't enjoy the feeling that they are in a 'ghetto' with other old people. When these adverse social circumstances are combined with failing physical health it is easy to see how psychiatric illness may be released. The same factors militate against quick recovery once disorder has occurred.

AETIOLOGY

While retirement is often portrayed as tranquil and undemanding – rather like an extended holiday – it is in fact beset with stresses. Losses occur as a direct result of retirement: loss of income, loss of an imposed timetable, and loss of the territory of work and the challenges, company, and status that were an integral part of the Monday to Friday battle. In their stead come new challenges: husbands and wives thrown upon one another's company for longer periods than they have been accustomed to, and survival on a limited budget that cannot be supplemented by increased effort. Work has come to be viewed as a scarce commodity not to be shared with the old. Time tends to be unstructured other than the alternation of night and day, the sequence of the seasons, and the *Radio Times*. Children and grandchildren may marry; grandchildren and great grandchildren may arrive. Even these happy events carry mixed messages. Inevitably, time brings further losses: bereavements, destruction of favourite haunts by redevelopment and, most significantly, loss of that sense of physical well-being that has hitherto been taken for granted. In its place come reduced mobility, impairments of the senses of sight, hearing, taste, and smell, and often pains associated with physical disease.

The most consistent characteristic of psychiatric disorders in old age is their association with physical illness and disability. This seems to apply across the whole range of psychiatric illness, including affective disorders and paranoid states as well as organic brain syndromes. Acute or subacute brain syndromes often complicate or act as presenting features of intercurrent physical illness, and dementing illnesses become progressively more common with increasing age.

Medical treatment prescribed for physical conditions may also produce psychiatric symptoms, and the intrusive attention from nurses and other carers which may become necessary are viewed as further humiliations.

There are therefore many stresses in old age which are capable of provoking mental disorder, although by no means everyone exposed to such stresses does break down. Sometimes it is possible to uncover a history of illness in earlier life or a history of similar conditions in close relatives. Sometimes it seems relevant that the patient has known no model of successful ageing in his or her own family. Certainly long-standing personality traits and coping strategies developed in earlier life are very important in determining how an individual will respond to difficulties encountered in old age.

SYNDROMES COMMON IN OLD AGE

Organic brain syndromes

TERMINOLOGY

You are likely to encounter a bewildering variety of terms for describing much the same thing. The alternative terminologies reflect the inadequacies of simple classifications to cope with the complexities and variability of organic brain syndromes in old age, where aetiology is usually determined by many factors. It is particularly important to be aware that organic brain syndromes that have been present for many months may be reversible when all the contributory factors have been identified and corrected, and the brain has had time to readjust.

Acute and chronic *'brain failure'* are, quite simply, terms that are best avoided: the brain is a very much more complex organ than the liver or the heart, and cannot be said to 'fail' in the same way. Acute and subacute *'confusional states'* are widely used terms which can be used interchangeably with acute and subacute brain syndromes: we prefer the latter terms, since 'confusion' is but one of the component parts of quite complex syndromes.

Acute and subacute brain syndromes ('confusional states')

CLINICAL FEATURES AND DIFFERENTIAL DIAGNOSIS (see pp. 140–46)

Acute brain syndromes have to be distinguished from other organic brain syndromes on the one hand, and from affective illnesses like depression and hypomania on the other.

1. The distinction between an acute brain syndrome and a **chronic brain syndrome** may present difficulties, since the presence of the latter makes symptoms of confusion and disorientation more likely when intercurrent illness strikes. This is sometimes referred to as 'decompensated dementia' (see p. 144).

2. Rarer conditions which should be distinguished from acute brain syndromes include **dominant hemisphere cerebrovascular accidents** in which there is a jargon aphasia but in which non-verbal tests are performed normally; and **transient global amnesias** related to bilateral temporal lesions.

3. Patients with **depressive illness** may appear confused and disoriented if they have impairments of vision or hearing as well; or if physical illness limits their ability to move.

It is usual for multiple pathologies to contribute to the development of both acute and subacute brain syndromes in old age.

In the elderly the majority of acute brain syndromes are due to intercurrent physical illness, but another important cause is intoxication by (prescribed) drugs. Elderly people are often prescribed combinations of drugs for various illnesses, and their reduced hepatic and renal function may impair their ability to metabolize these drugs. In addition the brain may be much more sensitive to their effects so that blood levels that would be therapeutic in younger patients become toxic.

Problems arise because the symptoms of an acute brain syndrome are often much more striking than the physical illness which has released them. Indeed, the latter may be relatively silent: pneumonia without pyrexia, and myocardial infarction or perforated peptic ulcer without pain. Hypothermia – which is virtually confined to the elderly – may also present in this way.

In younger adults, the combination of reliable information from the special senses and an intact brain protect us from illusions, misinterpretations, and hallucinations. In the elderly neither of these can be taken for granted. Failing eyesight and deafness are common; and increasing neural 'noise' in the ageing brain from random neural activity makes it progressively more difficult to decode 'signals' from the special senses. Thus a poorly defined signal might be further distorted to produce an illusion. The random neural noise may itself come about in a number of ways. Anoxic or toxic effects on neurons may disturb neurotransmitter activity, either by impairing synthesis, causing loss of re-uptake or inappropriate leakage. Such effects may be caused by events outside the brain, such as the effects of bacterial toxins or drugs. In addition, age-associated modifications to the blood–brain barrier make it more permeable to toxic substances, and structural changes to the brain itself make acute brain syndrome more likely to occur than in younger brains.

The other point to grasp is that many demented patients manage perfectly well in a protected environment which makes few demands of them, but they develop symptoms of acute confusion when they are stressed in some way. This is sometimes referred to as 'compensated' and 'decompensated' dementia. It is in this sense that stresses that produce symptoms of *depression or anxiety* can release a subacute brain syndrome in a previously apparently healthy old person, and thus depressive illness and anxiety states are included in the differential diagnosis. However, it must be appreciated that *social and psychological stress* without clear evidence of an affective illness can also cause a dementia to decompensate and manifest itself to doctors as a subacute brain syndrome: such stresses include anything that suddenly disrupts the environment: a spouse dying or being admitted to hospital, moving to a new house, being admitted to hospital for some other reason, or going on holiday.

Sometimes the cause seems to be loss of a familiar environment; sometimes it is too much stimulation from the environment. Thus a house with too much noise – perhaps dominated by the activities of teenage grandchildren – or a noisy ward with frightening machinery and frequent changes of staff may overload the patient with too much input.

Most acute brain syndromes resolve with identification and treatment of the underlying cause, but there may be a lag of several days or weeks between the resolution of the physical problem and the return of normal psychological functioning. During the recovery period the patient should be encouraged to walk, talk, remember things, and to exercise domestic and other skills. Rehabilitation including 'reality orientation' requires repeated practice and persistence to achieve one's full potential, and must take into account the patient's own baseline. However, sometimes even this can be improved if the patient's eyesight can be improved with new spectacles, hearing by providing a hearing aid or syringeing the ears, and discomfort from painful feet relieved by appropriate treatment. In the setting of an established dementia rehabilitation will aim at producing a sufficient improvement to allow a supported life style outside hospital.

Chronic brain syndrome ('dementia')

Dementia is highly associated with age: 5 per cent of the population above the age of sixty-five, 25 per cent of those aged above seventy-five, and 60 per cent of those aged over eighty-five show some of the impairments described below. It is very rare in younger people, in whom it is referred to as *'pre-senile dementia'* (see p. 148).

Only one in seven of the old people suffering from dementia are housed in institutions (hospitals, nursing homes, or residential homes): yet all institutions caring for old people carry a disproportionately large number suffering from dementia – somewhere between 40 and 60 per cent.

Multi-infarct dementia (or arteriosclerotic dementia) has an approximately equal sex incidence, and is more common among people aged between sixty-five and seventy-four than in those aged over seventy-five. On the other hand *Alzheimer's disease* (senile dementia of Alzheimer type, or 'SDAT'), tends to be seen more often in women, and is by far the most important dementia in those above the age of seventy-five.

AETIOLOGY (see p. 150)

A chronic brain syndrome can be produced by a number of pathological processes (see p. 153), but in old age it is not unusual for several processes to combine to produce it.

Remember the potentially reversible causes of chronic brain syndromes do occur in old age. *Hypothyroidism, vitamin B$_{12}$ deficiency, and anaemia* do not often produce dementia on their own, but they may each make a contribution to the causation, and certainly exacerbate the chronic brain syndrome produced by either Alzheimer's disease or multi-infarct dementia.

Chronic infections, constipation, impaired eyesight, reduced hearing, reduced mobility, depressions, and an understimulating environment are amongst the features that can contribute to a chronic brain syndrome. Finally, the effects of **drugs** deserve special mention and careful consideration in every case. They may have been prescribed in doses that are too high, they may be interacting with other drugs, or their side-effects may be contributing to the symptoms of the chronic brain syndrome.

DIAGNOSTIC CRITERIA (see p. 150)

There should be a history of progressive global deterioration of personality and intellect without associated impairment of level of consciousness, backed up by mental state findings indicating impairment of new learning. There are no absolute criteria for dementia: each individual's performance is judged relative to what might reasonably be expected of them, bearing in mind their past educational and occupational achievements.

DIFFERENTIAL DIAGNOSIS

1. **Distinction between Alzheimer's disease ('SDAT') and multi-infarct dementia:** the latter is distinguished from SDAT by the history of step-wise deterioration, and the presence of arteriopathic and focal neurological signs on physical examination.

2. **Other degenerative disorders:** Alzheimer's disease and multi-infarct dementia are relatively common, while *Huntington's chorea* (see p. 152), *Pick's disease* (see p. 152) and *Creutzfeld–Jacob disease* (see p. 152) are seen only occasionally.

3. **Primary and secondary cerebral neoplasms** are suggested by evidence of raised intra-cranial pressure and confirmed by CAT scan.

4. **Depressive pseudodementia** has already been described (see p. 154).

5. **Normal ageing:** Dementia must be distinguished from the effects of normal ageing described as *benign senescent forgetfulness*. In the latter condition patients forget part but not all of a task, retain insight into their disability, and respond well to cues. In dementia the patients may fill gaps by confabulation, and tend to mix up recent and past events.

COURSE

Alzheimer's disease often follows a more benign course in the senium than in earlier life with a slow development of both symptoms and disabilities. This means that many patients with Alzheimer's disease die of intercurrent illness before developing the more severe symptoms: however, others will develop both parietal lobe dysfunction and fits. **Multi-infarct dementia** is a very stressful illness, characterized by episodes of sudden loss of function, any of which may release symptoms of an acute brain syndrome for a time. However, the extremes of disinhibited anger, aggressiveness, and sexual activity which can be encountered in pre-senile dementias are much less often seen in the older age groups.

Schizophrenia and allied states (see pp. 164–75);

CLINICAL FEATURES

Most patients who develop schizophrenia in early adult life will survive into old age. Some of these will have predominant negative symptoms (see p. 166), while others will have combinations of negative symptoms and positive symptoms – most usually persecutory delusions accompanied by appropriate hallucinations.

Some patients develop schizophrenia-like psychoses for the first time in old age, and because of their special features these illnesses have been called *persistent persecutory states of the elderly*. The principal abnormality consists of auditory hallucinations which are accompanied by delusions of persecution. Other patients develop persecutory psychoses with marked depressive features.

AETIOLOGY

Genetic factors are less important than in schizophrenias of earlier life.

Persistent persecutory states are commoner in women, and patients tend to have previous life styles and personalities characterized by emotional and sexual coldness. Social isolation, often exacerbated by failing vision, failing hearing, or restricted mobility facilitate both the hallucinatory phenomena and the persecutory ideas.

TREATMENT

Formation of a reasonable therapeutic alliance is an essential, although often very difficult, first step.

Hallucinations can usually be suppressed with neuroleptic drugs: but compliance is always a major problem, and symptoms return when the medication is stopped. If the patient can be persuaded to persist with medication they often return to their former lives as competent, rather distant individuals. Life expectancy is not reduced, and treatment as an out-patient is usually possible. Old patients treated with neuroleptics for prolonged periods are often troubled by apathy and reduced drive, as well as the well-recognized symptoms of Parkinsonism. However, anti-Parkinsonian treatment should be avoided if possible, and the patient maintained on the smallest dose of neuroleptic that is effective in controlling their hallucinations.

AFFECTIVE DISORDERS

Depressive illness (see pp. 183–90)

Symptoms of anxiety and depression are found in 10–20 per cent of old people living at home, and even higher figures are found in those presenting for care to their general practitioner, to hospital out-patients, or to social services. Depressive illnesses are slightly less common than at earlier ages, and hypomania is rare.

Older patients are even more likely than younger patients to present with somatic symptoms when they are psychologically unwell (see Chapter 10). Those who will later be found to be suffering from a depressive illness will originally have sought help for complaints such as tiredness, weakness, palpitations, anorexia, constipation, breathlessness, and pains. It may be that physical pathology (for example, arthritis, a hemiparesis, or varicose veins) is indeed present and may account for some of these pains – but the symptomatology attributed to the physical disease is exaggerated by the mood disorder which itself may be hidden or denied.

Withdrawal from activities (*'Because I'm too old for them now and should give way to younger folk'*) and **reluctance to leave the house** (*'I'm not so good on my feet now, and if I fell I'd be such a trouble to everyone'*) may be presenting symptoms of a depressive illness, but the 'explanations' of the symptoms ar easily accepted by relatives. Indeed, the 'understandability' of symptoms of depression and anxiety is a great hazard for the elderly, since detection and treatment are made less likely. There are therefore parallels with the depressive states secondary to malignant disease (see p. 124): in both cases, symptoms may respond to treatment, and they should therefore be regarded as morbid phenomena rather than as 'understandable' reactions to circumstance.

The risk of successful **suicide** increases with age and must always be borne in mind with depressed old people, especially if they live alone or are physically ill. Although some make suicidal threats for the effect that such threats have on others, it must be remembered that suicide becomes more common with advancing age. Thus any hint that an old patient is contemplating suicide must be taken seriously, and the doctor must ensure that adequate supervision is available and must provide active treatment. In practice, this will usually involve admission to hospital. Old people who have survived a suicide attempt should certainly be admitted to hospital– voluntarily if possible, but on a compulsory order if necessary.

Psychotic depression (see p. 186)

In patients with psychotic depression, delusions of worthlessness, poverty, or nihilism occur at all ages, but delusions of infestation and cancer are also seen in the elderly. Psychomotor symptoms – either agitation or retardation – commonly accompany such delusions. Impaired concentration combines with a depressive conviction of failing memory to produce an apparent dementia:

> My brain's not what is was you know. I can't do the things I used to: I just can't take things in – my memory's hopeless, I'm going senile.

Such patients will perform poorly on tests of short-term memory during the mental state examination, leading inexperienced clinicians to conclude that they are indeed demented. The differentiation of *depressive pseudodementia* from degenerative dementias should be made by careful history-taking. In the former condition there will be a short time-scale of development with anxious and depressive symptoms predominating from the outset, and there may also be a history of earlier depressive episodes.

Even when the examination is confined to simple test material such as the Newcastle scale, the patient manages to communicate severe depression and self-doubt with his answers:

I don't know. I don't know. Oh, don't be bothering with me . . . it's all beyond me now.

In contrast, some demented patients produce inaccurate answers with confidence.

The differentiation of *Parkinson's disease* from psychotic depression can be difficult, since in both the patient may appear retarded: once more, correct assessment depends upon careful history taking.

Mania (see p. 190)

This occurs in old people, but it is less common than in early adult life. Mixed states with both depressive and hypomanic features may bewilder both the patient and his relatives: the typical picture of earlier adult life is unusual. Irritability, downright combativeness, and even paranoid sensitivity are more common than elation and a sense of well-being. There is a real risk that excessive activity combined with lack of both sleep and food may put life at risk by precipitating serious cardiac or respiratory problems.

ALCOHOLISM AND DRUG DEPENDENCE (see p. 197)

Some of those dependent upon alcohol in early adult life manage to survive into old age; and many more are now surviving into old age dependent upon sleeping tablets and 'minor' tranquillizers.

As such patients develop new pathology in their liver or brain they may lose their tolerance for alcohol or other drugs, and are therefore at higher risk for organic brain syndromes and other psychiatric disorders.

Some old people – mainly women – turn to drink or tranquillizers for the first time in old age. They have usually been prescribed such drugs for the symptomatic relief of symptoms of depression or anxiety, although in some dependence upon the drug has been released by the disinhibition of a dementing process. These patients typically come to medical attention through complications which include confusion, falls, and self-neglect; or the problem is reported by embarrassed relatives or home helps who have been prevailed upon to act as suppliers.

In theory treatment of those becoming dependent for the first time in old age should be straightforward, and should consist of withdrawal of the agent with appropriate treatment of the problem which has precipitated the dependence. However, in practice there are often real difficulties: partly because of the intractable nature of some of the associated social problems, but sometimes because of obstinacy on the part of the patient.

MENTAL HANDICAP (see pp. 229–34)

Those handicapped individuals who survive into old age are typically cared for by sisters or brothers after their parents' death. They may present as depressed or as 'confused' when death or illness of a carer confronts them with their own limitations in coping ability.

INVESTIGATIONS IN OLD PEOPLE

Home assessments

There are many advantages in making assessments in the patient's home. Not only is this convenient for the patient, but also it provides an opportunity for the doctor to see the patient functioning in the environment in which the problems have been identified. Information about current stresses and potential supports is readily available, as well as a great deal of useful information concerning the patient's personal life. If the patient is to be admitted to hospital, it is possible to make arrangements with relatives about how care will be resumed outside hospital when the time comes.

Physical examination

In addition to the usual physical examination including weighing the patient and testing the urine, it is important to remember to test eye-sight (with spectacles), hearing (with any hearing aid), to inspect teeth (and dentures), feet, balance, coordination, and to carry out a rectal examination.

A full blood count, biochemical profile, and chest film should be carried out in every case, together with any further special investigations which are indicated by the special circumstances of the case. If they are available, CAT scans should be carried out to investigate the possibility of intra-cranial pathology other than 'degenerative changes'.

TREATMENT OF THE ELDERLY PATIENT

It is of the first importance to build a trusting relationship between members of the multi-disciplinary team on the one hand, and the patient and his or her family on the other. Psychological treatments are usually exploratory or supportive. Dependence upon the therapist is unlikely to become intense, and can be sustained for relatively long periods while adjustment to new circumstances is achieved.

It is important that doses of psychotropic drugs are adjusted downwards, to take account of reduced body mass and reduced renal function in the elderly. High blood levels of drugs are easily attained, and may rise as the drug accumulates. The presence of other drugs, prescribed for other conditions, means that drug interactions may complicate the undesired effects of any psychotropic drugs that are prescribed. It is therefore important to make sure that all drugs being prescribed are really necessary, and that none are being prescribed in doses that are too high.

The problems described above should not lead to failure to prescribe necessary drugs: mental illness in old age causes much preventable suffering, and is also associated with premature death by suicide.

Interview techniques with old people

When approaching an interview with an elderly patient it is important to *take account of their relative slowness*, their tendency to tire easily, and the greater likelihood that they will have difficulty with memory as well as problems with eye-sight, hearing, and mobility. Making sure that your face is at the same level as the patient, that your eyes and lips can be seen, and that you speak slowly and clearly take little trouble and are much appreciated – for it provides extra cues to supplement fading or unreliable hearing.

Old people in particular have expectations about how a doctor will dress and behave: *a careful, polite approach is essential*. Repeated short interviews often achieve more than attempts to press on beyond the endurance of the patient. As in obstetric practice, two empty bladders are a good investment before you start.

Although you will encourage the patient to focus on their current problems as they give you the history, you should allow them to diverge from time to time to share a reminiscence with you – this shows an interest in them and their experiences, and will consolidate trust between you.

Since memory problems and confusion are common in elderly patients it is unwise to rely only on information from the patient, and you should always be sure to *talk to a relative as well*. It is not unusual for an elderly patient to be quite unaware of problems that others have noticed, and they may even deny that abnormalities reported by others have actually occurred.

Mental status examination in elderly patients

As with any other patient, this starts with *careful observation* and recording of the patient's appearance, behaviour, and spontaneous speech. If you are carying out an assessment in the patient's home remember to include the situation in which the patient is living. Thus there may be evidence of long-standing self-neglect or failure to cope; multiple locks and hostile messages may indicate a paranoid disorder.

There are occasions when this is all that can be achieved as more formal testing may be beyond the patient's ability. On these occasions be sure to obtain a history from a relative, and return to an assessment of the patient's cognitive state as soon as the patient's physical condition allows.

Examination of cognitive function is especially important as delirious states and dementing syndromes are common in the elderly. However, there are traps for the unwary. It is easy to elicit lack of awareness of current events and deficits in new learning in an old patient who is depressed, anxious, feeling physically unwell, in pain, or even just feeling uncomfortable in strange surroundings. You may conclude that the patient is demented or confused, when what is really wrong is that your test procedures were too fast, too long, too complex, or just badly presented. Short, simple tests that encourage the patient to do well with early items are better accepted and provide more worthwhile information. A number of question and answer tests have been developed that require the retrieval of knowledge acquired in the distant past and also require accurate recall of more recently acquired information. One such scale is Blessed and Roth's *Newcastle scale*, which has the advantage that it has been validated against post-mortem findings: patients with high scores are found to have normal brains, while those with low scores and a history suggestive of dementia are found to have degenerative changes in their brains. The severity of these changes has been shown to correlate well with the lowness of their scores.

ADMINISTERING THE NEWCASTLE SCALE

You will find the Newcastle scale on The Card (also reproduced at the end of this book). It is very easy to administer and score: jot down the actual responses with any comments of your own, and give one point for each correct answer. The 'recognition of persons' test is scored by asking the patient to identify other people in the room, or photographs of others which may be on the bedside table or mantelpiece.

INTERPRETATION OF THE SCORE

This is a rough and ready clinical test which should be looked upon as indicative of the state of cognitive impairment at the time of testing, rather than as diagnostic of a particular condition. Most old people without cognitive impairment will score within a few points of the maximum possible, and the best cutting point for discriminating between demented and non-demented subjects is 24/25.

FURTHER READING

Arie, T. (1981) *Health Care of the Elderly*. London: Croom Helm.
Blessed, G., Roth, M., and Tomlinson, B. (1968) The association between quantitative measures of dementia and senile changes in the grey matter. *British Journal of Psychiatry* 114: 797–811.
Blythe, R. (1981) *The View of Winter*. Harmondsworth: Penguin.
Bromley, D. B. (1977) *The Psychology of Human Ageing*. Harmondsworth: Penguin.
Hodgson, S. and Jolley, D. (1985) Psychiatry of the Elderly. In M. S. J. Pathy (ed.) *Principles and Practice of Geriatric Medicine*. Chichester: John Wiley.
Hodkinson, H. (1973) Mental Impairment in the Elderly. *Journal of the Royal College of Physicians* 7: 305–17.
Pitt, B. (1982) *Psychogeriatrics*. London: Churchill Livingstone.

PART 4
PSYCHIATRY FOR THE HOUSEMAN AND LEGAL ASPECTS

20 / PSYCHIATRY FOR THE HOUSEMAN

During your time in the department of psychiatry as a student you will learn to take your time and do things thoroughly: however, during your pre-registration year you are going to have to learn some short cuts. The patients you will see in the accident room, and those that you admit to the wards, have a high incidence of affective illnesses, acute brain syndromes, and alcohol-related problems, and they also present difficult psychological management problems. You will become a far better doctor if you learn to recognize and treat these disorders.

After an opening section on interview techniques (the short cuts!) we will deal with breaking bad news to your patient's relatives; dealing with the psychological effects of surgery; dealing with dying patients and with those recently bereaved. A final section will deal with emergencies in the accident room, including violent patients and those who have deliberately poisoned themselves.

WHEN TO SUSPECT PSYCHIATRIC DISORDER

In Chapter 2 we drew your attention to the **verbal and non-verbal cues** which indicate possible psychiatric disorder (see p. 14); learn to notice these, and to give such patients the opportunity of telling you how they have been feeling as you take the history. Get into the habit of asking **all** patients:

How have you been feeling in your spirits?
Have you been very worried about your health?
How have you been sleeping?

as you do the 'systems review' part of the interview: you will learn a great deal about your patients, and will often find yourself going on to the 'Short mental state for mood disorders', given below.

As you examine your patients, remember to observe their degree of **alertness**: if you have even mild doubts, carry out tests of **orientation** in order to detect acute brain syndrome. In elderly patients you will find the Newcastle scale useful as an indicator of current cerebral impairment; for younger adults use conventional memory tests – both will be found on The Card.

Now you are sitting down, writing up your notes. Are the patient's symptoms quite typical of some recognized physical disease, or are they atypical, and peculiar in some way? If the latter, consider giving the short mental state examination relating to mood (see below).

Has the patient got any potentially alcohol-related disease (see pp. 197–200)? If so, ask the 'CAGE' questions – also on The Card – and be prepared to go on to a drinking history (see p. 201).

A SHORT MENTAL STATE FOR MOOD DISORDERS

This should be given whenever you suspect a mood disorder. Many of the questions are perhaps those that you are used to asking anyway: but perhaps you are not used to allowing the replies to these questions to help you form a view about whether the patient is psychologically unwell. You will see that it consists of a set of rather general questions together with questions about anxiety and depression.

The **questions in emphasized type** should be asked of all patients, but it is necessary to give the questions in parentheses only if you have a positive reply to such questions.

Scoring and interpretation

The higher the score, the more likely is it that your patient has a mood disorder. The questions marked 'A' relate to anxiety, while those marked 'D' relate to depression. Ask yourself what relationship the disorder that you have elicited might bear to the somatic symptoms that have caused the patient to be admitted (see p. 124). Many patients who are anxious but not depressed will be found to have understandable anxiety symptoms that you can do a great deal to help. (For research purposes, diagnostic criteria for anxiety states and depressive illnesses are to be found on pp. 179 and 186.)

A short social history

Concentrate on the patient's present living conditions, rather than details of his or her past life.

> *Who is there at home ?*
> *Do you have any worries about them?*
> *How do you get on together?*

Anything happened to you recently that has upset you?
Any problems about the place you live in?
Any problems at work?
Any financial problems?

Seeing a relative

If you suspect a social or family problem, ask to see a relative. If you haven't time, or feel that the problem sounds too involved for you, ask the medical social worker for assistance.

Management

The management of the various disorders will be found on earlier pages. All require reassurance and explanation. If you haven't yet read the section on the management of somatization, maybe you ought to turn to p. 127 now.

BREAKING BAD NEWS TO RELATIVES

Telling a perfect stranger that her husband is dying is one of the most unpleasant tasks that may come your way. Perhaps because they are so uncomfortable about such interviews themselves, doctors often greatly increase the burdens that they impose on relatives.

1. Start by introducing yourself, and asking whether you can 'have a word' with them. Take them to an interview room where you can have some privacy, and settle them down.

2. Open by saying something like *'I expect you've been very worried about him'*. **Pause** to give them time to reply. If they agree, ask *How it has affected them – are they managing to sleep all right?* Ask any further questions that might be indicated: this is your opportunity to learn something about the relative, and you will need this information later in the interview.

   You will also gain some idea about whether they have already feared the worst, or whether you are about to shock them badly.

3. Make a clear **transition statement**, like *'Well, the reason that I've asked to see you is that we have found out more about your husband's illness'*. This has the effect of focusing the relative's attention on what you are about to say.
   Now, explain exactly what has been found, without using any jargon. If there is a positive side to the news (for example, that a tumour is operable) be sure to include it at this point, but do not go into details of treatment yet.

4. Now, **pause** again. This gives the relative an opportunity of absorbing what you have said, and asking you any questions. Don't hurry this part, it is important.

5. You have almost certainly been asked about treatment; but if not, explain this now. Almost certainly, the treatment has a good and a bad side. Be very sure that you **start with the good side**, saying what can be expected from treatment. If there is a chance of a cure, tell them what it is: otherwise explain what the treatment is meant to achieve. For example, if a loop of gut is to be made to by-pass an inoperable carcinoma of the head of the pancreas, explain what will happen if the operation *isn't* done, and what can be expected if it is.

   Once the positive objective of any proposed treatment has been grasped, *go on to explain the bad side* of any treatment: the mortality of an intended operation, or the side effects of radiotherapy. In those few cases where there is no treatment to offer or discuss, you must emphasize that you undertake to keep the patient comfortable.

6. At this stage you will often be asked to predict how long the patient has to live. *Never give a precise time*: you cannot possibly know. If there is even a remote chance of cure, remember to say so. If you have an idea of the sort of range, err on the side of optimism: *hope keeps people alive; and despair kills them.*

7. Finally, the issue will arise about *what the patient is to be told.* You must never swear a relative to secrecy: they will know the patient much better than you do. It is very helpful if you tell the relatives what has been said to the patient so far. Ask the relative if they think the patient would want to be told. If they intend to tell the patient and you feel that the patient is too weak to receive such news immediately after surgery, *then it is your duty to tell the relatives this.* The decision about what to say to the patient is discussed further on p. 291.

8. Finish by offering to see them again if they think of further questions for you. Remember that the relative is very anxious: they will not absorb everything that you have told them first time round. Be prepared to repeat it on another occasion. If you are in any doubt, ask them to say it back to you.

If you are seriously concerned about the relative's health, suggest that they go to see their family doctor, and offer to ring him or her up and explain the situation. The relative is not your patient.

THE EFFECTS OF MUTILATING SURGERY

There have been many studies of psychological problems and mental illness in patients who have undergone mutilating surgery, including mastectomy, hysterectomy, colectomy, and amputation. In each of these groups between 20 and 40 per cent of patients are found to be suffering from mental illness, mainly affective disorders and follow-up studies suggest that these disorders persist for at least one year. The changes observed are by no means limited to the effects of surgery as there are usually other major factors that influence the patients' mental state, including the effects of the disease – often malignancy – and the unwanted effects of any other treatment that the patient has already received.

The different ways in which relationships between physical and mental disorders may arise have been described in Chapter 10 and this section is concerned only with the psychological reactions to disease and its treatment.

Psychological reactions found after most mutilating procedures

1. **Uncertainty** regarding treatment procedures and their likely outcome and effect on the patient and her family give rise to **fear**.
2. **Helplessness** resulting from the sense of loss of control of one's own body and dependence on others.
3. **Guilt** and self-blame are often associated with the idea that the disease and its treatment are retribution for real or imagined imperfections.
4. **Sense of failure** is related to this and also to the idea that it may be too late to achieve past ambitions. (The above two phenomena may be part of a depressive illness.)
5. **Stigma** is anticipated due to disfigurement and its expected effect on others, for example that they will be contaminated. The fear of being shunned may result in social isolation.
6. **Isolation**, that is the patient avoids others to save herself and others from embarrassment and consequently may lose the support of others at a time when it is most needed.
7. **Anger and resentment** at the loss of part of oneself and the disruption to normal function that may ensue is often exemplified by the question 'Why me?'
8. **Sexual problems** are common after mastectomy (in one-third of subjects) when there are feelings of loss of femininity and loss of self-esteem. After colostomy sexual relationships are often disrupted by fear of noise, smell, and rejection.
9. **Effects of associated treatments** for malignant disease include fatigue, nausea, vomiting, hair loss, amenorrhoea, and impotence due to cytotoxic drugs and/or radiotherapy.
10. **Maintenance of abnormal illness behaviour** after recovery from physical disease may result in long-term disability due to the gains that have been derived from illness (see p. 222).

The causes of adverse reaction

Although it may seem obvious that most patients subjected to mutilating surgery will suffer at least some of these psychological effects, the fact is that only a substantial minority develop overt mental illness; the majority appear to adjust well although they may take some time to do so. What factors determine who will show the most adverse reactions?

The strongest predictor for the development of an affective disorder is the presence of the psychological problems described above. Those with a *family history* of affective disorder, or a *past history* are likely to be more vulnerable. Important aspects of the *pre-morbid personality* include the extent to which the subject has been able to adapt to previous stresses and to accept imperfections in herself: perfectionists tend to be more vulnerable.

Those who feel secure and have stable relationships are liable to maintain these and derive support, whereas those who tend to fear rejection will be more likely to isolate themselves and lack support.

A number of more immediate factors will also determine the nature of the response. Outward signs of disfigurement have a greater effect than when these are absent. The patient's knowledge of the likely outcome is also important: often uncertainty is more difficult to accept than a bad prognosis, although it is also important not to deny the patient some hope. Intercurrent problems, for example with finance, work, and housing, or in relationships, will also add to the burden and increase the risk of a poor adjustment.

Management

RECOGNITION

The majority of mental illnesses occurring in patients following mutilating surgery are unrecognized by medical and nursing staff and most patients do not spontaneously bring their anxiety or depression to the attention of staff unless specifically asked. The management therefore requires awareness of the nature and frequency of these problems and their causes, and **active enquiry** by staff (preferably including routine screening) to identify those patients most in need of help.

It has been shown that staff in general wards reward those patients who 'keep smiling' (however inappropriately) by spending more time with them and view them more positively; patients who openly display negative feelings are more likely to be rejected by staff, and are placed in beds on the periphery of the ward or furthest from the nursing station.

RESPONSE

This should include the opportunity to *ventilate feelings* without rejection; if you also provide *clear and accurate information* it will help to reassure the patient. At all stages, but particularly early on, it is essential to ensure adequate *relief from pain*. Positive measures are essential to provide *counselling* regarding practical problems such as the management of a colostomy, the availability and use of prostheses, or the management of *sexual and work problems*. Where there is evidence of symptoms of an affective disorder this should be treated in the same way as a similar disorder arising in a person who is physically fit, except that *tetracyclic antidepressants* appear to be better tolerated than tricyclics by patients on the general wards.

THE MANAGEMENT OF THE DYING

Many of the psychological problems and reactions that occur in those who have experienced malignant disease or mutilating surgery are also shared with the dying patient. The presence of these problems, and also of affective disorders, requires awareness by staff and active measures for management, in much the same way. Isolation in a hospital side-room surrounded by an aura of denial from staff and family is likely to increase fear and sadness and result in an undignified end.

Not all of those who are approaching death are aware of it but awareness is much greater than is generally supposed. Several surveys of patients who were dying suggest that *at least 75 per cent are fully or partly aware that they are dying*. However, most of these do not talk to hospital staff about it and only about half share this knowledge with their spouse. Patients sometimes express a wish 'to discuss their situation more fully', although not necessarily with a doctor. The following are some of the more important factors to be considered in the management of the dying.

1. **Relief from distressing physical symptoms** and the patient's clear knowledge that pain relief will be available *when necessary*, and not given on a four-hourly regime (see p. 137).

2. **A relationship with a doctor** who can be trusted to share the patient's values regarding the balance between trying to maintain life and reaching a comfortable and dignified end.

3. Provision of **counselling to relatives** who may have difficulty in accepting the patient's impending death and seek inappropriate and distressing treatments for the patient. They will also require help to face the patient, and to deal with their own grief, both before and after the patient's death.

4. Ensuring that the patient can **maintain close personal ties** with relatives and friends in order to share companionship and interests, and sometimes also the distressing experiences of grief. Explore the possibility that the patient might be discharged home, if the relatives say that they can manage, and the patient does not need hospital treatment.

5. **Symptomatic relief from extreme anguish** is necessary and available using tranquillizers or sedatives, and treatment with *antidepressants* should be based on the usual indications. However, avoid unnecessary and excessive sedation which may add to the patient's distress by cutting him off from contact with others and may also prevent him from active participation in religious rites that he regards as important. Also remember that not all patients fear death: much depends for example on age, religious beliefs, and the extent to which the patient feels he has accomplished his aims.

6. There are many factors that affect the decision as to **what and how much to tell a dying patient**. These can be dealt with only briefly here. However, you should be aware that there is increasing public opinion in favour of doctors' providing patients with the maximum information about themselves. This does not mean

that every dying patient should be informed that he is dying or that a direct reply should invariably be given to such questions as *'I will get better, won't I?'*. Much experience and tact is needed to deal with such questions sensitively depending on the needs of the patient and your knowledge of him or her. Even for the experienced it is usually best to avoid giving an immediate direct reply, although this may come later. Do not avoid the issue when a patient raises it but encourage him to talk about his knowledge of his condition and its likely outcome and what he has already been told. Often this will reveal that he is already aware of the truth and is some way towards accepting it; or conversely that he is at present denying the truth and wants you to share in this. The ultimate responsibility for the decision concerning what the patient should be told will, of course, rest with the consultant and general practitioner.

BEREAVEMENT

Immediately following the death of a close relative a person goes through several stages of a normal grief reaction.

Initially the person is in a state of shock during which although he knows intellectually that the person has died, he has not yet come to terms with it. He is able to function quite well while arranging the funeral and sorting out affairs. Others may notice that the person 'is taking it so well', but the person himself feels numb and may experience depersonalization. Others will have episodes of crying even in this stage, and panic attacks may be experienced. This stage of numbness and shock usually lasts between five and seven days.

It is followed by a realization of the loss with a sharp increase in affective symptoms. This acute grief lasts for four to twelve weeks and resolves during the next three months. The phenomena during this phase are:

1. Intense **pining** for the lost person, and **preoccupation with thoughts of the deceased**, accompanied by weeping. There is a tendency to concentrate on aspects of the environment associated with the lost person. A clear visual mental picture of the deceased is often retained and there may be dreams of the deceased. Initially the thoughts may be distressing, later they can be comforting.

2. **Illusions** are common and everyday household noises are misinterpreted as the deceased person coming in or moving about. Shadows in the dark or strangers may be fleetingly misinterpreted as the deceased person. **Visual or auditory pseudo-hallucinations** occur in which the person sees or hears the deceased. A sense of the *presence of the dead person* is common, which may be comforting. In abnormal grief reactions the sense of presence may be accompanied by talking to the dead person and preparing meals, and so on for him (see 'denial', p. 58).

3. **Depressive illness**. A triad of depressed mood, disturbed sleep, and weeping is seen in over 50 per cent of bereaved people. Other symptoms, such as anorexia, weight loss, tiredness, indecisiveness, anxiety, lack of interest and concentration, a

sense of futility, and guilty feelings also occur, so that many bereaved people will satisfy the diagnostic criteria for depressive illness (see p. 186).

4. **Somatic symptoms of anxiety** may predominate and severely distressed mourners may even express suicidal ideas because life seems hopeless without the deceased; they feel **guilty** about not having done more to prevent the death and may wish to join the dead person. The consultation rate for depressive or somatic symptoms of middle-aged widows increases three times in the six months following the bereavement. The somatic symptoms are sometimes similar to those experienced by the dead person.

5. The bereaved person may be **restless**, pacing the house, and unable to settle. Withdrawal from social contacts occurs and consolation may be rejected. The bereaved person sometimes **searches** for the deceased, by making frequent visits to the cemetery, and even calling out to him. She may constantly gaze at photographs of the dead person.

6. Feelings of **hostility** may be directed at other family members, God, or the doctor 'who let my husband die'.

All these phenomena should have largely subsided by six months after the death.

ATYPICAL GRIEF REACTIONS

These are commoner in women than men. They can be prolonged – an initial stage of numbness lasts more than two weeks and the whole grief reaction lasts over one year. It is also more severe, with *marked social withdrawal, inability to work, and suicidal acts.*

Persisting difficulty accepting the loss, *guilt* feelings, and *hostility* are severe. *Hypochondriacal symptoms* similar to those experienced by the deceased may occur.

Suicidal risk is raised two and a half times during the year following bereavement, with special risk at the *anniversary* of the death. Death from physical illness is also raised during the six months after bereavement, notably from cardiovascular disease.

Other forms of atypical grief include *delayed grief* where the individual functions normally for a while, and then has a grief reaction; *denial of grief* where the individual never appears to experience a grief reaction – but perhaps presents with otherwise inexplicable somatic symptoms much later. A psychotic form of denial was described on p. 58.

Atypical grief is more likely to occur when:

1. The death has been sudden and unexpected.
2. The person has been unable to view the body of the deceased, or to express appropriate grief at an early stage.
3. There was an ambivalent or hostile relationship with the deceased.
4. The loss involves a fully grown child.

5. The person experienced loss of their own parent as a child.

6. There are few relatives or other social supports.

ASSESSMENT AND MANAGEMENT

The aim of **assessment** is to decide whether the patient has a normal or atypical grief reaction. If it is the former, what stage has been reached and is the reaction proceeding? If the reaction is atypical, why is this so, at which stage has the reaction halted, and has the person developed a depressive illness? The presence of suicidal ideas must be assessed.

Management of those with an atypical grief reaction involves a special form of psychotherapy in which the person is guided through the remaining stages of grief. The patient brings photographs or belongings of the dead person and talks about him or her. The patient is thus confronted with the reality of the loss and the emotional expression of grief is facilitated. *Antidepressants* are prescribed if there is a depressive illness.

Grieving usually terminates naturally, but the patient may need encouragement to regain his former activities, or even start new ones, to combat loneliness and preoccupation with loss.

PSYCHIATRIC EMERGENCIES

This section is concerned with patients who present with violence or other disturbed behaviour and suicidal threats or acts. Although speedy action may be required don't forget to use the usual format of history followed by examination to reach a diagnosis. In the accident and emergency department there is usually a relative or at least a policeman with the patient if he or she is unable to give you a proper history; the nurses can give you valuable information on the general wards. Psychiatric emergencies present more commonly in the accident and emergency department than in the general wards, where they may be preventable.

Assessment and management

Don't panic! Remember that common things are common. In the general ward, a physically ill patient is most likely to have an acute brain syndrome; in the accident and emergency department, he or she is most likely to have a functional psychosis or an alcohol-related problem (including head-injury!). If the patient is very disturbed, restless, noisy, and abusive you must first assess the risk of violence. It is preferable to approach the patient quietly, introduce yourself by name, and attempt to get the patient to talk to you. If you succeed in starting a conversation, ask the patient to sit down.

Any such approach must be made **with other staff in the background**, who will retire if the patient settles (tell them not to go too far away), but will come to your assistance if necessary.

As soon as calm prevails, you will need to consider the possible causes of disturbed behaviour, using the scheme shown in *Table 15*.

Table 15 *Emergency assessment of patients with disturbed or violent behaviour*

Has the patient clouding of consciousness?

Clouding – **YES** – acute brain syndrome – check for head injury; check pupils; careful physical examination to find cause; sedate with care . . .

Clouding – **NO** – *Does the patient appear psychotic?* (that is show evidence of delusions or hallucinations)

Psychotic – **YES** – functional psychosis – check past history and attempt to identify features of schizophrenia or mania – consult psychiatrist. Avoid neuroleptics if possible. Sedate with diazepam and consider transfer to psychiatric ward

Psychotic – **NO** – *Does the patient have a mood disturbance?*
elation; depression; anxiety; anger; despair
Is there evidence of intoxication?
alcohol; drugs

THE MANAGEMENT OF VIOLENT BEHAVIOUR

Since psychotic patients are usually frightened try and be **non-threatening** in your approach: the presence of other staff nearby will often avert violence.

You must **appear in control** even if you don't feel it! This is why it is best to have spoken, however briefly, to some other informant before you approach the patient.

The decision to sedate is crucial. You should **avoid sedation if you possibly can**, since it may make diagnosis of the cause of the patient's problems very much more difficult. However, if violence has already occurred or seems imminent despite your attempts to calm the situation, you may have no alternative. If it has to be done use **intramuscular chlorpromazine**, 50–100 mg depending on the patient's size; carry out the injection rapidly with plenty of male staff. The more staff you have, the less likely is it that anyone will get hurt. If you are fortunate enough to have four people assisting you, assign one to each limb of the patient. Be prepared to repeat the dose if necessary.

If there is any question of epilepsy consider **haloperidol** or **paraldehyde** as alternatives.

The former does not lower the convulsive threshold in the way that chlorpromazine does, and is the treatment of choice for acute brain syndrome. The latter is an unpleasant drug since it is both smelly and painful; but it is safe, will not suppress the symptoms of a psychotic illness, and is itself an anticonvulsant.

The advice of the duty psychiatrist is necessary at an early stage regarding both sedation and possible transfer to a psychiatric ward.

Dealing with angry patients

Angry patients demand attention in two situations:

1. One is the normal person who **is overwhelmed with an intolerable stress**, often a life-threatening disease. Crises of confidence between the renal dialysis patient and his medical attendants can present in this form, when in deep frustration the patient rips the drips from his arms and thrashes out at anyone who approaches. The important first step is to understand the situation, usually by gaining information from the ward staff or those who bring the patient to casualty. A dialogue regarding the real problem is likely to lead to a reduction in the patient's tension:

   I can see that you're very angry. Would you like to tell me about it?

   Listen carefully to what the patient has to say. If he complains about other members of staff, hear him out but do not take sides. If sedation is necessary, try to get the patient's prior agreement: always tell the patient what you are doing, and why.

2. The other kind of angry 'patient' is the **antisocial personality** (see p. 65) who not uncommonly presents to casualty threatening violence or suicide. He may just have had a row with his wife and may seek refuge in a hospital bed: he will often drop the talk of violence once his real need to find alternative accommodation is discussed.

SOME COMMON EMERGENCIES

You should be familiar with those conditions which might lead to a psychiatric emergency and see whether you can identify patients at risk beforehand.

Acute brain syndrome (delirium) (see p. 140)

The emergency will typically arise in the middle of the night, when the patient's psychotic experiences are most intense and disturbed behaviour ensues. Patients at risk are all those who have serious physical illness, but keep a special eye out for **drowsiness** and early signs of **clouding of consciousness** which are detectable during the day with careful examination. The nursing staff are likely to pick this up before you and they may be alerted to it by the patient's relatives, who notice that the patient is less alert at visiting time. Take special note of the following:

1. The elderly patient on many drugs is especially at risk as are those who develop a chest infection.

2. The patient who has been a heavy drinker prior to admission (for example for a hernia operation) may go into a withdrawal state, whose early signs of tremor, anxiety, and insomnia should be detected before delirium tremens develops.

3. The post-operative patient who is 'going off' represents a high risk. Take brisk action to correct electrolyte or acid-base disturbance, anaemia, or infection.

Treatment is of the delirium (see p. 145) but the patient who is up and pulling his drip out or trying to leave the hospital will require sedation as well as the special nursing care: **remember that *haloperidol* is the drug of choice.**

Functional psychoses

A relapse of schizophrenia or affective psychosis may occur while the patient is on a general ward as a result of the stress of the concurrent physical illness and its treatment. This is a good reason to ask about previous psychiatric as well as physical illness in your routine history-taking.

Any psychosis may present as disturbed behaviour especially if the patient experiences persecutory delusions. The mood disturbance of mania or depression should become clear if it is possible to engage the patient in conversation.

Treatment of the functional psychosis is along usual lines; but an early decision is needed, in consultation with the psychiatrist, regarding possible transfer to a psychiatric ward.

Panic attacks (see p. 177)

These can present as an emergency because the patient experiences sudden and intense fear (often of impending death) together with somatic symptoms of anxiety. The presence of medical personnel is often sufficiently reassuring to the patient. Rebreathing into a paper bag may help if hyperventilation is pronounced. A single dose of a benzodiazepine given orally or interavenously will bring the anxiety under control if other measures fail.

SUICIDE AND SELF-POISONING

The characteristics of those who successfully commit suicide and those who deliberately harm themselves without the intention of death may seem separate. The elderly man who takes himself to a lonely place with a lethal dose of barbiturates represents a different phenomenon from the young girl who impulsively takes a handful of tablets in front of her boyfriend in the context of a row. However, there is an area of overlap between these extremes.

Most of those who poison themselves have social problems, and many have psychiatric illnesses – usually affective illnesses. Most will have seen their doctors in the week preceding the episode, and may well have been given the tablets which have just been taken for an 'illness' that they do not even have.

Approximately 1 per cent of patients seen at hospital following an episode of self-poisoning eventually kill themselves, and this represents an increased risk of 100 times compared to the general population. Approximately half of successful suicides have previously deliberately harmed themselves.

The other problem is repetition. Such patients often cause great problems of management and they elicit resentment among those who try to help. Up to 20 per cent of self-poisoners seen at the hospital repeat the act within one year. The aims of assessment are therefore:

1. To identify those who are at greatest risk of suicide. The characteristics of these groups are given in *Table 16*.
2. To treat underlying disorders.

Table 16 *Factors associated with increased suicidal risk*

Demographic and social
    Male
    Over forty-five years
    Separated, divorced, or widowed
    Social isolation
    Unemployment
    Recent bereavement

Medical
    Severe or chronic physical illness
    Depressive illness
    Alcoholism
    Antisocial personality disorder
    Previous episode of self-poisoning

Evaluation of suicidal risk

Patients seen in casualty or admitted to the general wards who have taken an overdose or deliberately injured themselves may present acute problems of management.

When such a patient is seen in casualty there are two separate assessments to be made:

1. What is the severity of the physical damage resulting from the deliberate self-harm (or is about to occur if the patient has ingested a drug whose adverse effects have not yet become apparent)?
2. What is the risk of further suicidal behaviour in this patient and what is the likelihood that he may successfully commit suicide? Risk factors are shown in *Table 17*.

INTERVIEWING

The **history from a relative** or other informant is especially important. If the patient is drowsy or in a coma, do this right away; otherwise after you have seen and examined the patient. This covers the same areas as the interview with the patient.

Table 17 *Characteristics associated with repetition of self-poisoning*

Demographic and social
- Previous episode
- Not living with relative
- Lower social class
- Unemployed
- Criminal record

Medical
- Alcohol and drug problems
- Previous psychiatric treatment
- Antisocial personality disorder
- Histrionic personality disorder
- Passive dependent personality

When **interviewing the patient** you need a quiet private place for the interview and to allocate a sensible amount of time for it. *Do not attempt to interview a patient drowsy after an overdose and expect to get a clear history.*

The patient is often an adolescent who is shy and reluctant to talk. She may be preoccupied with guilt about the episode of self-poisoning, still be angry after a row (this anger can be displaced on to you!), or depressed and retarded. These will exercise your interview skills and may appear as apparent refusal to cooperate with you or refusal to see the psychiatrist. However, *an assessment must be made* and it is usually best to make this clear to the patient: be polite, but firm.

The **history** is taken in the usual way but the following are the points most directly related to assessment of suicidal risk.

1. **Detailed description of the episode of self-poisoning:**

   Objective:
   - Exactly what was taken, where and when, and was anyone else present? Were there any precautions to avoid discovery?
   - Was there a **suicide note**? (If so, could you see it, please? The content may indicate increased or decreased risk.)
   - Was there any other act in anticipation of death?
   - Was action taken to alert potential helpers after taking the overdose?

   Subjective:
   - What was the patient's stated intent?
   - What was the patient's **estimate of lethality** of the substances taken? (Even though you consider ten diazepam tablets relatively harmless the patient may have thought that dose would kill her: it is what the patient thinks that is important.)

2. Evidence of recent/current **psychiatric illness**, notably symptoms of depressive or psychotic illness.

3. Is there a **past history** of psychiatric illness or previous episodes of self-poisoning?
4. Is there any evidence of **alcohol or drug abuse**?
5. Recent **precipitating life event**, such as bereavement, redundancy, break-up of a close relationship. Are there job problems or unemployment, marital, family, or other interpersonal conflicts? Are there financial or other social difficulties?
6. Is there a **family history** of mental illness or self-poisoning? Does the patient **live alone**; if so can he go and stay with someone for a while if necessary?

The **mental state examination** is performed in the usual way but evidence of depressed mood and continuing suicidal ideation is sought. Is the patient relieved or sorry to find himself still alive? The presence of psychotic phenomena and brief assessment of cognitive functioning are also important.

Now record your opinion about the whole episode. Why did the episode occur? What was the seriousness of suicidal intent? Who may continue to care for the patient?

> **Opinion:** *Self-poisoning with 10 'librium' tablets taken from mother's handbag following a row with boyfriend. Episode seems to have been demonstrative, and without real suicidal intent: told mother what she'd done almost at once; elder sister known to have taken 25 librium without ill effect. Discharge to care of mother.*

Does the patient need to be seen by a psychiatrist? Some hospitals have a policy that all self-poisoners are seen by a psychiatrist but this is gradually changing. Compare the above patient with this one:

> **Opinion:** *Self-poisoned with 50 aspirin, having hidden herself in garden shed. Increasing depression since death of husband last year, and pain from rheumatoid arthritis. Left note saying she could take no more, and disposing of her property. Discovered by son on chance visit to the house. Seems severely depressed with nihilistic ideas. She lives alone.*

It is necessary to make your assessment sufficiently detailed for a decision regarding discharge to be made if there is no continuing suicidal risk. Clearly, the last note should end with the words: 'Will psychiatrist please advise on further management?'

If in doubt, or if there is continued suicide risk, psychiatric illness, or the possibility that the patient may have to be compulsorily detained it is essential to request advice from a more senior doctor on your own unit, or from a psychiatrist.

THE PATIENT WHO TRIES TO LEAVE BEFORE YOUR ASSESSMENT IS COMPLETE

If you have grounds for supposing that the patient may be a risk to him/herself you may detain him/her with an Emergency Order. This requires agreement of the nearest relative or an approved social worker (see p. 306).

LONG-TERM MANAGEMENT

This will be determined by your senior colleagues, the social worker, and possibly the psychiatrist. The patient may be discharged to the care of the GP and local social services or other agency in which case it is essential that you inform that person of the episode and the patient's discharge. This is best done by a phone call by either yourself, the ward sister, or social worker, in addition to your letter.

The patient may be discharged with an appointment for the medical clinic. If this is to review social or psychological factors it is best done quickly (one or two weeks) or the patient may not attend.

Responsibility for the patient may be transferred to the psychiatrist. If this is transfer to a psychiatric ward it is usually straightforward. But if the patient is being discharged, ensure that the appointment and any instructions regarding prescription are understood by the patient, psychiatrist, and GP before the patient leaves your ward. Do not prescribe potentially lethal drugs like tricyclic antidepressants unless you have taken steps to reduce the risk of a repetition (see p. 189).

FURTHER READING

Creed, F. and Pfeffer, J. (1982) *Medicine and Psychiatry, a Practical Approach*. London: Pitman Medical.

Hinton, J. (1967) *Dying*. Harmondsworth: Penguin.

Kubler-Ross, E. (1969) *On Death and Dying*. London: Tavistock.

Parkes, C. M. (1972) *Bereavement*. Harmondsworth: Penguin.

21 / LEGAL ASPECTS OF PSYCHIATRY

The law is now increasingly affecting the practice of medicine as a whole, but for many years there have been legal regulations about psychiatric work. The Mental Health Act (1983) controls the compulsory admission of patients to hospital, and there are legal principles which are vital in considering patients' fitness to appear in court, their responsibility for offences that they commit, their ability to make valid wills, and many other matters.

Most doctors will at some time in their working lives need to prepare a court report, perhaps in a case involving compensation for personal injuries, or to give evidence in court, most likely a Coroner's Court, or to have to deal with a disturbed patient who may require detention in hospital for treatment. Although forensic work is more frequent for those who take up psychiatry, some acquaintance with legal aspects of psychiatry is essential for all doctors who undertake clinical work.

FITNESS TO PLEAD

You cannot have a fair trial unless you are 'fit to plead', and for this you must:

1. Be aware of the charge against you – for example, that you are accused of burglary.
2. Know the difference between pleading guilty and not guilty.
3. Be able to follow the proceedings in court and challenge a juror (in practice, the solicitor or barrister for the defence does much of this).
4. Be able to advise lawyers about your defence, or to defend yourself.
5. Understand the verdict of the court – for example, 'Guilty and sentenced to six months in prison'.

However, let us suppose that you have been arrested and charged with burglary, but there is doubt as to whether you are fit to plead. A jury at a preliminary trial, at which the evidence is usually psychiatric, decides if you are 'under disability'. If you are found fit to plead, a second trial takes place later, with a fresh jury, to determine whether you were guilty of the burglary.

If you are found 'under disability' this has the same effect as an order under Section 41 of the *Mental Health Act (1983)*, and the Home Secretary directs your admission to a specified hospital within two months. It may take months or years to achieve your discharge even if you make a rapid recovery – and this prolonged detention happens to someone who has never had a proper trial, and who indeed may not have committed the burglary at all! For this reason it is best to avoid a patient being found 'unfit to plead' whenever possible – usually by delaying the court hearing to allow treatment of the mental disorder to take place so that the patient will be fit to plead and thus get a fair trial. Permanent 'unfitness to plead' is usually due to severe mental handicap or brain damage.

If someone standing trial *refuses to speak* in court, there is a similar procedure to determine whether he or she is 'mute of malice' – which means keeping quiet to save your skin. If muteness is caused by mental illness ('mute by visitation of God': for example, catatonic schizophrenia or psychotic depression) the individual is also 'under disability', and is dealt with as if unfit to plead.

CRIMINAL RESPONSIBILITY

You cannot be convicted of most crimes in an English court unless two ancient Latin requirements are satisfied.

1. **Actus reus**: it must be proved than the offender did the illegal act (for example, stole some meat from a supermarket), and
2. **Mens rea**: it must be established that he did the act in a certain state of mind – with a guilty intent (for instance, that he took precautions to avoid being detected, and did not just absent-mindedly carry the meat out of the shop).

You may be exempted from criminal responsibility by:

1. **Mistake** – about fact, or the situation; not about the law (for example, you buy stolen property in all innocence).
2. **Accident** – a child runs in front of your car and is seriously injured when you are driving with due care and attention, and within the speed limit.
3. **Duress** – with a gun in your back you are forced to open your employer's safe and hand over his money.
4. **Necessity** – killing in self-defence.
5. **Age** – you cannot be tried and punished for an offence, even if you have committed it, before you reach the age of ten. Between ten and fourteen you are

doli incapax, and it has to be proved that you knew that what you did was wrong. By the age of eighteen you become liable to the full rigours of the law.

6. **Drink and drugs** – to be acquitted you must be 'so drunk as to be incapable of forming an intent' (too drunk or drugged to be able to decide to offend). A habitual heavy drinker is usually expected to be able to forecast the deleterious effects of alcohol on himself, and should have decided to limit his drinking if he knows he may become violent after, say, eight pints of beer.

7. **Automatism** – post-epileptic automatism or confused behaviour in a hypoglycaemic state rarely provides a defence. (And if it succeeds, you are likely to be committed to a Special Hospital such as Broadmoor for a long period!)

8. **Insanity** – the **McNaghten Rules**. These state that a defendant must be 'labouring under such defect of reason due to disease of the mind, as not to know the nature and quality of the act, or, if he did know it, that he did not know he was doing wrong'. These are difficult conditions to satisfy. However, if you are so mad that you either do not know what you are doing, or do not know that it is wrong – then you will be found 'Not guilty by reason of insanity', and the Home Secretary will direct your admission to a specified hospital within two months of your trial.

The **Homicide Act (1957)** allows a person to be convicted of manslaughter rather than murder if he 'is suffering from such abnormality of mind . . . as substantially impaired his mental responsibility' for the killing. (Abnormality of mind may include mental handicap, mental illness, psychopathy, or head-injury – although these conditions are described in legal rather than medical terms in the Act.)

Amnesia does not exempt you from criminal responsibility: forgetting the details of an offence, whether because of intoxication with alcohol, head-injury, hysterical dissociation, or for other causes, is not a defence!

COURT REPORTS

These should be clear, free from jargon, and systematically set out using headings:

1. An **introduction** which states the evidence on which the report is based – the number of interviews you have had with the defendant, the documents that you have read, and the other professionals whom you have consulted.

2. A section giving the defendant's **background**, and stressing the psychiatric aspects. (In serious cases, a full **history** goes in here.)

3. A cautious comment on the **offence**, concentrating on the defendant's **mental state and circumstances** 'at the material time'.

4. A summary of his **mental state** at the time of your examination, with a clear indication of whether you consider him to be suffering from a psychiatric disorder.

5. A **conclusion**, which sums up what has gone before, and deals with questions of

criminal responsibility and **fitness to plead** where these are relevant, and ends if possible, with a **recommendation to the court** such as:

I therefore recommend that the Court considers dealing with the case by placing Mrs Smith on probation, with a condition of attending the City Hospital's psychiatric out-patient department for treatment.

APPEARING IN COURT

The doctor giving evidence in court should be formally dressed, should speak clearly and simply, avoiding or explaining medical jargon, and remember that he is trying to explain technicalities with which he is familiar to laymen to whom they may be new. The English legal system is an *adversarial* one, so questions may be asked first by the side which has asked you to appear (for instance, the defence). This is known as the *examination in chief*, and is followed by *cross-examination* by the opposite side (for instance, the prosecution), and then *re-examination* by the original questioner.

The judge or magistrates may also question the witness. Remember that the truth will often lie somewhere between what is being put forward by the opposing sides, and that it is important not to be drawn by the questioning too far over to either the defence or the prosecution view, unless you wholeheartedly endorse that idea. Useful phrases are 'I cannot comment on that'; or 'I cannot go that far' – followed, if possible, by a restatement of your view.

THE MENTAL HEALTH ACT

Until the Mental Health Act (1959) almost all psychiatric in-patients were compulsorily detained. Since then the proportion has fallen progressively, so that now the vast majority are informal, with the same rights and freedoms as any other hospital patients. Only about 5 per cent are now compulsorily detained, and there are restrictions on the powers of psychiatrists to treat them without their consent.

The Mental Health Act (1983) is like most Acts of Parliament in that it is a lengthy and forbidding document, and like other Acts its paragraphs are numbered. This leads to potentially confusing references to 'Section 37' or to 'Sectioning' for compulsory detention. It is preferable and more intelligible to refer to each section by name: to a 'Treatment Order' rather than Section 3, a 'Hospital Order' rather than Section 37, and so on.

There are complex and varying conditions for the making and renewal of each section: an 'Assessment Order' (Section 2), and a 'Treatment Order' (Section 3) are used most often, and will be used as examples in what follows.

Assessment Order

An Assessment Order (Section 2) requires two medical recommendations, one from a qualified psychiatrist (approved under Section 12 of the Act) and one from another doctor, who may be the patient's general practitioner. The consent of the nearest relative – or an approved local authority social worker – is also needed (except for orders made by the courts or the Home Office). This kind of admission is used when a patient:

1. Is suffering from a mental disorder (the type need not be specified),
2. Is unwilling to be admitted to hospital,
3. But needs to be admitted *either for his own health and safety and/or for the protection of others.*

The admission is for assessment, but this can be followed by treatment. It lasts up to twenty-eight days, and the patient may appeal within the first fourteen days to a *Mental Health Review Tribunal.* This is a small informal court with three members: a legally qualified president, an independent psychiatrist (in practice this means from another health district), and a lay person. The tribunal has the power to discharge the patient from the order, so that he could then decide to leave or to remain as a voluntary patient.

Treatment Order

If the patient needs to be kept in for longer than twenty-eight days a Treatment Order (Section 3) can then be made, detaining him or her for up to six months. Because this order deprives the patient of liberty for much longer, there are more stringent requirements:

1. The patient's mental disorder must be specified as either *mental illness, severe mental impairment, mental impairment, or psychopathy,* and details of the disorder must also be given.
2. It must be *of a nature or degree which make it appropriate for him to receive treatment in a hospital,* and
3. Treatment cannot be provided unless he is detained.
4. In the case of the milder disorders (mental impairment and psychopathy), treatment must be likely to 'alleviate or prevent a deterioration of his condition.'

Tables 18 and 19 deal with commonly used compulsory admissions, with longer-term admissions (you must be sure to be well acquainted with these), and with orders involving Courts.

The Mental Health Act Commission

The Mental Health Act Commission has about ninety members, including psychiatrists, psychologists, nurses, social workers, lawyers, and lay people. These are appointed by the Secretary of State for Health and Social Services for up to four years, and they have generally supervisory responsibilities for detained patients, including:

1. Reviewing the **use of powers of detention**.

Table 18   *Compulsory emergency admission under the Mental Health Act (1983)*

Section number	description	signatures needed	patient in	maximum detention
4	Emergency Order	any doctor, nearest relative or social worker	not specified	72 hours
5(2)	Admission Order	doctor-in-charge	hospital	72 hours
5(4)	Holding Order	qualified nurse	hospital	6 hours
136	admission by police	police constable	public place	72 hours

Table 19   *Longer-term admission under the Mental Health Act (1983)*

Section number	description	signatures needed	patient in	maximum detention
2	Assessment Order	two doctors (one approved); nearest relative or approved social worker	unspecified	28 days
3	Treatment Order	two doctors (one approved); nearest relative or approved social worker	unspecified	6 months
37	Hospital Order	two doctors, magistrates or Crown Court	unspecified – but often in prison	6 months
		to a Section 37 may be added: (when the patient's behaviour presents a serious risk to the public)		
41	Restriction Order	Crown Court judge	unspecified	indefinite

2. Interviewing and visiting detained patients and **investigating their complaints**.

3. Supervising **consent procedures**. (Detained patients can be treated against their will only in a serious emergency, or if independent doctors and lay members of the Commission agree.)

4. Preparing **Codes of Practice** on admission procedures and on the medical treatment of mentally disordered patients.

TESTAMENTARY CAPACITY

Any doctor may be asked to assess testamentary capacity, meaning the ability to make a valid will. A patient's general practitioner is much more likely to be asked to do this than a psychiatrist. If a patient is seriously ill, or even dying, he may decide to make a will, and may ask the doctor attending him to witness it. If the doctor does this he is said to have 'attested the will', and should have considered the patient to be of *sound disposing mind*. If the will is subsequently contested, he may have to answer questions in court about the patient's mental state.

Anyone over the age of eighteen who is not 'of unsound mind' can make a will. Mild dementia would be unlikely to affect a simple will, although it might invalidate a complex one. However, someone who is confused, forgetful, or even deluded may be able to draw up a will with legal assistance.

Having a *'sound disposing mind'* involves:

1. Knowing what property you own.
2. Knowing who has claims on it: you should know the names of your nearest relatives.
3. Being able to form a judgement on the relative strengths of these claims, without undue distortion due to mental abnormality.

FURTHER READING

The English Legal System (1975) London: HMSO.
The Mental Health Act (1983). London: HMSO.
Trick, K. and Tennent, T. (1981) *Forensic Psychiatry – An Introductory Text* London: Pitman.
Report of the Committee on Mentally Abnormal Offenders (1975) London: HMSO.

GLOSSARY

Acute dystonia consists of muscle spasms, often painful and alarming in appearance, which may have their onset within the first week of starting a neuroleptic drug. They may include spasms of the tongue, neck, back, and extrinsic ocular muscles ('oculogyric crisis'). They respond rapidly to anti-cholinergic anti-Parkinsonian drugs.

Agitation is a state of increased motility which accompanies tension and is seen in some depressed patients. It may take the form of poorly organized but purposeful activities such as cleaning, in which the patient starts the same activity frequently, becomes distracted, starts an alternative activity, and so on. There may be repetitive hand wringing leading to excoriation of skin, or head rubbing resulting in hair loss. Behaviour may be importunate. For example, a patient may knock at a door, start to ask a question, break off and walk away, only to repeat this behaviour each time the door is closed. The inexperienced commonly fail to recognize that such behaviour may be caused by agitation and use meaningless terms such as 'attention-seeking' or 'hysterical' to describe the patient. The degree of agitation is not directly related to the severity of subjective anxiety, and a retarded patient may also describe inner feelings of great tension.

Akathisia is a state of increased motility accompanied by a subjective feeling of restlessness and is an extrapyramidal effect of neuroleptic drugs.

Akinesis is a reduction in motor activity particularly affecting muscles of facial expression, and accessory movements such as arm swinging when walking. It is a feature of Parkinsonism and is commonly drug-induced. Thus there is a particular risk of failing to differentiate this treatment side-effect from depressive retardation and of consequent inappropriate treatment.

Ambivalence. Refers to vacillation of motivation. Also used to mean vacillation between complying and refusing when asked to do something.

Approximate answers or 'answering past the point'. Replies to questions which are almost (but not) correct and imply a knowledge of the correct answer, for example: *'How many legs has a sheep?' 'Five.'*

Automatism. A simple or complex motor act, often inappropriate to the circumstances, (for example, undressing in a supermarket) carried out while apparently unaware of the environment and without conscious motivation. Associated with organic cerebral disorders, particularly epilepsy, and with hysteria.

Blunting of affect is a disorder that may be seen in schizophrenia, particularly in those with a chronic disorder. The usual modulation of mood is lost, and the patient lacks warmth, but does not convey the lowering of affect seen in severely depressed patients.

Catatonic symptoms. A collective term for a variety of motor behaviours, including ambivalence, negativism, posturing, and waxy flexibility.

Compulsions are closely related to obsessions, but are repetitive acts rather than thoughts. They may be simple actions, such as repeated checking, for example to see whether a door is locked before going to bed, or there may be complex rituals involving sequences of actions, each of which the subject feels compelled to repeat for a 'magical' number of times. For example, a patient may feel compelled to wash his hands seven times to avoid contamination, then he thinks this must be repeated in case he touched the sink, which might have been contaminated, and so on. Sometimes, as with obsessions, there is an attempt to resist compulsive actions. However, some patients practise compulsive acts in order to relieve the distress caused by an obsessional thought. For example, compulsive handwashing may be welcomed and practised to avoid the obsessional idea of contamination. The patient knows the actions are his own and based on his own will, even though they distress him and he may struggle to avoid them. In this respect they differ from passivity phenomena from which they must be distinguished.

Depersonalization is an unpleasant perception of change in mental functions or body image. The patient may no longer experience usual feelings towards others. Parts of his body may look unfamiliar, although correctly identified as his own. The experience may be accompanied by **derealization**, in which the external world seems altered and unfamiliar: the experience is unpleasant. Both can occur as isolated symptoms – especially due to fatigue – but they commonly accompany affective illnesses, or any other mental illness higher in the hierarchy.

Depressive delusions. Delusions of guilt, self-blame, poverty, infestation, and infection are associated with depression and reflect the low self-esteem and hopelessness for the future which are characteristic of that mood. Of course such ideas occur commonly in depressed patients without necessarily being delusional in quality. Nihilistic delusions are extreme variants, in which the patient believes that he is losing his physical or mental functions due to disease, or that he is already dead. For example, a depressed patient insisted that his head was shrinking, that his forehead was growing smaller so that he no longer had a place to wear his glasses, and that this state would soon be incompatible with life.

Fugue. A disturbance of behaviour characterized by wandering, without conscious motivation, in a state of altered or diminished consciousness; subsequently there may be amnesia for the event. Associated with organic (including epileptic) and hysterical states.

Grandiose delusions include beliefs that the patient has special powers, is chosen by God, or has been sent to save the world. For example, following laminectomy a greengrocer believed he was in hospital because he was a famous neurosurgeon, was there to operate on the other patients, and that the staff were there to assist him. He strutted about the ward issuing imperious commands and held his hands as though 'scrubbed up'. Such beliefs are particularly likely to occur in manic patients, but are also found in schizophrenics and those with organic cerebral disorders.

Hysterical amnesia is differentiated from other memory defects by the characteristic loss of personal information, both recent and long term. For example, the patient is unable to remember his name and address, whether he has family, and fails to recognize close relatives. By contrast, he appears to have no difficulty in recognizing, naming, and using equally familiar objects, such as food and drink. Such profound and selective memory loss does not occur in other disorders.

Incongruous affect is a display of affect which is inappropriate to the patient's subjective mood state. For example, a patient may smile to himself briefly when describing a recent bereavement. Never assume that this is inappropriate, based on your own expectation of what the patient's mood should be. Ask the patient why he smiles. He may say he feels sad and does not know why he smiles, in which case this is probably an example of incongruous affect. However, he may say he was remembering an amusing incident at the funeral or thinking of the legacy he expects to receive. Inappropriate affect is a characteristic of schizophrenia.

Labile mood is when fluctuations occur in response to circumstances, but show rapid and excessive variation with loss of control. It is strongly suggestive of organic brain disease and may be a feature of dementia, but can also occur in histrionic personalities and in some manic-depressive illnesses.

Mannerisms. All people have certain mannerisms, which are habitual and meaningless movements, such as stroking the face or hair or clearing the throat, which tend to increase when they are tense. They imitate purposeful movements and can be brought under voluntary control.

Mutism is total absence of speech. It may occur as a feature of stupor in depressive illness, schizophrenia, or organic brain disease. Occasionally it may be a hysterical symptom. **Elective mutism** is seen mainly in disturbed children and is characterized by mutism which occurs in some settings but not in others. For example, the child may speak normally at home, but is mute at school.

Negativism. The response to a request which is the opposite to that which is required. Sometimes also used to mean failure to carry out a task.

Obsessions are repetitive thoughts which the subject feels are forced into his conscious mind against his wishes, that is he feels compelled to have them. The nature of these thoughts is unpleasant and, therefore, he tries to resist having them. Both the thoughts and the attempt at resistance are associated with anxiety. An essential feature is that the patient knows these are his own thoughts, that is they originate in his own mind, even though their content is contrary to his own wishes. For example, the patient may find the idea forced into his thinking that his hands are contaminated by faeces, that he has failed to wash his hands properly, and that he may poison others for whom he is preparing food. It is also important to note that the idea is not a delusion: the patient is not convinced that his hands are contaminated, but fears that they might be and is unable to put this fear from his mind, although he may know intellectually that it is 'foolish'.

Over-activity becomes a problem when the actions are either inappropriate or are not completed. Manic patients may display considerable energy, start many activities, but fail to complete them. **Loss of inhibition** may also lead them to inappropriate activities, such as spending sprees or sexual excesses.

Passivity. Delusions of passivity are included in the phenomena that characterize schizophrenia, which appear to be based on a breakdown of 'ego-boundaries', that is the normal awareness of the boundaries between ourselves and other people in the world outside ourselves. Included are beliefs that one's body is under the control of other people or forces, that other people control one's thoughts, are able to place thoughts into or remove them from one's mind, can read each thought as it goes through one's mind or that the thoughts in one's mind do not belong to oneself. These beliefs are extremely concrete, that is that a thought can actually be taken out of one person's mind and placed in another mind. The subject may feel physically controlled, like a marionette. It is easy to identify such beliefs incorrectly by asking inaccurate questions.

Perplexity. A mood state of bewilderment, with uncertainty about the nature of immediate experience of the environment. The subject usually appears puzzled.

Phobias are fears of specific objects or situations which are not generally regarded as dangerous, such as spiders, mice, heights, crowded or enclosed places. The phobic person will tend to avoid the feared situations, but will not always do so. It is crucial to the definition of a phobia that the subject is aware that the fear is irrational, because the object of fear is not dangerous. Thus it must be differentiated from a delusion. For example, an agoraphobic patient may be housebound, but will know that there is nothing harmful outside the house. A patient with persecutory delusions may also fear to go out, but this is because he believes there is danger, for example a gunman waiting to kill him, and that it is, therefore, a sensible precaution to remain in the house.

Posturing. Used to refer to abnormal body posture. Manneristic posture is a stilted exaggeration of normal posture. Stereotyped posture is non-adaptive, rigidly maintained, and often uncomfortable.

Pressure of speech describes the rapid outpouring of ideas which is characteristic of mania. This is accompanied by an increase in the quantity of speech and often in the volume. It may be difficult to interrupt, to ask questions, or to direct a conversation successfully with a patient who shows this disorder. The continuity of thinking is often, but not necessarily, also affected.

Reference. Ideas (or delusions) of reference involve beliefs that events in the environment have special meaning for the subject and refer particularly to him. For example, the news reader on television mentions an epidemic of fever, and the patient knows that this is a message specially intended for him rather than others and that it is a warning to guard himself against infection; the patient hears laughter from a nearby room and is sure that people are laughing at him; a stranger on a bus is overheard saying 'He's gay', and the patient knows he is referring to him. Ideas of reference occur in a wide range of disorders, including depression, mania, and schizophrenia, and have little diagnostic specificity.

Retardation of movement involves delay in initiating movement, slowness in subsequent performance of the movement and also a reduction in the total quantity of movement. It is usually accompanied by retardation of speech (see next entry) and is most commonly seen in depressive illness.

Retardation of speech is often associated with retardation of movement. It is characterized by delay in the initiation of speech, for example in response to a simple question, as well as by a slow rate of speech production. The volume of speech may be so low as to make it difficult to hear what is said. The quantity of speech may be greatly reduced. Retardation is usually symptomatic of depressive illness. Depressed patients who show retardation of speech do not usually experience slowness of thinking, but often describe their thoughts as being in a state of turmoil. The examination of the mental state of a retarded patient calls for great tolerance and patience on the part of the interviewer.

Secondary delusions. This refers to delusions which are secondary to some other abnormality, such as a hallucination. If you hear voices of spies planning to kill you, you may develop the belief that such plans exist! Other examples of secondary delusions would be those that can be understood in terms of abnormal emotion, or those which can be attributed to coarse brain disease, such as a cerebral tumour.

Stereotypies. Utterances or movements which are monotonously repeated, non-goal-directed, executed in a uniform way, and have no obvious significance for the subject, for example rocking to and fro on a chair, endlessly repeating the same oath, or the same barking noises.

Stupor is characterized by total immobility, except for following movements of the eyes, and mutism. (Confirm by moving the patient's head yourself, and seeing whether he moves his eyes to continue to fixate points in the visual field.) It can occur in depressive illness, in which it appears to be an extreme form of retardation. However, it can also be found as a catatonic feature of schizophrenia or due to organic cerebral disorders.

Tardive dyskinesia is a syndrome which may include many different rhythmic or jerking movements and tremors; these may be multiple, affecting most of the body, and are then disfiguring and extremely distressing. Most commonly they have their onset several months after the start of neuroleptic drugs. They are liable to become worse initially when the drug is stopped, and there is at present no reliable treatment.

Thought block is experienced by the patient as an interruption in the flow of thinking, so that thoughts are totally absent for a period of a few seconds. It is common in anxious people – for example, students during vivas. In psychotic illness the patient may suddenly go silent, for example in mid-sentence, look blankly, and then continue on the same or a different theme. It is important to ask the patient what he noticed during this interlude, and what he was thinking about. Often it emerges that he was distracted by other thoughts, sounds, and so on, rather than experiencing total absence of thoughts, in which case thought block did not occur. This phenomenon must also be differentiated from *petit mal epilepsy*. Thought block occurs in some schizophrenics and is often associated with secondary delusions of interference.

Thought broadcasting. The delusion that one's private thoughts are being made known to others, perhaps throughout the world.

Thought echo. The experience of thoughts being repeated or echoed with very little interval between the original and the echo.

Tics are sudden involuntary twitchings of muscle groups often mimicking expressive movements and particularly involving the face, for example frowning or 'screwing up' the eyes. They occur commonly in children at times of tension and may persist into or emerge during adult life.

Torpor. A state of pathological drowsiness with a tendency to fall into a dreamless sleep.

Twilight state. Conscious awareness is narrowed down to a few ideas and attitudes which dominate the subject's mind.

Tremor at rest is a common feature of anxiety. Static tremor may also occur in Parkinsonism. All tremors, both static and intentioned (due to cerebellar disorders), are exacerbated by anxiety, and tremor in an anxious patient may, therefore, be due to an organic cerebral state in addition to the anxiety.

Volition is the state of energy and drive which directs our purposeful activity. Loss of volition is, therefore, a state of inertia in which a person fails to carry out necessary or usually enjoyable activities although the ability to carry them out is in other respects preserved. It is often difficult to assess during an interview.

Waxy flexibility. On moving parts of the patient's body into a new posture the examiner notes a plastic resistance, and the posture may subsequently be maintained.

INDEX